PERSPECTIVES IN Ambulatory Care Nursing

Caroline Varner Coburn, DNP, MS, APRN, ANP-BC

Clinical Associate Professor
Emory University Nell Hodgson Woodruff School of Nursing
Atlanta, Georgia

Deena Gilland, DNP, MSN, RN, NEA-BC, FAAN

Vice President and Chief Nursing Officer, Ambulatory Care,
Emory Healthcare
Clinical Instructor, Emory University Nell Hodgson Woodruff
School of Nursing
Atlanta, Georgia

Beth Ann Swan, PhD, RN, FAAN

Clinical Professor
Associate Dean and Vice President, Academic Practice Partnerships
Emory University Nell Hodgson Woodruff School of Nursing
Atlanta, Georgia

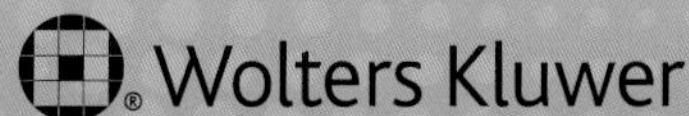

Philadelphia • Baltimore • New York • London
Buenos Aires • Hong Kong • Sydney • Tokyo

Vice President and Publisher: Julie K. Stegman
Manager, Nursing Education and Practice Content: Jamie Blum
Acquisitions Editor: Michael Kerns
Senior Development Editor: Julie Vitale
Senior Editorial Coordinator: Emily Buccieri
Editorial Assistant: Molly Kennedy
Marketing Manager: Brittany Clements
Production Project Manager: Catherine Ott
Design Coordinator: Steve Druding
Art Director: Jennifer Clements
Manufacturing Coordinator: Karin Duffield
Prepress Vendor: S4Carlisle Publishing Services

9 8 7 6 5 4 3 2 1

Printed in China

Library of Congress Cataloging-in-Publication Data

Names: Coburn, Caroline Varner, editor. | Gilland, Deena, editor. | Swan, Beth Ann, 1958- editor.
Title: Perspectives in ambulatory care nursing / Caroline Varner Coburn, Deena Gilland, Beth Ann Swan.
Description: 1st edition. | Philadelphia: Wolters Kluwer Health, [2021] | Summary: "The impetus for Perspectives in Ambulatory Care Nursing came when Dr. Deena Gilland and I initiated a new course at the Nell Hodgson Woodruff School of Nursing at Emory University, titled "Ambulatory Care Nursing.""—Provided by publisher.
Identifiers: LCCN 2020044356 | ISBN 9781975104641 (paperback)
Subjects: LCSH: Nursing. | Ambulatory medical care.
Classification: LCC RT120.O9 P47 2021 | DDC 362.12—dc23
LC record available at https://lccn.loc.gov/2020044356

shop.lww.com

To my sons, Charlie Morgan and David.
I'm so happy to see the adults you've become.
To my husband Charles for his unfailing,
unflagging, and unconditional love and support.

—Caroline Varner Coburn

To Susan Grant who gave me the opportunity
to step into the world of ambulatory nursing.
To Linda McCauley who had the foresight to see the
importance of adding ambulatory nursing to BSN curriculum.
To Sharon Pappas for her continued support and promotion
of the value of ambulatory nurses to the population and healthcare.
To Dan, Alison, and Alex who are my strength and forever supporters.

—Deena Gilland

To my parents, Elizabeth and John H. Reck,
for raising me to believe that anything is possible.
To my daughters, Erica and E. Connor Swan,
for being impossible.
To my husband, Eric J. Swan, for making
everything possible, you're my inspiration.

—Beth Ann Swan

About the Authors

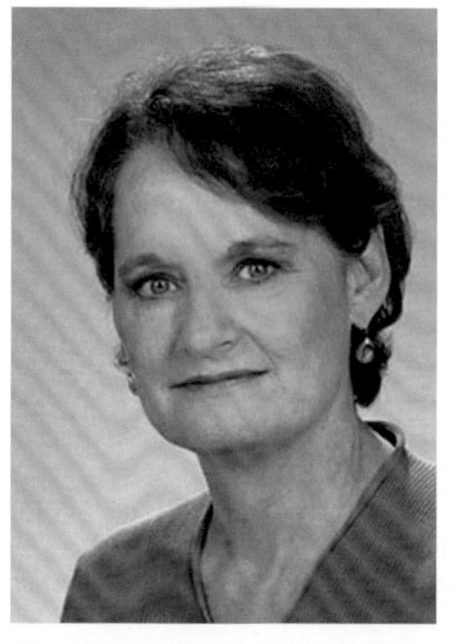

Caroline Varner Coburn, DNP, MS, APRN, ANP-BC

Caroline Varner Coburn earned her BSN from Duke University, MS from Georgia State University, Adult Nurse Practitioner certification from Emory University, and DNP from the University of Alabama at Birmingham. She currently holds the position of clinical associate professor at Nell Hodgson Woodruff School of Nursing, Emory University, Atlanta, GA. Her academic focus is ambulatory nursing and interprofessional collaboration for education of undergraduate, graduate, and postgraduate nurses in a domestic and global context. In support of these academic interests, she is actively involved in a collaborative relationship between the Emory School of Nursing and a nongovernmental organization in The Bahamas. As part of a national taskforce for the American Academy of Ambulatory Care Nursing, she participated in the development of guidelines for academic–clinical collaboration in ambulatory care.

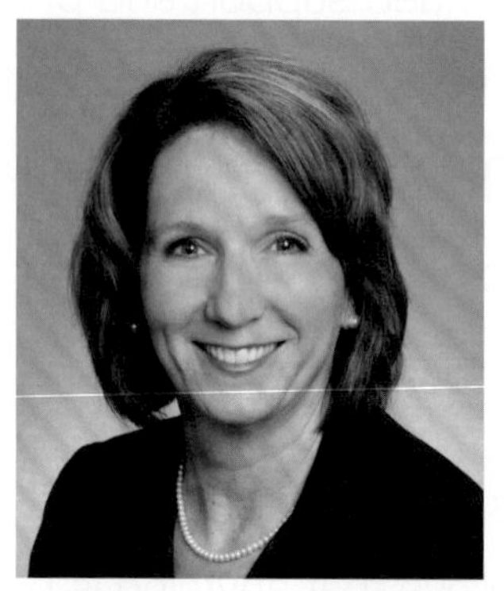

Deena Gilland, DNP, MSN, RN, NEA-BC, FAAN

Deena Gilland is the vice president of Patient Services and chief nursing officer of Emory Healthcare's Ambulatory Practice and an instructor at the Nell Hodgson Woodruff School of Nursing at Emory University. Prior to her current role she served as the director of Oncology Services for the National Cancer Institute (NCI)-designated Winship Cancer Institute of Emory University.

Gilland has dedicated the past decade to establishing a national model and structure for nursing practice in an ambulatory care setting. Her work centers on nursing optimization and illuminating the value of nursing. Gilland impacted nursing practice by developing an ambulatory nursing organizational structure with senior nursing options, optimizing the ability of nurses to impact the health of our population. Her innovative work to develop a prelicensure nursing student path into ambulatory nursing, along with creating methods to induct them through a nurse residency, has advanced the profession nationwide and forged a path for nurses in the ambulatory care.

Gilland received her Doctor of Nursing Practice in Health Systems Leadership and her MSN in Healthcare Leadership from the Emory School of Nursing, and her BSN was obtained from Georgia College. She completed the Managing Healthcare Delivery program at the Harvard Business School and is a fellow of the CNO Academy. She currently serves on the board of directors for the American Academy of Ambulatory Care Nursing (AAACN).

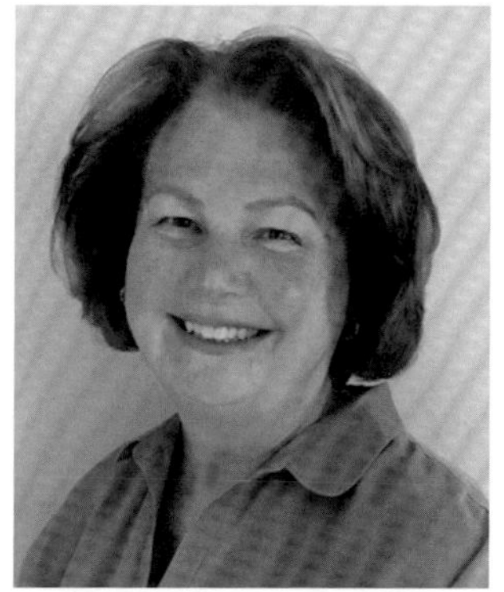

Beth Ann Swan, PhD, RN, FAAN

Beth Ann Swan earned her BSN from Holy Family College, and her MSN and PhD from the University of Pennsylvania School of Nursing. She is a fellow of the American Academy of Nursing, past president of the American Academy of Ambulatory Care Nursing, and a 2007–2010 Robert Wood Johnson Executive Nurse Fellow. She is nationally and internationally known for her research and work in health care and nursing. As an expert clinician, she was an early leader in exploring the impact of changing health care delivery models on outcomes of care. Throughout her career, Dr. Swan has been an advocate for engaging consumers in their health care, promoting ambulatory and primary care, and creating innovative evidence-based practices to improve care. She was a member of the Veterans Health Administration Choice Act Blue Ribbon Panel and was a member of the Josiah Macy Jr. Foundation Planning Committee for Preparing Registered Nurses for New Roles in Primary Care. Her numerous publications cover a wide range of topics focused on ambulatory and primary care, innovations for practice and education, and health care policy.

Contributors

Karen Alexander, PhD, RN
Assistant Professor
Jefferson College of Nursing, Thomas Jefferson University
Philadelphia, Pennsylvania

Harriet Udin Aronow, PhD
Research Scientist IV, Nursing Research
Professor, Medicine and Biomedical Sciences
Cedars-Sinai
Los Angeles, California

Helen Baker, PhD, MS, MSc, BSN, FNP-BC
Assistant Clinical Professor and Global and Community Engagement Coordinator
Lillian Carter Center for Global Health and Social Responsibility
Emory University Nell Hodgson Woodruff School of Nursing
Atlanta, Georgia

Noreen Bernard, EdD, MS, BSN, RN, NEA-BC, FAAN
Chief Nursing Officer
Longs Peak Hospital and Broomfield Hospital
University of Colorado Health
Denver, Colorado

Mary Blankson, DNP, APRN, FNP-C, FAAN
Nurse Executive; Chief Nursing Officer
Community Health Center, Inc.
Middletown, Connecticut

Diane Brown, PhD, RN, FNAHQ, FAAN
CALNOC Board of Directors Member
Kaiser Permanente Northern California Executive Director, Medicare Strategy & Operations
CALNOC, Walnut Creek CA
Kaiser Permanente
Oakland, California

Caroline Varner Coburn, DNP, MS, APRN, ANP-BC
Clinical Associate Professor
Emory University Nell Hodgson Woodruff School of Nursing
Atlanta, Georgia

Mary Coffey, PhD, MPH, RN, CNE-BC
Director of Ambulatory Nursing
Virginia Commonwealth University
Richmond, Virginia

Debra L. Cox, MS, RN
Nurse Administrator
Center for Digital Health
Mayo Clinic
Rochester, Minnesota

Rocquel Crawley, DHA, MBA, BSN, RNC-OB, NEA-BC
Sr. Director of Operations
Children's Hospital of Richmond at VCU
Richmond, Virginia

Cindy J. Dawson, RN, MSN, CORLN
Chief Nurse Executive and Associate Director
University of Iowa Hospitals and Clinics
Iowa City, Iowa

Cyndy Banik Dunlap, DNP, RN, NEA-BC, FACHE
Vice President of Nursing Services and Chief Nursing Officer
Ascension Providence
Waco, Texas

Michele Farrington, BSN, RN-BC
Program Manager
University of Iowa Health Care
Iowa City, Iowa

Deena Gilland, DNP, MSN, RN, NEA-BC, FAAN
Vice President and Chief Nursing Officer, Ambulatory Care, Emory Healthcare
Clinical Instructor, Emory University Nell Hodgson Woodruff School of Nursing
Atlanta, Georgia

Mary Elizabeth Greenberg, PhD, RN-BC, C-TNP, CNE
Associate Clinical Professor
School of Nursing
Northern Arizona University
Tucson, Arizona

Lynda R. Hardy, PhD, RN, FAAN
Associate Professor, Director
Data Science and Discovery
The Ohio State University College of Nursing
Columbus, Ohio

Anne T. Jessie, DNP, RN
Senior Director of Population Health Management and Clinical Innovations
Gorman Health Group
Chicago, Illinois

Beckie Kronebusch, MS, APRN, AGCNS-BC
Clinical Nurse Specialist
Mayo Clinic
Rochester, Minnesota

Ann Marie Matlock, DNP, RN, NE-BC
Chief, Medical Surgical Specialties Service
Captain, United States Public Health Service
National Institutes of Health Clinical Center
Bethesda, Maryland

Nancy May, DNP, RN-BC, NEA-BC
Chief Nurse Executive
University of Michigan Health System
Ann Arbor, Michigan

Linda A. McCauley, PhD, MN, BSN, RN, FAAN, FAAOHN
Dean and Professor
Emory University Nell Hodgson Woodruff School of Nursing
Atlanta, Georgia

Carrie McDermott, PhD, APRN, ACNS-BC
Corporate Director
Nursing Professional Practice
Emory Healthcare
Clinical Assistant Professor
Emory University Nell Hodgson Woodruff School of Nursing
Atlanta, Georgia

Aleesa M. Mobley, PhD, ANP-BC, CPHQ
Assistant Professor, Clerkship Director
Neuro Musculoskeletal Pain Management
Rowan University School of Osteopathic Medicine
Stratford, New Jersey

Cynthia L. Murray, BN, RN-BC
Clinical Nurse Advisor Primary Care
Veterans Health Administration
Office of Nursing Services
Washington, District of Columbia

Sharon Pappas, PhD, RN, NEA-BC, FAAN
Chief Nurse Executive
Emory Healthcare
Clinical Professor
Emory University Nell Hodgson Woodruff School of Nursing
Atlanta, Georgia

Susan M. Paschke, MSN, RN-BC, NEA-BC
Retired Senior Director, Ambulatory Care
Cleveland Clinic
Cleveland, Ohio
Part time Faculty
Nursing Administration and Health Systems Leadership
Kent State University
Kent, Ohio

Carol Rutenberg, MNSc, RN-BC, C-TNP
President and CEO
Telephone Triage Consulting, Inc.
Hot Springs, Arkansas

Roy L. Simpson, DNP, RN, DPNAP, FAAN, FACMI
Assistant Dean, Technology Management
Clinical Professor, Doctoral Program: Doctorate Nursing Practice
Emory University Nell Hodgson Woodruff School of Nursing
Atlanta, Georgia

Rachel E. Start, MSN, RN, NEA-BC, FAAN
Director
Ambulatory Nursing and Nursing Practice
Rush Oak Park Hospital
Oak Park, Illinois

Beth Ann Swan, PhD, RN, FAAN
Clinical Professor
Associate Dean and Vice President, Academic Practice Partnerships
Emory University Nell Hodgson Woodruff School of Nursing
Atlanta, Georgia

Barbara E. Trehearne, RN, PhD
Chief Nurse and VP
Quality & Safety for Kaiser Permanente WA (retired)
Seattle, Washington

Sharon Tucker, PhD, APRN-CNS, NC-BC, FNAP, FAAN
Grayce Sills Endowed Professor in Psychiatric-Mental Health Nursing, College of Nursing
Director, DNP Nurse Executive Track
Director, Implementation Science Core, Fuld EBP Institute
Nurse Scientist, Wexner Medical Center
The Ohio State University
Columbus, Ohio

Mary Hines Vinson, DNP, RN-BC
Associate Chief Nurse, Ambulatory (Ret.)
Duke University Health System
Consulting Associate, Duke University School of Nursing
Durham, North Carolina

Stephanie G. Witwer, Ph.D., RN, NEA-BC, FAAN
Nurse Administrator—Primary Care
Mayo Clinic
Rochester, Minnesota

Reviewers

Judy L. Borgen, MSN, RN, CNE
Instructor
School of Nursing
Oregon Health & Science University
Monmouth, Oregon

Mary T. Bouchaud, PhD, MSN, CNS, RN, CRRN
Director FACT 1 BSN Program and Associate Professor
Jefferson College of Nursing, Thomas Jefferson University
Philadelphia, Pennsylvania

Julia Bucher, PhD, RN
Associate Professor
York College of Pennsylvania
York, Pennsylvania

Donyale Childs, PhD, RN
Associate Professor
Albany State University
Albany, Georgia

Lucus Christoffersen, Ed.D(c), MSN, APRN-CNP, RN, ACNPC-AG, CEN, CPEN, CCRN, TCRN
Nurse Educator
Bingham Memorial Hospital
Blackfoot, Idaho

Kim Clevenger, EdD, MSN, RN, BC
Associate Professor of Nursing
Morehead State University
Morehead, Kentucky

Vera Dauffenbach, EdD, MSN, RN
Associate Professor
Bellin College
Green Bay, Wisconsin

Mary K. Donnelly, DNP, MPH, FNAP, ACNP-BC, ANP- BC, CNL
Assistant Professor
Program Director, RN-MSN Hybrid
University of San Francisco School of Nursing and Health Professions
San Francisco, California

Celeste Dunnington, RN, PhD
Associate Professor
Brady School of Nursing
Shorter University
Rome, Georgia

Matthew J. Fox, MSN, RN-BC
Associate Professor of Nursing
Ohio University Zanesville
Zanesville, Ohio

Donna Guerra, EdD, RN
Clinical Assistant Professor
College of Nursing
The University of Alabama in Huntsville
Huntsville, Alabama

Lillian J. Jones-Bell, MS, RN, PHN
Program Director and Faculty
RN Transition to Practice Program in Ambulatory Care
University of San Francisco School of Nursing and Health Professions
San Francisco, California

Margaree Jordan-Amberg, MSN, RN
Adjunct Professor
St. Catherine University
St. Paul, Minnesota

Bonny Kehm, PhD, RN
Faculty Program Director
Excelsior College
Albany, New York

Angela Kouri, MSN, RN-BC
Instructor
Saint Francis Medical Center College of Nursing
Peoria, Illinois

Jennifer Manning, DNS, ACNS-BC, CNE
Associate Dean for Undergraduate Nursing Program
LSUHSC School of Nursing
New Orleans, Louisiana

Donna E. McCabe, DNP, GNP-BC, PMHNP-BC
Clinical Associate Professor
NYU Rory Meyers College of Nursing
New York, New York

Mary Beth McCloud, PhD, RNC-OB, NPD-BC, CNE, FCN
Assistant Professor
Frostburg State University
Frostburg, Maryland

Andreea Meier, DNP, MSN, RN
Dean, College of Nursing
Charleston Southern University
Charleston, South Carolina

Donna Molyneaux, PhD, MSN, BSN, RN, CNE
Associate Professor
Gwynedd Mercy University
Gwynedd Valley, Pennsylvania

Debra M. G. Murray, DNP, RN, PHCNS-BC, CPNP-PC
Norfolk State University
Norfolk, Virginia

Montra E. Reinhardt, MSN, RN
Associate Professor and Dean
School of Nursing
Ivy Tech Community College–Bloomington
Bloomington, Indiana

Karen Robertson RN, MSN, MBA, PhD candidate
Associate Professor, Co-Chair Nursing Department
Rock Valley College
Rockford, Illinois

Lynette Scianna-DeBellis, MA, RN, CMSRN
Nursing Faculty
Mount Saint Mary College
Newburgh, New York

Lisa South, RN, PhD
Professor
Walden University
Minneapolis, Minnesota

Dawn Stone, PhD, RN, ANP-BC, COHN-S
Associate Professor
Director, MSN Program
Director, Ambulatory Care Nursing
Pomona, California

Misty Stone, MSN, RN
Clinical Assistant Professor
The University of North Carolina at Pembroke
Pembroke, North Carolina

Lori Sullivan, DNP, MSN, RN
Associate Professor of Nursing
Finlandia University
Hancock, Michigan

Kristin E. Wade, MSN, RN, CMPE
VP of Nursing & COO for Baylor Medicine
Baylor College of Medicine
Houston, Texas

LeAnne Wilhite, DNP, APRN, ACNP-BC
Associate Dean of Undergraduate Nursing
Union University College of Nursing
Jackson, Tennessee

Portia J. Zaire, MSNED, BSN, RN-CCCTM
Partner Liaison
The Ohio State University College of Nursing
Columbus, Ohio

Preface

"The difficulty lies not so much in developing new ideas as in escaping from old ones."

John Maynard Keynes

Background

The impetus for *Perspectives in Ambulatory Care Nursing* came when we (Dr. Deena Gilland and Dr. Caroline Coburn) initiated a new course at the Nell Hodgson Woodruff School of Nursing at Emory University, titled "Ambulatory Care Nursing." In planning for this course, we found that existing textbooks on population or public health did not capture the perspectives of ambulatory care nursing. At every available nursing conference, we asked if publishing houses had any textbooks in progress on this subject, and when the answers were negative, we decided to submit our own book proposal.

The contributors to this book represent some of the outstanding leaders in ambulatory nursing. Among them is Dr. Beth Ann Swan, who agreed to join us as third editor and provided invaluable expertise and resources.

Why a separate ambulatory care course? Current courses in most prelicensure nursing programs generally include at least one course on population or public health, which is valuable content. However, it is our contention that both population health and public health generally view individual care from a larger perspective, whereas ambulatory care addresses care on an individual and family level.

We also found that the broad spectrum of ambulatory care more than provided enough content for a stand-alone course, without significantly overlapping with an existing course in population health. The different sites of ambulatory nursing offer a myriad of experiences, from primary care to same-day surgery to specialty clinics to infusion centers, dialysis, urgent care, and telehealth, to name a few.

Perhaps most important, over the time we have taught ambulatory care as a separate course, it has become increasingly apparent that many students have a persistently acute and episodic care focus. We believe it does them a disservice when we fail to immerse them fully in an understanding of healthcare delivery across the care continuum. Even if they know their interest lies within the acute care setting, it is essential for them to understand the full spectrum of an individual's and family's care and its impact on the success of not only inpatient treatment but also overall health. Students and registered nurses (RNs) need to be knowledgeable about and understand where an individual and family came from and where they are going, in order to holistically provide care across the continuum rather than in silos.

How to Use This Book

This book is intended to be useful in both academic and practice arenas. As the U.S. healthcare system turns toward preventive care and keeping individuals out of the hospital, schools of nursing also will turn to more content to prepare students for this shift. For these schools, this book can provide structure and substance for courses that address these topics. Certainly, it is our hope that courses focused specifically on ambulatory care nursing will find appropriate content in these chapters. But as care across settings comes into clearer focus across the entire nursing education curriculum—in courses on public and community health, population health, issues and trends, adult health, medical-surgical nursing, and fundamentals, to name a few—we believe the perspectives offered in this text will help all nurses become more practice-ready. In particular, Chapter 15 addresses the need for and incorporation of ambulatory care content into nursing curricula.

Additionally, this book can provide resources for nonacademic settings. Ambulatory care sites are hiring new graduates in increasing numbers and seeing acute care RNs shift to ambulatory settings. These RNs will need a full understanding of ambulatory care, and this text can serve as an orientation tool as well as a reference for nursing management in implementing practice change. Chapter 16 discusses professional development of the ambulatory care nurse within the perspective of the general healthcare system.

Whether used in stand-alone ambulatory care courses, across the nursing education curriculum, or as a further resource for practicing RNs, to support the different uses of this book, a table is located at the end of this introduction that maps the main content topics found in this book to the appropriate chapter. Also, each chapter contains a case study with accompanying questions for class discussion or individual responses.

A word about the use of *individual*: In the writing of this book, there was discussion about the best way to describe those who receive care in an ambulatory setting. We decided on the word *individual* rather than *patient* or *client* for several reasons. *Patient* is most often descriptive of someone in an acute setting or within a clinic. This leaves out those who are cared for in health fairs, homeless shelters, workplaces, schools, and the many other settings where individuals work, play, or worship.

Client often is used in the ambulatory setting in place of *patient*. However, this word can be rather impersonal and almost implies a delivery of service rather than a collaboration in care. For all of those reasons, we chose *individual*, both to remain as neutral as possible in the description and because, ultimately, care should be focused on individuals and their families.

COVID-19 Impact

As this introduction is being written, our world is going through an extraordinary time coping with the Coronavirus (COVID-19) or severe acute respiratory syndrome coronavirus 2 (SARS COV-2) pandemic. In 2020, the Year of the Nurse and the Midwife, the role of nurses in every country has never been more acknowledged and appreciated. The skill and commitment of RNs in acute care settings is undeniable and well documented; however, because this book is about RNs in nonacute settings, we would like to say a few words about the impact of COVID-19 on ambulatory care nursing.

Within this book, the impact of COVID-19 is discussed in the chapter on telehealth in respect to long-standing changes. However, because current information may quickly become outdated, we chose not to address this specific topic in other chapters.

The role of the ambulatory RN was thrust into the spotlight in this health crisis, and ambulatory RNs were positioned into roles that made a substantial impact in the response to COVID-19. For example, in at least one university system, ambulatory care RNs were deployed as the public-facing team on the COVID-19 hotline. These RNs ensured that individuals, employees, and community contacts were appropriately educated, triaged, and, as needed, scheduled into COVID-19 screening clinics. Other ambulatory RNs were utilized in nurse practitioner and RN-led virtual care clinics where COVID-19–positive individuals were cared for via telehealth visits through daily symptom management.

Ambulatory RN care coordinators assumed the role of managing all COVID-19–positive individuals discharged from inpatient units through transition management visits

(Landor et al., 2020). This both enhanced individual outcomes and contributed to the financial sustainability of the health system. In addition, RNs and advanced practice registered nurses (APRNs) led drive-through and independent screening and testing sites, supporting the epidemiologic response to this crisis.

The need for home healthcare does not disappear in the face of quarantines, and ambulatory care RNs in that field faced the same issues related to personal and client protection as did their acute care counterparts. Like hospitals and ambulatory care settings, home health organizations also faced difficulties in retaining RNs who would work with COVID-19–positive patients and hurdles in acquiring sufficient personal protection equipment. Mental health support for these RNs was an ongoing challenge, as it was in other ambulatory and acute settings.

Arguably, the field of telehealth will be the one most profoundly changed because of this forced shift in care delivery. Even the darkest cloud can have a silver lining, and because of these changes, RNs and APRNs are finding and enhancing their skills in virtual care. Reimbursement models are being modified and it is to be hoped that these changes will continue and expand to allow for full RN compensation in this growing arena. Additionally, as both providers and individuals become comfortable with some form of remote care, true person-centered care may include adapting for problems with face-to-face encounters, whether the challenges be distance, transportation, or physical impairment.

In a final note, the following observation was made by Susan Mitchell Grant, who was chief nurse executive at Emory Healthcare during the Ebola crisis when those patients were being admitted to Emory University Hospital. Her comments at that time are equally relevant today:

> … People often ask why we would choose to care for such high-risk patients. For many of us, that is why we chose this occupation—to care for people in need.… We can either let our actions be guided by misunderstandings, fear and self-interest, or we can lead by knowledge, science and compassion. We can fear, or we can care. (from an op-ed in the *Washington Post*, August 11, 2014. http://news.emory.edu/stories/2014/08/community_responds_oped/campus.html)

Reference

Landor, M., Schroeder, K., & Thompson, T. (2020). Managing care transitions to the community during a pandemic. *Journal of Nursing Administration, 50*(9), 438–441. https://doi.org/10.1097/nna.0000000000000913

Caroline Varner Coburn
Deena Gilland
Beth Ann Swan

Content Map

Using this content map: some topics, such as roles of advanced practice nurses and nurse leaders, are woven throughout most chapters and are not specifically noted here. Also, care coordination is not listed here because it is a separate chapter and also is integrated into most chapters.

Key Content	Chapter(s)*
Accreditation	5*
Advocacy	4*, 7
Behavioral and mental health, integrated care	2, 3, 10, 12, 14
Care delivery and payment models	2*, 3, 6
Community and public health	1, 3, 10, 13, 14
Continuum of care	1, 8*, 10*, 13
Cultural and literacy considerations	3, 7, 14*
Education and self-care management	7*
Elements and history of ambulatory care nursing	1*, 2*, 8, 10, 15
Health Information Technology/informatics	2, 6, 8–10, 16
Healthcare delivery models	2*, 5
Home health	1, 11*
Nurse executives/nursing leadership	6, 16
Nurse navigation/case management	8*
Nurse residency/professional development	16*
Nurse-sensitive indicators/nursing economic impact	5*, 6, 10
Nursing workforce and education	15*, 16*
Payment models and care delivery methods	1, 2*, 5*, 10
Policy/regulation	3*, 4, 7–9, 11, 13, 14
Practical nurses and unlicensed personnel	4*, 5
Primary care/patient-centered medical homes	2*, 5, 6, 10*
Protocols and delegated orders	9, 10
Quality measurement/evidence-based practice	5*, 6*, 16
Scope of practice	4*, 7, 9, 11, 13
Social and economic influences on health	1, 2, 3*, 14*
Specialty and episodic care	1, 11*, 12*
Team-based/interprofessional care	6, 10*, 16
Telehealth and virtual care	1, 6, 9*
Veterans, women, school, prison, occupational health	3, 13*
Vulnerable populations	2, 3*, 13, 14*

*Content is primary in this chapter.

Acknowledgments

Dr. Coburn would like to express her appreciation to Dr. Linda McCauley, dean of the Emory University Nell Hodgson Woodruff School of Nursing, and Dr. Sandra Dunbar, senior associate dean for academic advancement. Without the first Writing Retreat sponsored by Dr. McCauley and without the ongoing support provided by these two nursing leaders, this book may never have come to be. Appreciation also goes to the members of the Ebbtide writing group: our fearless leader Kylie Smith, and Dorothy Jordan, Lisa Thompson, Sharon Vanairsdale, and Kelly Wiltse Nicely—for reminding us all to hang in there and it will happen!

Contents

UNIT 1

Changing Landscape of Healthcare in the United States

1

Ambulatory Nursing: An Overview

Caroline Varner Coburn and Deena Gilland

PERSPECTIVES

"Our ability to invest in the ambulatory care nurse workforce requires that we recognize the need for change in our current care delivery model. This change can be achieved through the continued support of nursing programs that are currently in existence, and an investment in new educational opportunities. Through this educational commitment and with improvements to the regulatory practice of nurses, we can sustain our nurse workforce and position nurses to practice across all settings in an effort provide care to those in need."

Jeannie Cimiotti, PhD, RN, FAAN, Associate Professor, Emory University Nell Hodgson Woodruff School of Nursing, Atlanta, Georgia

LEARNING OBJECTIVES

Upon completion of this chapter, the reader will be able to:

1. Describe the historical basis of ambulatory care nursing.
2. Understand the defining elements of ambulatory care, especially in the context of individual, environment, and nursing role.
3. Compare similarities and differences between ambulatory care, population health, and public health.
4. Explain the social, economic, and policy influences leading to and having an impact on the current state of ambulatory care nursing roles and practice.
5. Understand the general arenas of nursing roles in the various ambulatory care settings.
6. Compare and contrast the roles of nursing in the acute care and ambulatory care settings.

KEY TERMS

Ambulatory care nursing
Care coordination
Community care
Home visitation
Ongoing care
Specialty and episodic care
Transition management
Virtual care

History

If the fictional nurse Cherry Ames, from the 1950s' era series of mystery novels written by Helen Wells, had followed her career path, she may have become an office or clinic nurse after 25 years of working in a hospital setting. Why? Being a clinic nurse was viewed as being easier, slower paced, and less stressful than a hospital nurse.

Fast forward to the 21st century, and the nurses with the same expectation are in for a shock. **Ambulatory care nursing** has evolved as a career specialty of its own, not simply a junior version of care delivered in the acute setting. Ambulatory care nurses coordinate care for individuals with multiple, complex health issues; address the health and economic implications of hospital readmissions, adherence to treatment, and the impact of being underserved/underinsured; and help individuals navigate a system that sends them home with increasingly complicated needs. How did the profession evolve to this point?

Timeline of Nursing in Ambulatory Care

A variety of events and advances have led to the field now defined as ambulatory care nursing. Although nursing/midwifery in the generic sense has been practiced in the home and community for centuries, the concept of trained nurses caring for strangers became more acceptable through the work of Florence Nightingale. From her time of primarily hospital- and combat-based settings, nurses then began to move into the community.

This movement took many forms, from a community-based focus, as illustrated by Lillian Wald in the Henry Street Settlement, to the home-based care by the Visiting Nurse Service, still in existence today, or to the many roles in both settings of public health nurses. However, although community nursing and home-based nursing are elements of ambulatory care, the majority of nursing roles in this specialty evolved from a background of physician-based practices. Traditional office care was physician driven, often with a single nurse—registered nurse (RN), licensed practical or vocational nurse (LPN or LVN)—or possibly no nurse at all. An unlicensed medical assistant (MA) might be trained by the physician to assist as needed, with the majority of care being provided by the physician directly.

In the early 21st-century United States, there are fewer small-office practices and fewer physicians whom provide the majority of care for their individuals. In part, this is due to workplace constraints such as regulatory and payer requirements, limited ability to negotiate fees, and stressful lifestyle demands (Association of American Medical Colleges, 2019). Also, although primary care and disease prevention have long been recognized as important concepts, it is only in recent years that the U.S. health system has begun to increase support for those efforts in educational and financial terms. Finally, individuals are presenting to the outpatient setting with multiple, complex health issues. All of these factors combine to set the stage for a transformation in delivery of ambulatory care. As healthcare delivery has evolved, so has nursing practice in ambulatory care settings.

Evolving Roles for Nurses

In the evolution of the traditional practice of doctor of medicine (MD) and MA described earlier, the RN role is often more supervisory or administrative than one incorporating implementation of care. MAs are allowed to perform any tasks that the physician assigns or delegates to them, and LPNs provide basic nursing care as their education allows. On the face of it, this practice design often appears to be more economically practical than an enhanced use of RNs for individual care and coordination. Therefore, RNs may not be fully recognized for the value of their education and expertise, possibly because of habit and tradition and/or lack of knowledge about data supporting the value of RN **care coordination** in ambulatory care.

Although it has been a challenge to educate providers and health systems, a growing body of research supports the value that RNs bring to ambulatory practice, especially in the areas of health-related outcomes and patient satisfaction in the care of chronic conditions (Bauer & Bodenheimer, 2017; Chan et al., 2018; Hass & Swan, 2014). However, the economic value of the RN has been more difficult to establish unequivocally, arguably because of the limited amount of billable services that are tied to nursing-specific activities. However, as evidence continues to demonstrate the economic value of RNs in ambulatory care, there is support for increased visibility of this value through more billable services and identified nurse-sensitive indicators of quality improvement (Mastal et al., 2016; Needleman, 2017; Zolotorofe et al., 2018).

In conjunction with establishing intrinsic value for the field of ambulatory care nursing, this specialty has faced the challenges of defining itself, elevating the role of nursing in this setting, and providing support for the use of RNs at their full scope of education and practice. In 1987 the American Academy of Ambulatory Care Nursing (AAACN), the professional organization for this specialty, formalized the scope and standards of practice for ambulatory care nursing. This first description of ambulatory care practice scope and standards was followed in 1997 by the first formal definition of ambulatory care nursing practice and by subsequent publications of scope and standards for professional ambulatory care nursing (AAACN, 2017a).

Defining Ambulatory Care

The AAACN logo includes the words "Many Settings. Multiple Roles. One Unifying Specialty." This phrase encapsulates both the strength and the challenge of ambulatory care. Even within the field of ambulatory care, definitions have been blurred. For example, primary care is a specialty within ambulatory care, but for some practitioners the terms "primary care" and "ambulatory care" have been used interchangeably when discussing competencies. Also, some competencies, such as care coordination, **transition management**, and telehealth, have been carefully delineated, but primary care and other settings under the ambulatory care umbrella may need further clarification.

Ambulatory care is a relatively new nursing specialty and one that continues to refine and clarify its position in the profession. To provide an overview, AAACN places the elements of ambulatory care into three general categories: the individual, the environment, and the nursing role, which are illustrated in Figure 1.1. These are discussed further on, as is the specific role of nursing in this specialty.

In addition to the general overview, ambulatory care consists of numerous specialty areas. Nursing has precedent for capturing subspecialties under one overarching professional specialty. For example, medical–surgical nursing is established both in the academic and in the clinical setting as a field of nursing, even though that field includes the many and diverse specialty areas that might fall under the categories of "general surgery" or "general medicine."

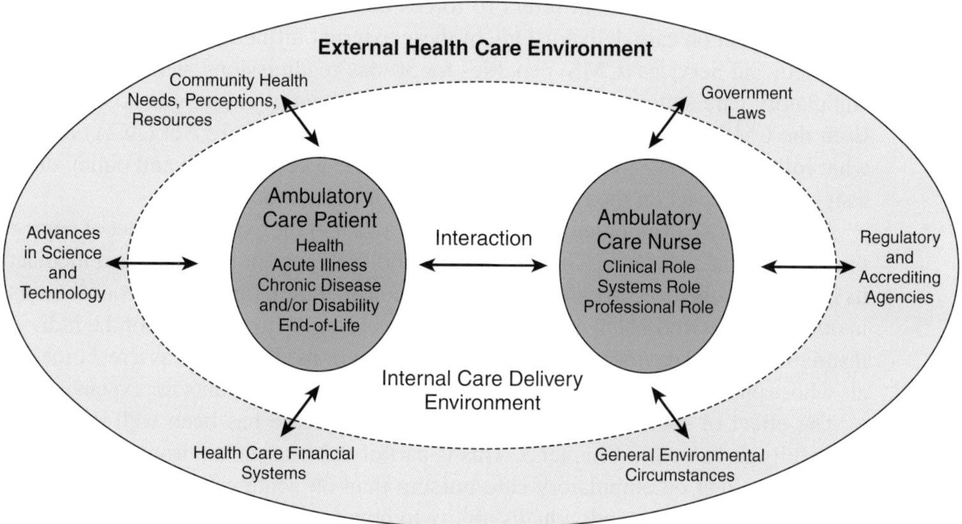

FIGURE 1.1 Framework of ambulatory care nursing. (Used with permission of American Academy of Ambulatory Care Nursing [AAACN], aaacn.org)

Similarly, ambulatory care includes a range in age from newborn to geriatric, and a range of care delivery settings from primary to episodic to urgent care. As the field evolves, further subspecialties in ambulatory care will become more defined.

Individuals

Individuals are the focus of ambulatory care, whether they are technically ambulatory or not. The infant in arms, healthy teenager, young mother, older individual, veteran, and individual with a mobility disability are all members of the ambulatory nurse practice. They and their significant others are supported at whatever point in their health continuum they are in when they reach out for care.

Possibly one of the defining elements of ambulatory care is locus of control. In ambulatory care, the individual is in charge of their treatment regimen, and the RN role is one of consultant and collaborator. This concept is discussed in more detail later in this chapter; however, an understanding of individual control is exemplified by the ways individuals enter the ambulatory care system. In general terms, encounters in ambulatory care are initiated by the individual and are brief, less than 24 hours, and allow for a high volume of individuals in a short time.

Often, it is difficult for the RN new to ambulatory care to let go of the control they may be used to in acute care or may have experienced as a student. In ambulatory care, any treatments, medications, or lifestyle changes are essentially completely under the control of the individual, not the MD, nurse practitioner (NP), physician assistant (PA), RN, or any other member of the staff. It is important to respect and support that control, realizing that treatment success depends on the individual's willingness and/or ability to understand and adhere to the recommended regimen.

Environment

As illustrated in Figure 1.1, the environment that defines ambulatory care nursing can be divided into internal and external. Internal environment refers to the setting where the individual receives care. In ambulatory care, the internal environment may be wide ranging: episodic care such as an urgent care clinic or same-day surgery, an ongoing primary care practice, a virtual or telehealth setting, or an infusion/oncology facility, to cite only a few examples. This is in contrast to an acute care setting, in which the internal environment has less variability. Regardless of the illness, surgery, or health challenge, the acute care environment is within a hospital setting.

The external environment refers to forces outside the practice setting that, nevertheless, have an impact on care delivery. One of these external influences is the Centers for Medicare and Medicaid Services (CMS) penalties for 30-day readmissions, which caused hospitals and ambulatory care settings to focus on addressing potential causes for hospital readmissions. Both the CMS penalties and the impact of the Affordable Care Act (ACA) are discussed in what follows. However, on both a national and state level, political and policy decisions have a significant impact on the external influences of ambulatory care.

Arguably, RNs in ambulatory care are more aware of the external impact of payment sources than are RNs in acute care. The individual's ability to pay for treatment and medications, with its impact on adherence to care, is an ongoing consideration for RN care coordinators. As noted in other chapters, the RN in ambulatory care may serve as an advocate for the individual whose insurer has denied payment for a specific treatment or medication or as a resource for individuals whose pharmaceutical company may offer coupons or discounts for expensive medications.

The effect of socioeconomic influences on healthcare has been well documented and is more fully discussed in Chapter 3. This is part of the external environment that has considerably more effect on ambulatory care nursing than on acute care nursing, primarily because in ambulatory care, the individual's ability to obtain and afford treatment has a direct impact on the success of treatment. Other points of contrast between acute and ambulatory care are discussed in more detail next.

To summarize, the internal environment of ambulatory care may be defined by its variety of locations. However, the external environment is complex and wide ranging and affects individual care in multiple ways. In general, the acute care setting is less varied and is less affected by external environmental influences than is the ambulatory care setting.

Social, Economic, and Policy Influences

Much has been written to account for the decrease in the length of inpatient hospital stay over recent years, with adjusted reimbursement protocols and concerns for hospital-related adverse events arguably being two of the most powerful reasons. Whatever the reasons, individuals go home sicker than they used to. In addition, the downstream effect of early discharge may be hospital readmission, with resulting financial penalties for hospitals on that end as well. This situation alone provides a strong argument for a robust support system, one that helps individuals in the hospital to transition home or elsewhere and provides resources to keep them from returning unnecessarily to the emergency department or hospital.

Drivers of Change

Change in the U.S. healthcare system has come from both negative and positive drivers. Related to ambulatory care, one of the most powerful negative drivers for change has been penalties imposed on hospitals by the CMS for unnecessary rehospitalization (CMS, n.d.). As a result, all players in the healthcare system are forced to consider the causes of rehospitalization and how to address them, with significant implications for the role of providers outside of the acute care setting.

In the past, hospitals were not forced to follow individuals after discharge. With the readmission penalties, this has changed, and new strategies are constantly being implemented. In an ambulatory setting that is part of a hospital system, the rewards for decreasing unnecessary readmissions can be implemented more easily. The clinics associated with that hospital can be provided with encouragement and incentives to address posthospitalization issues. However, a clinic–hospital connection is not always present or seamless, so additional interventions are needed for hospitals to ensure that these individuals are appropriately followed after discharge.

One approach to the unnecessary readmission challenge is the use of effective transition management at discharge. The concepts of care coordination and transition management (CCTM) are discussed in more detail in Chapter 8, but from a hospital perspective, transition management provides a mechanism for following recently discharged individuals to ensure both their understanding of posthospital care and their access to appropriate follow-up.

Although not the result of a specific penalty, hospital expense also may be considered a negative driver for insurance companies. Insurance companies, which arguably have the strongest financial incentive to reduce hospitalizations, have taken steps with the use of care coordinators and lifestyle coaches to support their individuals and decrease hospitalizations of all kinds. This role may be filled by an RN or by another trained healthcare professional.

In combination with disincentives (ie, financial penalties and concerns for in-hospital events), incentives also have been offered to address the conditions resulting in hospitalizations of any kind. Disease prevention, healthy lifestyle, optimal wellness: these terms reflect a shifting mindset in the healthcare community from treatment to prevention, and financial incentives are available to support these incentives. Through the use of bundled payments, capitation, and other cost-saving measures, practices may be rewarded for providing the most appropriate care, even including interventions that might not be billable under traditional fee for service. Patient-Centered Medical Homes, Accountable Care Organizations, and other collaborative arrangements have supported and enhanced these developments, and these are discussed in more detail in Chapter 2.

Although initiation of the CMS penalties for readmissions was a driver for change within hospitals, the Patient Protection and Affordable Care Act (PPACA) addressed the need for affordable preventive and urgent care on an individual level and initiated change in the ambulatory care world. As noted by the AAACN, "A number of evolutionary societal, legislative, regulatory, technological, and health industry trends form the context of the ambulatory care environment, effecting change in both care delivery systems and practice of professional nursing. Today ambulatory care has evolved into sophisticated, highly complex organizations and systems" (Mastal et al., 2016, p. 94). The healthcare delivery shift from traditional inpatient settings to ambulatory care settings has been caused largely by economic factors, such as a decrease in inpatient admissions, reduced average length of stay, and increase in total outpatient visits (Mastal et al., 2016).

The financial shift of emphasis by the CMS on preventive care has also provided support to providers in primary care settings and created an opportunity for ambulatory care nurses. In 2015, the U.S. Health and Human Services announced plans that future Medicare payments would be linked to value (Bauer & Bodenheimer, 2017). The CMS has introduced fee-for-service add-on payments that RNs can provide, such as annual wellness visits and chronic care management services. Couple this with pay-for-performance and person-centered medical home (PCMH) rewards that support team-based care models, and the value of the RN in ambulatory care is magnified.

In summary, rather than having a health crisis as a person's first introduction to the healthcare system, focus is now increasingly placed on pulling individuals into healthy living habits before they become ill. Alternatively, if an illness has already occurred, then the goal is to employ all possible resources to minimize the long-term effects and maximize the best possible quality of life. RN education, with its emphasis on individual-centered, holistic care through the life span, is a natural fit for the current national emphasis on keeping people as healthy as possible and in the hospital as little as possible.

Nursing Impact and Response

The educational background of nurses is based on an understanding that care of the individual includes all health influences: economic, physical, emotional, psychosocial, as well as any barriers to care or adherence. This places nurses in an excellent position to fully understand and implement a system of care that is focused on optimal health rather than illness. RNs represent the largest profession within the U.S. health workforce, with expectations that demand for RNs will continue to increase over the next decade (U.S. Bureau of Labor Statistics [BLS], 2012). In addition, a larger percentage of the growth in demand for RNs is estimated to come from needs outside the hospital in response to the ACA (Spetz, 2014).

Settings such as ambulatory care surgery, infusion centers, and urgent care centers have flourished in response to these drivers to shift care out of the hospital. As more individual care moves with this shift and as the individuals being cared for become increasingly complex, RNs with the skills and knowledge to implement a complete plan of care become essential to the success of the healthcare system. All of these factors have led to an increased awareness of the value RNs bring to the field, a contribution that continues to be documented in studies and analyses (Bauer & Bodenheimer, 2017; Ensign & Hawkins, 2017; Salmon & Echevarria, 2017). It has been called the beginning of a "golden age for ambulatory care nursing" (Swan & Haas, 2011, p. 331).

Ambulatory Nursing Roles: An Overview

For many people, the words "ambulatory care nurse" bring to mind only the setting of the office nurse providing care under the supervision of a physician. Understandably then, defining and explaining this increasingly complex field is a challenge. Although the roles of RNs in ambulatory care are not easily defined, the value of RNs in ambulatory care is becoming increasingly recognized. In 2016 the Josiah Macy, Jr. Foundation sponsored a conference to explore the contributions of nurses in this changing healthcare world. The published proceedings from the conference, *Registered Nurses: Partners in Transforming Primary Care*, make a strong case for the current value of RNs in ambulatory care, as well as the need to reevaluate the current roles and responsibilities of these RNs (Bodenheimer & Mason, 2017).

To provide an overview of current roles in ambulatory care, the general and varied responsibilities of the ambulatory care nurse will be considered, followed by a discussion of the specific roles that are commonly found in this multifaceted field. All of these topics are addressed in further detail in other chapters of this book.

It may be helpful to discuss RN responsibilities as a separate category from specific RN roles. Regardless of the role, the responsibilities of an ambulatory care RN may look quite different depending on the setting, the job requirements, and the RN experience. However, these responsibilities may generally be placed into the following three categories:

- Clinical: This may be the most visible RN responsibility, one in which the nurse provides care and/or education to individuals or groups along the continuum of health needs.
- Management and/or organization: RNs who participate in the direction and coordination of the practice or who are responsible for the supervision of personnel, workload, or legal, regulatory, and fiscal issues.
- Professional excellence: This is a responsibility that frequently overlaps with all other roles and responsibilities. On a practice level, it may include participating in quality improvement or ensuring evidence-based practice, whereas on an individual level, the RN may initiate or participate in professional development of self or staff.

Regardless of RN responsibilities, it is also important to define the role of registered nursing in this field. In 2017, the AAACN produced a white paper that provides a broad definition of the role of the RN in ambulatory care. In this document, the organization describes the importance of RNs in this field, especially as it relates to continuum of care:

- RNs provide high-quality, evidence-based care across the life span to enhance individual safety; reduce adverse events; impact and improve individual satisfaction; support and promote optimal health status; track admissions and readmissions; and manage costs within and among continually expanding, diverse, and complex populations. Therefore, RNs are essential to the delivery of safe, high-quality care and should not be replaced by less-skilled licensed or unlicensed members of the healthcare team.
- RNs are the team members best prepared to facilitate the functioning of interprofessional teams across the care continuum, coordinate care with individuals and their caregivers, and mitigate the growing complexity of transitions in care.
- RNs play a critical role in the delivery of telehealth services and **virtual care**. The development of the art and science of telehealth nursing practice has improved and expanded coordination of healthcare services, reduced individual risk, and contributed significantly to care management models (AAACN, 2017a).

An additional report by the AAACN on scope of practice for ambulatory care nurses describes professional ambulatory care nursing as a specialty practice of nursing that focuses on "quality care across the life span to individuals, families, care-givers, groups, populations, and communities" (Murray, 2017, p. 6). This description and the previous role definitions provide a wide-ranging view of what it means to be an ambulatory care nurse. However, it is also useful to mention the most common ambulatory care settings and RN roles for those settings.

The areas discussed next are covered in detail in other chapters; however, they provide an overview of the various settings included under the umbrella of ambulatory care. For the purposes of description, this overview will categorize ambulatory care roles with an individual-based focus of **ongoing care, specialty and episodic care, community care, home visitation,** and virtual care. It is important to emphasize that the distinctions made are not meant to be mutually exclusive; in each setting, the RN will apply skills and competencies that are mirrored in other settings.

Ongoing Care

The category of ongoing care encompasses the most traditional view of ambulatory care: the physician-led clinic (see Chapters 8, 10, 13, and 14). But it may also include ongoing care provided through areas such as school and employer clinics, the Veterans Administration, Public Health Service clinics for Native Americans, nurse-led and NP clinics, or healthcare for incarcerated individuals, as a few examples.

The common factor for these various settings is that care is delivered to an individual who is considered part of the practice population. Whether the individual is seen only rarely or on a regular basis, this clinic would generally be the individual's first stop for a health issue, which may sometimes then lead to referral to another resource.

The nursing role in ongoing care settings varies widely. For example, within the health maintenance organization or individual-centered medical home, the nurse may deliver care at a high level of autonomy. In a school or prison clinic, there may be more specific limitations on the nurse's scope of practice. However, in all of these settings, care is being delivered to an individual who is considered a recurring individual for the practice.

Specialty and Episodic Care

The specialty clinics include areas such as cardiology, oncology, pulmonary, and other disease-specific clinics. Episodic care refers to either settings that individuals are likely to visit only once (urgent care centers or ambulatory care surgery, for instance) or areas like infusion centers, where they may come multiple times but only for a specific treatment (see Chapters 11 and 12).

The common factor in these examples is that they are established clinics, often connected to a health system, but are secondary to the individual's primary care provider. In fact, in many cases, individuals are referred to these clinics by their primary care provider. Although for some individuals their specialty provider may serve in many ways as a primary care provider (examples include women's health, oncology, and chronic conditions like heart failure and asthma), the distinction remains that this setting is meant to focus on a specific area of the individual's health picture.

These settings may provide the most skills-intensive setting for ambulatory care nurses, particularly in ambulatory care surgery and infusion, but also in areas such as cardiology and pulmonology. In these areas, the nurse's contribution is often as intense as that of nursing care delivered in the hospital setting, the focus being on a single procedure or health challenge.

Community Health and Public Health

Many of the responsibilities, tasks, and competencies that are needed for community health nursing are the same as those in the category of ongoing care, described earlier. One difference is that community health is often delivered outside of the traditional site-specific clinic setting. Some examples of community health are pop-up clinics; faith-based nursing; or clinics that serve homeless, refugee, or underresourced individuals (see Chapters 10, 13, and 14).

In the context of community care, the ambulatory care nurse is functioning outside the traditional clinic setting for a population that may include either individuals or groups. These settings are not formally connected to the individual's primary care network, may include both groups and individuals, and may include individuals who have no primary care provider at all. The RN role may be one of direct care or may consist primarily of educational and screening activities.

Public health, in comparison with community health, over time has been established and refined as a specific entity. Public health nurses are part of a state's healthcare system and have a well-defined set of roles and responsibilities. However, although public health may fall into a distinct category, it is considered by the AAACN to be under the umbrella of ambulatory care nursing and shares similarities with community health nursing. The distinctions between community health and public health nursing are more easily defined on paper than in practice because, although public health nursing operates under a different organizational structure, many of the nursing functions are similar in the two settings.

One similarity between the two areas is that the nursing focus can be either on groups or on individuals. In both public health and community health, activities may include presentations on risk reduction for common health issues like heart disease or cancer or outreach to vulnerable populations to mitigate socioeconomic influences on health. On the individual level, they may include primary care functions such as complete physical examinations or chronic disease management.

Care delivery modes may become blurred between the categories of public health and community care even though the settings may be distinct and separate. For example, both community clinics and public health clinics may be either episodic or ongoing. A temporarily homeless person or someone needing vaccination services may need the community or public health services only for a short time. However, in some cases such as clinics for indigent or underserved individuals, the clinic may serve as the primary source of care.

Because the role of the public health nurse is well documented and explored in many textbooks, the emphasis in this book will be on the community health nursing aspect of ambulatory care, avoiding a discussion of the separate field of public health nursing.

Home Health

In the discussion of ambulatory care so far, there has been a common element: the individual comes to the place providing care. In the category of home health, however, the reverse is the case: care comes to the individual (see Chapter 11).

Home health may include chronic or palliative care conditions involving ongoing visits, follow-up after an acute episode that may require only a few treatments, or end-of-life care. Because individuals are discharged from hospitals with more complex problems, a stronger need has emerged for nurses who can care for individuals with a variety of challenges such as intravenous lines, respiratory ventilators, or cardiac support machines. For instance, in the past, it would have been unlikely for an individual to be discharged from the hospital with ongoing treatments such as intravenous inotropic medications or a ventricular assist device. Now, however, this is a fairly common practice.

Home health nurses may have a wide variety of roles and responsibilities, including oversight of assistive personnel, evaluation of a home for safety risks, evaluation of the individual for ongoing or new care needs, and collaboration with other healthcare providers and resources. Arguably, more than in any other area of ambulatory care, the home health nurse also interacts more intimately with the individual's family or support system for data and information regarding the individual, as well as for adherence to care.

Virtual Care

Telehealth and virtual care (Chapter 9) are part of all the foregoing categories; in almost any ambulatory care setting, there is some kind of virtual care, either through telephone conversations that might include triage, assessment, and care or through the monitoring of remotely collected data. Telehealth and virtual care may also be provided in a stand-alone setting with a telephone or video connection to a bank of individuals.

The nursing role for virtual care includes specific competencies that require skill and education to master. One of the most challenging competencies of telehealth is that of having to assess the individual without being able to use visual or tactile information. In other types of virtual care, such as remote data collection or visual remote care, the nurse has greater access to objective and observational data. For example, data may be collected remotely for a variety of parameters such as blood pressure, pacemaker functioning, or blood glucose. In all of these situations, however, the RN must be equipped to evaluate the data and act on the information that is gained without physical access to the individual.

The RN in telehealth and remote monitoring is guided by protocols and decision support tools to make clinical changes. In the situation of video virtual care, an advanced practice RN or an MD is often making the clinical decisions. However, ideally, the RN is with the individual on the other end, providing the physical assessment data and supportive information. The RN in this role is able to use skills and competencies at the top of their licensure and further demonstrate the value of RN education in ambulatory care.

Overview

More comprehensive discussions of these roles are addressed in subsequent chapters of this book. The key point of this overview is that ambulatory care nursing is evolving, refining, and defining itself as one that applies the principles of preventive and holistic care to every ambulatory setting. The initiative, persistence, and vision of nurse leaders have brought the field of ambulatory care nursing to where it is now: positioned to lead in a healthcare setting that needs the skills and knowledge that are fundamental to nursing education.

Comparison: Ambulatory and Acute Care Nursing

Many nurses in ambulatory care have come from the acute care setting: hospital, long-term care facility, or a similar environment. Traditionally, they have had the impression that ambulatory care nursing would be both slower paced and easier than working in a hospital. Additionally, in the past, those hiring for ambulatory care clinics required some experience in acute care before transitioning to ambulatory care. The assumption was that ambulatory care required a degree of independence and clinical skill that could be gained only in an acute care setting.

Both of these assumptions have been challenged in the current ambulatory setting. Many former hospital nurses are surprised to find that they are working equally hard and are having to draw upon expert knowledge for clinical judgment, care coordination, and interprofessional collaboration to an equal or greater extent than they did in the acute care setting. Ambulatory care can no longer be considered an easier job than acute care; furthermore, there is evidence that knowledge and skills required in acute care do not necessarily transfer to ambulatory care; new knowledge, skills, and perspectives are required (Ashley et al., 2016; Swan, 2007; Walshe Allen, 2016). Additionally, new RN graduates are successfully starting their careers in ambulatory care, especially with the initiation of new graduate residencies in this area (Fritz, 2017; Gilland et al., 2019).

To consider the differences between ambulatory and acute care nursing, it may be helpful to place these differences in three general categories: treatment management, individual encounters, and organizational roles. The competencies of care coordination and transition management are essential to all of these areas and are addressed separately.

Treatment Management

As has been noted previously, a primary difference between ambulatory and acute care nursing lies in locus of control; in the acute care setting, the RN holds a high degree of control over delivery of care. Even tasks that the individual may have previously performed, such as medication administration, are taken over by the RN. In ambulatory care, success of a treatment regimen is dependent on the individual's adherence and commitment, as well as external factors that might support or interfere with the plan of care. The healthcare team may have little to no control over those factors, or indirect control at best.

In the acute care setting, treatment is initiated, implemented, and observed by the healthcare team. In the ambulatory care setting, implementation of a treatment regimen is in the hands of the individual, outside the observation of the healthcare team. Additionally, modifications to the treatment plan may be made by the individual without the knowledge of the healthcare team.

Another difference in treatment management has to do with timing. In an acute care setting, the individual's treatment period is defined: admission to discharge. The nursing treatment of this individual also is shaped and limited by a specified diagnosis or diagnoses. In contrast, an ambulatory care individual may be seen only intermittently over a period of years, or may have a cluster of visits followed by a long period of inactivity, or any combination of those. Over that more flexible period of time, medical issues may be added or resolved, and the nurse must adapt to different individual needs.

Finally, the overall treatment management perspective differs between ambulatory and acute care nursing. In most cases, an ambulatory encounter is viewed in the context of the individual's total healthcare picture. For instance, in primary care, all aspects of the individual's care are considered, from preventive to chronic to end of life. Even in an episodic setting such as same-day surgery or specialty clinics, the care is coordinated and information shared with the primary provider, which, ideally, provides the continuity of care characterized by ambulatory care.

In an acute care setting, the focus is on the specific issue that brought the individual to the hospital; the nurses caring for an individual may have very limited knowledge of the individual's situation outside of the hospital or even all elements of their past history unless it were relevant to the current admission diagnoses. Box 1.1 illustrates the difference in treatment management between ambulatory and acute care.

Individual Encounters

In most ambulatory settings, care is initiated by the individual who comes to the clinic or setting for delivery of care. In hospitalization, the initial event may have been out of the individual's control, and for delivery of care the healthcare team comes to the individual. In both settings, the family or support group may be included in the plan of care, but in ambulatory care, these resources are even more important as part of the individual encounters.

As noted earlier, in a hospital setting, the nurse has direct and continuous observation of the individual, whereas the ambulatory care nurse must rely on intermittent observations to gain a full picture of the individual's health status. In addition, the ambulatory care nurse may have to rely to a greater degree on indirect or second-hand information. For instance, to evaluate the effectiveness of an intervention to reduce smoking, the nurse may have to depend on the individual's or family member's honesty and accuracy in reporting as well as observations from family or friends.

BOX 1.1 Acute and Ambulatory Comparison: Treatment Management

Acute Care	Ambulatory Care
An RN on a cardiac unit delivers or oversees a complicated regimen of medications and treatments for the individuals on that unit. One of the individuals is feeling nauseated and unable to take oral medications. The nurse is able to administer an antiemetic and return at a later time to give the oral medications. Although there was a slight delay, the schedule for these interventions was fairly firm.	An RN in the cardiac clinic meets with an individual about heart failure. The nurse finds that this individual has not been consistent in obtaining daily weights or reducing dietary sodium and counsels on the importance of adhering to diet and reducing sodium. This has been a challenge in the past, so the nurse tries a different intervention tactic in the hope that the result will be improved at the next visit.

Note. RN = registered nurse.

The actual encounter time in ambulatory care is shorter, which means that the ambulatory care nurse may have only a few minutes to assess and evaluate an individual. Also, there is generally no opportunity to return to an individual later in the day to reevaluate or follow up on an assessment.

Role Definition

Organizational roles are less clearly specified in ambulatory care than in the acute or hospital setting. This may in part be explained by the evolution of ambulatory care nursing, as described earlier. For many years, the "nursing" role in a physician's office had been carried out by an MA or even someone with no prior healthcare education who was trained by the physician. This may have contributed to some of the blurring of roles between unlicensed personnel, LPNs or LVNs, RNs, and advanced practice RNs such as NPs.

Whatever the background cause of the difference, it may be observed that nurses in acute care settings have specific responsibilities that help define their roles more clearly. Medication administration, for instance, is the sole responsibility of the hospital nurse, unlike an ambulatory setting in which medications and injections such as flu shots or vaccines may be administered by non-nurses. The flexible nature of ambulatory care also broadens the range of activities carried out by the nurses in that field. The ambulatory care nurse may provide triage for walk-in individuals, or advocate for an individual with an insurance provider, or answer telephone questions about health concerns, potentially all in the same day. Although this may exemplify the need for the education and skills that RNs bring to ambulatory care, it also illustrates the challenge in defining this specialty for those who are more familiar with the hospital-based roles of nurses.

Another aspect of organizational differences between ambulatory and acute care nursing has to do with workload. Although hospital nursing may have an element of unpredictability in terms of numbers and acuity of individuals, the physical restrictions of a hospital unit limit that unpredictability to some degree. However, in ambulatory care, variations in workflow may be more significant because of issues like walk-in individuals, individuals who are no-shows or who are considerably late for an appointment, urgent visits, and numbers of telephone calls, which in theory might have no limitations.

Care Coordination and Transition Management

CCTM crosses multiple roles within all three categories of treatment management, individual encounters, and organization. These are also defining roles for ambulatory care nursing and are discussed in more detail in Chapter 8. However, the following is intended to be a general overview of the similarities and differences between care coordination in the acute and ambulatory care settings.

In acute care, CCTM is incorporated within the larger goal of helping an individual progress to discharge. In ambulatory care, these are primary aspects of the nursing role. For the hospital RN, the need for care coordination ends when the individual is discharged; for the ambulatory RN, care coordination is an ongoing element of individual care along the continuum of health and may also be a distinct specialty role.

In acute care nursing, the RN's care coordination activities are tied to the individual's needs for that specific hospitalization. Care coordination within the hospital is related to in-hospital services such as procedures, diagnostic testing, and supplemental services such as physical or respiratory therapy and may be a small part of the RN's responsibilities. However, in ambulatory care, coordination and transition management activities incorporate the full healthcare needs of the individual, including, but not limited to, referrals between medical specialties and specialty services such as home care or mental health. Care coordination in ambulatory care may be incidental to the RN's primary role or may fully occupy that role. A title such as

BOX 1.2 Acute and Ambulatory Comparison: Care Coordination

Acute Care	Ambulatory Care
Over the course of a shift, an acute care RN coordinates care for a postoperative cardiac surgery individual by balancing the timing of interventions with the radiology and physical therapy departments, guiding a nursing assistant, and updating physical assessment information with the individual's medical team.	A nurse navigator in the oncology clinic has contacted an individual newly diagnosed with breast cancer. The RN gathers the appropriate radiology, pathology, and medical history information to help educate the individual; coordinates visits with the appropriate surgical, medical, and radiation oncologists; and organizes a team meeting to ensure the individual is supported.

Note. RN = registered nurse.

care coordinator or nurse navigator is a familiar one in ambulatory care clinics, particularly in a specialty like oncology.

Transition management is closely linked to care coordination and refers to seamless transition and follow-up from one setting to another. Because these competencies are so closely aligned, CCTM is offered by the AAACN as a single certification.

In the acute care setting, the importance of transition management has become more recognized as hospitals try to avoid rehospitalizations and in some hospitals may be supported with a specific position. Nurses designated as transition managers or coordinators in this setting are focused on transitioning the individual to an assisted living or home setting and generally providing follow-up for a designated period after discharge.

In addition to the role differences in care coordination for acute versus ambulatory care, a difference in perspective should also be noted. As has been discussed, in acute care the essential role of care coordination revolves around diagnostic and therapeutic responses to a primary diagnosis. However, in ambulatory care, this perspective shifts to one of maintaining optimal overall health. In that context, the RN coordinates the diagnostic and treatment services that may address specific health issues or may provide insight on potential health risks or may prevent a particular disease or infection. Even in episodic or specialty clinics, care coordination is implemented through communication between these clinics and the individual's primary care provider.

The knowledge, skills, and competencies of RNs in both acute and ambulatory care are essential to the healthcare system and to individual individuals in that system. In the end, there are more similarities than differences in the ways that RNs care for their individuals, but a fuller understanding of the differences that do exist can only help to support improved communication and teamwork between the different specialties. Box 1.2 illustrates the difference in care coordination between the ambulatory and acute care setting.

Summary

As discussed earlier, ambulatory care nursing can be seen to have a wide scope that is not confined to one type of practice setting or type and requires specific education and knowledge based on the practice setting and care being delivered. For these reasons, the role of the RN in ambulatory care is complex and requires critical reasoning and judgment in order to deliver the most appropriate care.

As with many nursing specialties, ambulatory care has core attributes but also encompasses subspecialties. Because it is a nursing specialty that is growing in significance and impact, it also continues to refine and define its role in the delivery of healthcare.

Ambulatory care nursing has roots in the work of nursing pioneers who led the way in providing direct community healthcare. It has built on those roots to produce a specialty that draws on the entirety of nursing education coupled with the skills of care coordination, collaboration, transitional care, and virtual health to address the challenges of episodic, preventive, and chronic care. Regardless of the eventual shape of healthcare in the United States, the importance of primary and preventive care will not diminish, and the role of healthcare outside of the hospital setting will continue to grow. Therefore, RNs who have the education, skills, competence, and judgment to collaborate with individuals and families to achieve the highest possible level of health will remain valuable members of the healthcare team.

Case Study

Transition from Acute to Ambulatory Care

Janet Johnson is a 25-year-old RN who has worked in hospital medical–surgical units since her graduation from nursing school. She and her husband recently had their first child, and she has been seeking a job that provides more regular hours from Monday through Friday. She is currently employed at a large academic medical center and has heard of job openings at the primary care clinic affiliated with the hospital.

In her previous jobs, she has been a shift leader, responsible for making individuals' assignments and delegating jobs to the unlicensed assistive personnel. She also worked with some of the physicians, advanced practice nurses, physician assistants, and social workers to initiate weekly meetings to discuss individuals with complex issues related to treatment and discharge.

Janet plans to highlight her leadership in quality improvement related to reducing infections from central line dressing changes and to note that during her shifts the individual's transfer time from the emergency department to the unit is significantly less than average.

She is known for being a very efficient nurse, always delivering medications and treatments on time. She believes that she can best serve individuals by ensuring that they adhere to the prescribed treatment plan and is kind but firm in explaining what they need to do and why.

In general, she believes that transitioning from her unit to primary care will be very easy and that ambulatory care nursing will not be as challenging as her current position.

Consider the following questions:

1. Which of Janet's skills and talents will be most helpful in the ambulatory care setting and why?
2. Which will be less helpful and why?
3. What would you say to Janet regarding her impression of ambulatory care nursing?
4. What might be the greatest personal challenge she will face in the new environment?

Key Points for Review

- Ambulatory nursing, although present for many years, has recently evolved into an integral role as the focus of healthcare delivery has moved from the inpatient to the outpatient setting and has shifted from treatment to prevention.
- Current economic and policy trends support the need for a robust system of primary and preventive care, which provides an ideal opportunity for the knowledge, skills, and competencies of RNs.
- A variety of roles outside the traditional acute care hospital exist under the overarching description of ambulatory care, including the areas of community health, public health nursing, telehealth, and virtual healthcare.
- Both acute and ambulatory nursing practice have common elements but with different perspectives in care delivery.

REFERENCES

American Academy of Ambulatory Care Nursing. (2017a). *American Academy of Ambulatory Care Nursing position paper; the role of the registered nurse in ambulatory care.* https://www.aaacn.org/sites/default/files/documents/PositionStatementRN.pdf

Ashley, C., Halcomb E., & Brown, A. (2016). Transitioning from acute to primary health care nursing: An integrative review of the literature. *Journal of Clinical Nursing, 25*(15–16), 2114–2125. https://doi.org/10.1111/jocn.13185

Association of American Medical Colleges. (2019). *The doctor is out. Rising student loan debt and the decline of the small medical practice.* Statement for the Record Submitted by the Association of American Medical Colleges (AAMC) to the House of Representatives Committee on Small Business, June 11, 2019. https://www.aamc.org/download/498034/data/aamcstatementtothehousesmallbusinesscommitteeregardingmedicaled.pdf

Bauer, L., & Bodenheimer, T. (2017). Expanded roles of registered nurses in primary care delivery of the future. *Nursing Outlook, 65*(4), A1–A10, e1, 351–488. https://doi.org/10.1016/j.outlook.2017.03.011

Bodenheimer, T & Mason, D. (2017). *Registered nurses: Partners in transforming primary care.* Proceedings of a conference sponsored by the Josiah Macy Jr. Foundation in June 2016; New York: Josiah Macy Jr. Foundation. https://macyfoundation.org/publications/registered-nurses-partners-in-transforming-primary-care

Centers for Medicare and Medicaid Services. (n.d.). *Hospital readmissions reduction program.* https://www.cms.gov/medicare/medicare-fee-for-service-payment/acuteinpatientpps/readmissions-reduction-program.html

Chan, R. J., Marx, W., Bradford, N., Gordon, L., Bonner, A., Douglas, C., Schmalkuche, D., & Yates, P. (2018). Clinical and economic outcomes of nurse-led services in the ambulatory care setting: A systematic review. *International Journal of Nursing Studies, 81*, 61–80. https://doi.org/10.1016/j.ijnurstu.2018.02.002

Ensign, C. M., & Hawkins, S. Y. (2017). Improving patient self-care and reducing readmissions through an outpatient heart failure case management program. *Professional Case Management, 22*(4), 190–196. https://doi.org/10.1097/ncm.0000000000000232

Fritz, E. (2017). Transition to practice in ambulatory care nursing. *Journal for Nurses in Professional Development, 33*(5), 257–258. https://doi.org/10.1097/NND.0000000000000376

Gilland, D. E., Muirhead, L., Toney, S., & Coburn, C. (2019). Building a workforce pipeline: Development of an ambulatory nurse residency program. *Nursing Management, 50*(7), 32–37. https://doi.org/10.1097/01.NUMA.0000558520.60241.1f

Haas, S. A., & Swan, B. A. (2014). Developing the value proposition for the role of the registered nurse in care coordination and transition management in ambulatory care settings. *Nursing Economic$,* 32(2), 70–79. PMID: 24834631.

Mastal, M., Matlock, A., & Start, R. (2016). Ambulatory care nurse-sensitive indicators series: Capturing the role of nursing in ambulatory care—The case for meaningful nurse-sensitive measurement. *Nursing Economic$,* 34(2), 92–97, 76. PMID: 27265952.

Murray, C. L., (ed.) (2017). *Scope and standards of practice for professional ambulatory care nursing* (9th ed.). American Academy of Ambulatory Care Nursing.

Needleman, J. (2017). Expanding the role of registered nurses in primary care: A business case analysis. *Journal of Medical Practice Management, 32*(5), 343–351. PMID: 30047709.

Salmon, S. W., & Echevarria, M. (2017). Healthcare transformation and changing roles for nursing. *Orthopedic Nursing, 36*(1), 12–25. https://doi.org/10.1097/NOR.0000000000000308

Spetz, J. (2014). How will health reform affect demand for RNs? *Nursing Economic$, 32*(1), 42–44. PMID: 24689158.

Swan, B. A. (2007). Transitioning from acute care to ambulatory care. *Nursing Economic$, 25*(2), 130–134. PMID: 17500502.

Swan, B. A., & Haas, S. A. (2011). Health care reform: Current updates and future initiatives for ambulatory care nursing. *Nursing Economic$, 29*(6), 331–334. PMID: 22360110.

U.S. Bureau of Labor Statistics. (2012). *National employment matrix.* https://data.bls.gov/projections/nationalMatrixHome?ioType=o

Walshe Allen, J. (2016). Transitioning the RN to Ambulatory Care. *Nursing Administration Quarterly, 40*(2), 115–121. https://doi.org/10.1097/NAQ.0000000000000151

Zolotorofe, I., Fortini, R., Hash, P., Daniels, A., Orolini, L., Mazzoccoli, A., & Gerardi, T. (2018). Return on investment for the baccalaureate-prepared RN in ambulatory care. *The Journal of Nursing Administration, 48*(3), 123–126. https://doi.org/10.1097/nna.0000000000000586

2

Healthcare Delivery

Nancy May, Cyndy Banik Dunlap, and Susan M. Paschke

PERSPECTIVES

"As transformation continues across healthcare, care delivery places nurses at the center for innovative, person-centered, coordinated care. Nurses in all care settings are uniquely poised to support individuals and families in successful engagement and self-care management and to advocate for shared decision making. Nurses are central to person-centered care that advances healthcare's Quadruple Aim of better culture, better care, better health, and lower costs."

Nancy Howell Agee, President and CEO of Carilion Clinic and Chair of the American Hospital Association

LEARNING OBJECTIVES

Upon completion of this chapter, the reader will be able to:

1. Describe the development of the ambulatory nursing model from a historical perspective.
2. Discuss ambulatory care delivery models that have evolved as payment has moved from volume to value.
3. Understand the many roles of registered nurses in ambulatory care.
4. Explain the importance of national reports in guiding enhanced and emerging roles for registered nurses in ambulatory care.
5. Describe the future roles of ambulatory registered nurses in transforming care.

KEY TERMS

Ambulatory care | **Care delivery models**

The 19th Century

Nursing was a relatively young profession in the 19th century when public health and home care nursing debuted. The more recent movement of care provision from the hospital setting to the **ambulatory care** environment dates back to the public health nursing tenets found in the writings of Florence Nightingale. In *Notes on Nursing: What It Is and What It Is Not* (1859), Nightingale described the home as the location for providing care to individuals, including requirements for the necessities for a "healthy house—pure air, pure water, efficient drainage, cleanliness and light" (p. 14). These environmental concepts eventually led to the establishment of public health and visiting nurse societies providing care for those individuals experiencing extreme poverty in tenements and other public housing developments in urban areas across the country in the late 19th century. Based on Nightingale's work in the Crimea, former school teacher Clara Barton organized the American Red Cross in 1881 as a permanent relief organization to provide nursing care and supplies in times of war or other conflicts.

Care of those individuals experiencing extreme poverty was mostly unknown until Lillian Wald and Mary Brewster set up the Henry Street Settlement House in New York City in 1895. The goal was to provide care in the home for those who were ill, regardless of insurance or ability to pay. Individuals of all ages were cared for, including children sent home from school owing to illness. As the number of children missing school continued to grow, Lillian Wald helped establish school nursing in 1902 in an effort to prevent children going home with minor ailments or the need for first aid. Hospice care also began during the end of the 19th century. The Sisters of Charity adopted the term "hospice" as a place of shelter or rest for weary or ill travelers on a journey. They began to care for the terminally ill, who were in need of shelter or rest for their journey, in designated "hospice homes" in Ireland and England.

The 20th Century

The arrival of the 20th century brought forth changes in the concepts of healthcare provision and responsibility. Advancements in biology, chemistry, and other related sciences led to the near eradication of diseases such as tuberculosis, yellow fever, diphtheria, cholera, and others owing to the development of better diagnostic tests and vaccines. The discovery and development of immunizations in the 1930s helped shift the focus to prevention of illness rather than treatment. Penicillin, first discovered in 1928 by Sir Alexander Fleming, was the first naturally occurring antibiotic and remains the most frequently used worldwide. During the early part of the century, most ambulatory care was provided in physicians' offices or via home visits or "house calls" by physicians. The majority of nursing care continued to be provided in public health, school, or home health settings.

1960s

In the 1960s, social programs to aid in the care of older persons and the poor were created by the U.S. government. Medicare is a federal insurance program that provides for hospital and ambulatory care for older individuals and some persons with disabilities. Medicaid is an assistance program designed to serve lower income individuals of all ages and includes coverage of some medical expenses. The inception of these two programs presented opportunities for healthcare to those previously without or unable to pay for insurance. Consequently, visits in ambulatory care clinics began to increase.

1970s

In 1978, the World Health Organization (WHO) proposed a definition of primary healthcare as "essential health care … made universally accessible to individuals and families in the community" (p. 1). Around the same time, the Institute of Medicine (IOM, 1978) defined primary care as "personal health services that emphasized prevention, removing barriers to care, coordination, continuity and the inclusion of patients and families in decision making" (p. 16). These concepts promoted nurse–patient and provider–patient relationships over time as the basis for continuity of care and initiated the care coordinator role for the registered nurse (RN) in ambulatory care settings.

The 1970s also saw the development of health maintenance organizations (HMOs) based on a prepaid medical plan developed by Henry J. Kaiser for employees of the Kaiser Shipbuilding Company in 1941. The health plan, Kaiser-Permanente, strongly supported preventive medicine and education of members about maintaining their own health with the goal of providing quality healthcare services at lower costs. This concept was the impetus for HMOs that continued to develop through the 1980s as more organizations sought to decrease costs while improving quality. Managed care is a concept derived from HMOs and focused on furnishing an array of healthcare services through a provider network, emphasizing preventive care, and utilizing quality improvement practices and financial incentives for increased efficiency in the healthcare system through capitated payments (Fillmore et al., 2014). Care coordination and transition management (CCTM) are key roles in the managed care system and have been an integral aspect of the role of the ambulatory care nurse.

1980s

By the mid-1980s, concern about quality of care and rising costs led to an amendment to the Social Security Act. Initially intended as a framework to monitor quality of care and appropriate utilization, diagnosis-related groups (DRGs) were established by an amendment to the Social Security Act in 1983 as the national payment system for those on Medicare. The impact of the DRG system dramatically changed the healthcare reimbursement system from a retrospective cost-based system to a prospective payment system (PPS) and created incentives to encourage decrease in hospital utilization, decrease in length of stay, and transition of care delivery from the inpatient to the ambulatory care setting (Rhodes, 1988).

1990s

Quality of care continued as a critical focus nationally into the 1990s. The National Committee for Quality Assurance (NCQA), founded in 1990, developed statistical measures to assess and track the quality of managed care and other healthcare plans. The Healthcare Effectiveness Data and Information Set (HEDIS) is a tool used to measure a plan's performance on specified dimensions of care and service, such as control of high blood pressure, comprehensive diabetes care, breast cancer screening, childhood and adolescent immunization status, and body mass index (BMI) assessment. This data collection and analysis allows for organizational internal benchmarking, as well as comparisons with other similar organizations.

The Children's Health Insurance Program (CHIP) was signed into law in 1997 and provides matching funds to states to provide health coverage for children of families that do not qualify for Medicaid but cannot afford other coverage. CHIP coverage includes inpatient and ambulatory care medical benefits, dental benefits, and well child care, including immunizations.

The 21st Century

The shifting perspectives regarding health and the healthcare system in the latter part of the 20th century have had significant implications for ambulatory care and ambulatory care nurses into the 21st century. Ambulatory care delivery sites have expanded to include many nontraditional sites such as drug stores, department stores, telehealth, and virtual clinics. The role of the ambulatory care nurse has expanded to include provision of care and education, advocacy, and care coordination in these varied settings. Ambulatory care nurses work independently and in collaboration with other healthcare providers with the individual as the focus and driver of their care (American Academy of Ambulatory Care Nursing [AAACN], 2017).

Healthy People

Beginning in 1990, and following with new targets every 10 years, the U.S. Department of Health and Human Services introduced the Healthy People initiative in the United States. These national goals are meant to guide national health promotion, disease prevention, and preventive services in an effort to improve the health of everyone living in the United States (Centers for Disease Control and Prevention, 2018). The tracking mechanisms were also expected to help identify emerging public health issues at the local, state, and national levels. Healthy People 2000 included 22 health status indicators, such as infant mortality, motor vehicle accidents, suicides, homicides, and deaths from cancers and cardiac disease. Data were collected every year to determine progress toward each indicator. Unfortunately, none of the indicator goals had been reached by that year.

In 2000, Healthy People 2010 included many of the same indicators but also included, for the first time, increasing the quality and number of years of healthy living and the elimination of health disparities. There were 28 objectives, each having a target to reach by 2010, and 10 leading health indicators (LHIs) identified as measures of public health, including physical activity, obesity, tobacco and substance abuse, mental health, responsible sexual behavior, injury and violence, environmental quality, immunization, and access to healthcare. Some of the LHIs demonstrated significant progress, but all of them were included in the target goals for the initiative for the next 10 years.

Healthy People 2020 was published in December 2010 with four overarching goals for the population:

- Attain high-quality, longer lives free of preventable disease
- Achieve health equity and eliminate disparities
- Create environments that promote good health
- Promote healthy development and behaviors across all life stages

The 2020 LHIs remain the same as the 2010 initiatives as they continue to reflect the major health concerns of the country today.

Ambulatory care nurses have the ability to impact these indicators for the individuals they care for in any of the settings that comprise ambulatory care. Nurses partnering with individuals and other members of the healthcare team have played a key role in the evolution of care delivery in the ambulatory setting from the basic care provided in homes and schools in the 19th century to the highly technical and sophisticated care provided in ambulatory settings today.

Quality Versus Quantity, Value Versus Volume

An ongoing challenge in the U.S. healthcare system is the rising cost of care and insurance premiums. The increasing costs have threatened the ability of individuals and their families to access care, jeopardized the ability of businesses to provide health insurance coverage, and stressed the budgets of government entities (Pulcini & Hart, 2014). Healthcare costs have grown dramatically from 1980 through 2010 and are projected to continue to increase through 2023. In comparison with other developed countries, the United States has the highest expenditures per capita, at $8,422 compared with Norway, which spends approximately $3,000 less as the second highest country per capita costs. Despite such expenditures, the average life expectancy of a U.S. citizen is 1.3 years less compared with citizens of other developed countries; furthermore, the United States ranks 28th in male life expectancy, 26th in female life expectancy, and 36th in infant mortality (Berwick et al., 2008; Public Broadcasting Service, 2012).

Several factors have contributed to the increased cost of U.S. healthcare. Providers, including physicians and hospitals, have benefited financially from the incentives created by the fee-for-service (FFS) payment programs. A higher percentage of specialists compared with primary care physicians along with practicing medicine to reduce malpractice litigation has made tests and procedures more expensive. Additionally, rising costs of healthcare technology and drugs, increased administrative burden of providing services, and lack of consumer knowledge have contributed to the higher cost of care in the United States. With these rising costs, Medicare and Medicaid are threatened with a financial crisis, Medicare's trust being estimated to run out of money in 2030 and Medicaid recording the second largest expenditure in most states, behind education costs (Pulcini & Hart, 2014).

A key driver of the increased costs was the reimbursement for care by Medicare and Medicaid, initiated by the private employer insurance plans, with the FFS methodology (Pulcini & Hart, 2014). Moreover, the outcomes of the healthcare delivery system were dismal, as reflected by the IOM reports on quality. Historically, the structure of healthcare delivery and financing in the United States has driven the increasing volume of procedural and diagnostic care compared with other countries' providers (McClellan et al., 2017). Payment to providers has been based on the quantity, extent, and frequency through the FFS reimbursement (Werner et al., 2011). Physicians and hospitals were paid on the basis of the number of services rendered to an individual, whether the services actually improved the quality of care or outcome of health for the individual. Consumers, health plans, and businesses questioned this approach of paying for volume of tests and procedures without consideration of the quality or outcomes of the care delivered.

The argument grew that the FFS model was flawed. Individuals, especially those with chronic health conditions, often had multiple physicians and other healthcare providers and encountered frustrations associated with fragmented and disconnected care. Diagnostic tests and other procedures were duplicated because of lack of coordination and decision-making between providers, including primary care providers, specialists, and hospitals. Care processes were not grounded with the known evidence-based practices; therefore, testing and procedures might be ordered even though the intervention may not improve the illness or diagnosis. Individuals experienced lost or unavailable medical records between providers and therefore had to share the same information over and over as they sought care. The result of the FFS methodology of reimbursement was a significant lack of value of the care provided to the individual.

Many strategies and tactics to control costs have been deployed by federal and state governments, businesses, and other stakeholders throughout the years with limited success to improve quality and discourage unneeded services. Use of regulations, forced competition, managed care programs, and incremental changes from FFS to prospective payments have been attempted to decrease the growth curve of costs in the last 40 years (Pulcini & Hart, 2014). These attempts to reform healthcare and decrease costs were thwarted by a fragmentary approach to address a very complex healthcare delivery system. Some of these approaches, employed over time, are important for their relevance to ambulatory care and for the enhancement of the delivery system of today and the future.

Pay-for-Performance Demonstration Projects

In the late 1990s, the concept of linking quality outcomes to drive cost reduction and efficiency was examined. To promote quality improvement and public reporting of quality metrics and outcomes, the Centers for Medicare and Medicaid Services (CMS) worked in partnership with stakeholders to launch the Hospital Quality Alliance: Improving Care Through Information program. With this initiative, public reporting of quality metrics and outcomes became available online at the website *Hospital Compare* for consumers to view the performance of hospitals and their partner physicians (CMS, 2009).

Additional steps were taken by the federal government and CMS to further drive value within healthcare. The Executive Order by President George W. Bush in 2006 directed federal agencies to collect and compile quality and cost results and publicly report these findings to beneficiaries and enrollees (Kurtzman & Johnson, 2014). The first Medicare hospital pay-for-performance program was announced in 2007 and outlined potential incentives for hospitals to improve care and costs (Kurtzman & Johnson, 2014).

CMS, as the largest payer for healthcare, also began to link payment incentives with improved quality with the introduction of pay-for-performance incentive programs (CMS, 2009). The initial experiment in pay-for-performance was a partnership created by CMS with Premier Inc. and its 414 Premier hospitals in 2003. Known as the Premier Hospital Quality Incentive Demonstration project, the goal was to determine whether financial incentives were effective in improving quality of hospital care in 33 metrics of care. During the 2-year project, process-based quality metrics saw improvement in some diagnoses. Additional studies indicated that health outcome metrics based on evidence-based practices were not as easily achieved in diagnoses such as acute myocardial infarction, community-acquired pneumonia, and knee and hip replacements (Werner et al., 2011).

From this inaugural pay-for-performance demonstration project within the public sector, over 40 projects were developed within the private sector as of 2011, with limited evidence of improving the quality of care for inpatients. Although pay-for-performance hospitals outperformed nonparticipating facilities in the first 3 years of the project, one study indicated that the discernible differences in quality metrics between the two groups of hospitals were not observable at 5 years (Werner et al., 2011). Key characteristics of hospitals that were successful in pay-for-performance projects were those that had larger financial incentives, limited community competition, and a healthy financial position (Werner et al., 2011).

Physicians, too, were impacted by pay-for-performance models. The Physician Quality Reporting Initiative (PQRI) was initiated with reporting of 74 quality metrics in the second half of 2007, with reimbursement paid to the individual providers in 2008. This model was established as a low-risk payment model to physicians with no penalties for poor performance and supported the engagement of providers in reporting metrics (Stulberg, 2008). Although this experiment was a tool to prepare providers and their staff in the process of quality reporting, a study of providers indicated the lack of belief that the work had any true impact on outcomes (Federman, 2011). An additional concern raised by providers participating in the pay-for-performance payment models was the focus that specific quality metrics may deprive providers of the incentive to address other key care tactics that were not being rewarded (de Bruin, Baan, & Struijs, 2011).

In another pay-for-performance model for physicians, the Medicare Physician Group Practice Demonstration (PGPD) created the ability for a group practice of physicians to receive incentives if certain quality metrics were achieved with lower costs. Group practices were eligible to receive up to 80% of any savings produced from improvement of 32 quality metrics. A study of 10 physician practices found that quality metrics did improve but had mixed results in improving costs. Some of the organizations realized significantly lower costs, whereas others demonstrated little or no cost savings (Colla et al., 2012).

Undaunted, CMS continued to coordinate pay-for-performance initiatives with other agencies and organizations. To forge continued improvement in cost and quality, CMS added additional metrics using unique reporting periods and linking incentive payment schemes with the Medicare physician fee schedule. Based on the results of these pay-for-performance models with hospitals and physicians, new models were and are being developed and proposed through legislation and pilot projects (CMS, 2009).

Triple/Quadruple Aim

With healthcare in a fiscal crisis, a challenge had been introduced and embraced by key national and state stakeholders to increase the value of care by improving not only health outcomes for individuals but also the cost of care received. Built on the concept of providing value to the healthcare system, the *Triple Aim*, a framework developed by the Institute for Healthcare Improvement (IHI) and widely known through the work of Donald M. Berwick, took the definition of value an extra step. Healthcare system improvement could be achieved only by concurrently improving the health of a population and the experience of the individual in regard to quality, access, and reliability and decreasing the per capita cost of care (Berwick et al., 2008). To achieve the *Triple Aim*, three foundational goals needed to be achieved: (1) enrolling a certain population into a cohort for care, (2) engaging all members of that identified population to improve their health, and (3) coordinating services through an organization that is accountable for the entire care and costs of a defined population. To achieve this, certain key functions would have to be addressed, including the following:

- Individuals and their families would need to be knowledgeable about the influences and choices related to their daily life and the drawbacks of relying on tests and procedures for care.
- Resources would need to be appropriately allocated and positioned by the organization to the affected population.
- The cost per individual within the identified population would need to be calculated and shared with all stakeholders.
- Primary care should focus on individuals and the inclusion of community resources.
- Organizations would need to adopt reliable evidence-based practices (Berwick et al., 2008).

As the *Triple Aim* was embraced by the healthcare industry, the pressures of attempting to adopt all three goals to practice led to concerns about provider and staff burnout. The challenges of adopting new care strategies into daily practice created frustrations for the team, resulting in disengagement in the work to drive improvements. With the shift of the delivery model into improving quality, reducing costs, and driving individual satisfaction, providers and healthcare professionals required a supportive environment to practice person-centered care. Therefore, a fourth goal has been adopted to ensure the well-being of the care team. Now known as the *Quadruple Aim* to improve the work life of clinicians, certain activities can be implemented to support team-based care: (1) maximizing the knowledge, skills, and competencies of all team members; (2) staging the scheduling and planning of individual visits; (3) enhancing documentation techniques within the electronic health record (EHR); and (4) locating space for the team to work together (Bodenheimer & Sinsky, 2014; Sikka et al., 2015).

Value-Based Purchasing

The concept of value-driven healthcare was shaping the next phase of pay-for-performance by CMS to improve the quality of care and maintain or reduce costs. Value-based purchasing (VBP) programs were initiated in 2012 to model the *Triple Aim*'s goals of better care of individuals and populations at a lower cost (CMS, 2018a). VBP, as an initiative, was made mandatory for almost all hospitals and physician practices to restructure care practices from quantity to quality of care. Based on the *Triple Aim*'s goals of improving care for individuals and populations and driving to lower costs, VBP required the adoption of evidence-based practices and processes leading to improved outcomes for individuals. Key measures of outcomes included mortality, complications, hospital-associated infections, and safety. In addition, this program pushed hospitals to improve the experience of care being received by individuals and families (CMS, 2018a).

With value-based programs, hospitals had a certain percentage of Medicare funds withheld with the intent of using these same funds to provide incentive payments to facilities demonstrating improvements. Those hospitals not improving were penalized by not receiving their funds withheld (CMS, 2018a). In addition, these programs were developed to demonstrate transparency of the results to the consumer. Through these practices and processes implemented within the delivery of care, those hospitals with improvement in quality and costs were recognized compared with their peers (CMS, 2018a).

Patient Protection and Affordable Care Act

The continued exponential growth in healthcare costs, the inability to improve quality for healthier outcomes, and the unabated increase in the numbers of uninsured marked a turning point for policy makers that could not be ignored. On March 23, 2010, the Patient Protection and Affordable Care Act (PPACA) was signed into law to address the crisis of the healthcare system with the confluence of rising costs, poor accessibility by all, and the questionable quality of services rendered (Hoffman, 2014).

The foundational approach through this law was to expand healthcare coverage and carry out necessary reforms to the care delivery system. By aligning incentives with providers throughout the continuum of care instead of the individual providers of care, the PPACA aimed to create coordinated, accessible services to reduce costs (Blumenthal et al., 2015). Through this law, the tactics subserving this strategy were to create an accountable system with providers owning the outcomes and the costs of care (Guterman et al., 2010).

One strategy identified in the PPACA to drive the redesign of current reform projects and create future **care delivery models** and payment methodologies was the establishment of the CMS Innovation Center (CMMI) for the purpose of testing, studying, and evaluating innovative person-centered practices that reduce expenditures and improve the quality of care. In addition to being tasked with developing new payment and service models, CMMI's key priorities also included creating opportunities for quality improvement and studying the outcomes of the models tested. In addition to evaluating the results, sharing of identified best practices in current demonstration projects with other payers and seeking input from stakeholders to establish future models of care were critical. The work of CMMI extends beyond the beneficiaries of Medicare, Medicaid, and the government-sponsored CHIP. The outcomes of its studies have implications and potential adoption of practices within the private health insurers of the nation (CMS, 2018a; Shrank, 2013).

Healthcare for the Uninsured and Underinsured

As national demonstration projects moved forward to improve care and costs, an important deliverable of PPACA was improved coverage for the uninsured and underinsured. Previous federal policies relied on the ability of employers to provide health insurance benefits and/or on individuals to acquire their own health insurance, whereas other industrialized countries adopted policies to provide healthcare for all individuals (Reinhardt, 1997). Within the United States, most individuals older than 65 years are covered by Medicare. Of those employed, approximately 50% have coverage through their employer. Unless individuals can qualify for Medicaid or CHIP, they are left without healthcare coverage. In 2008, 46 million U.S. citizens younger than 65 years did not have health insurance, a population that grew steadily each year by approximately 1 to 2 million. The affordability to acquire coverage was beyond the reach of these citizens (Hoffman, 2014). These Americans found themselves uninsured.

The inability to have health insurance coverage drives the health outcomes of individuals. Health improves with health insurance; improved health leads to better incomes and labor force participation (Hadley, 2003). When individuals postpone or sacrifice care owing to its unaffordability, untoward health problems can occur, leading to increased costs of care, poorer outcomes, and even death. Choices made by people in regard to whether or not to get needed care, getting needed care on time, and where they go to receive care make a difference in health outcomes (Hoffman, 2014; Reinhardt, 1997).

In addition to risking health outcomes, the financial security of the uninsured is also jeopardized by the concern of how to pay for care when needed. Lower income families consist of many uninsured who have constrained assets and savings, leaving them without a safety net when health problems occur. A study in 2009 demonstrated that one out of five uninsured used their entire savings to settle a medical bill (Hoffman, 2014).

Estimates in 2015 revealed that 7 to 16.4 million uninsured had been able to secure health insurance coverage because of key provisions in the law, leaving a projected 32 million to be covered by 2019. Many of these newly insured individuals came from groups such as Hispanics and Blacks, low-income households, and young adults. A key element of the law to decrease the number of uninsured was the extension to young adults up to 26 years of age to remain on a parent's coverage plans. Federal subsidies to other individuals allowed the affordability of the purchase of plans within the healthcare marketplace. Lastly, the law supported the expansion of Medicaid for states to include uninsured individuals (Blumenthal et al., 2015; Hoffman, 2014).

Shift to Ambulatory and Primary Care in Support of Population Health

Important deliverables from the PPACA dramatically increased the number of insured citizens, escalating the demand for value and quality of care delivered beyond the hospital walls in ambulatory and primary care. The PPACA focused access to care on primary care. Placing primary care as the point of access led to the identification of significant benefits for individuals and providers, including the following:

- Improving access to care
- Coordinating care across providers and settings
- Decreasing hassles in the administrative work of care
- Improving health maintenance and care coordination for chronically ill individuals

These key provisions of primary care in ambulatory settings were identified as the means to improve the overall health of not only each individual but also the population of a group of individuals or communities. Therefore, provisions had been made within the PPACA to include improvement in payment schedules to primary care providers, expansion of the primary care workforce, opportunities for creating new care delivery models and processes, and redress of the imbalances in the value of resources between specialists and primary care (Davis et al., 2011; Goodson, 2010).

Subsequently, the recognition of the importance of primary care and ambulatory care within healthcare reform led to the examination of the roles for RNs in these settings and the conclusion that RNs are essential providers in current and future care delivery models. Therefore, the PPACA had a significant impact on supporting expanded roles for RNs in ambulatory and primary care, thus contributing to improved care and reduced cost.

Care Delivery Models

To further advance the design of a more effective healthcare delivery system, PPACA drove necessary reforms through the provision of a variety of models for providers to affect the quality and cost of care rendered. Mandated payment model reforms or new advancements in demonstration projects served as catalysts to new generations of care delivery systems. These reform models included the incorporation of the evaluations and results of the prior decade's demonstration projects. VBP programs for providers and hospitals, patient-centered medical homes (PCMHs), accountable care organizations (ACOs), pilot or demonstration payment projects spanning the local to federal levels, and penalties for poor performance are examples of the reform mechanisms embedded within the PPACA. Initial estimates were that these types of design models could lead to over $692 million in cost reductions within the first decade of implementation (Guterman et al., 2010). In addition to the models described in this chapter, telehealth practice and virtual care and technologies are discussed in Chapter 9, and Federally Qualified Health Centers (FQHCs) are discussed in Chapter 10.

Patient-Centered Medical Homes

Office practice redesign to improve quality and provide value had been discussed, studied, and promoted through pilot projects from as early as 1970. The advent of computers with their potential to streamline operational activities and the exploration of research studies to manage patient flow presented medical office practices with the opportunity to improve quality and costs within a clinic setting. Through these redesign studies, PCMHs became a conceptual model of care to support the health of individuals in primary care settings. The term "patient-centered medical home" was developed and adopted through guiding principles established by the American College of Physicians, American Academy of Family Physicians, American Academy of Pediatrics, and the American Osteopathic Association in 2007 (Kilo & Wasson, 2010).

Essentially, PCMHs are an enhancement of the current primary care office and are recognized as a significant strategy in improving quality, costs, and care experiences of individuals and their providers (Arend et al., 2012). Whereas the primary care office provides episodic care, PCMHs focus attention on the individual and inclusion of the individual with the provider in shared decision-making while providing comprehensive care that includes acute, chronic, and/or preventive health activities or management (David et al., 2018). PCMHs embrace the qualities of primary care, including continuity of care, accessibility for services at the right time and place, inclusion of all of the individual's health needs and concerns, and the coordination of all services required for a positive outcome. In addition to these core qualities, PCMHs contain the foundational attributes for innovation and payment reform (Arend et al., 2012).

Team-based care supports the concept of PCMHs with all members of the team supporting clinical activities (David et al., 2018). A wide array of healthcare professionals are members of the team, including advanced practice registered nurses (APRNs), nurse case managers, social workers, pharmacists, nutritionists, clinical educators, community health workers, psychologists, population health analysts, and information technologists. Navigators, an emerging role for RNs within PCMHs, serve as the primary point of contact for the individual, coordinating and integrating the team's efforts and providing oversight to the care rendered (Dunlap et al., 2017). As a result of this interprofessional, collaborative care model, research has demonstrated reductions in costs, improvements in the care experience, and increased quality and staff satisfaction (NCQA, 2018).

Although widely embraced by healthcare practices, the verdict of PCMHs improving quality and costs is currently unclear. Early indications are that PCMHs produce modest savings and improved outcomes (Arend et al., 2012). However, to ensure the future success of PCMHs, this care delivery model needs to receive support through further payment enhancements and reformation of other aspects of overall healthcare delivery models. Moreover, PCMHs are threatened by the lack of trained healthcare professionals, including physicians, APRNs, and physician assistants (PAs), creating challenges to this model of team-based care. Another means of ensuring the success of PCMHs is to engage their population to become more knowledgeable, accountable, and interested in managing their own health. Mechanisms to make that relationship bidirectional should be studied, evaluated, and rapidly adopted into care redesign (Kilo & Wasson, 2010). Lastly, the PCMH model of care needs to be given time to gauge its effectiveness and efficacy as relationships need to be nurtured and supported over time between individuals, the practice team, specialty care, and the hospital (Nichols et al., 2017).

Regardless of these challenges, CMS continues to support the concept of this care delivery model. Through the Medicare Access and CHIP Reauthorization Act (MACRA) of 2015, PCMHs that become certified enjoy full credits in the MIPS incentive program. This National Committee on Quality Assurance (NCQA) recognition program, seen as the most widely used across the nation for PCMHs, requires that medical home practices be evaluated for the achievement of such status. Functions crucial to obtaining this recognition are patient tracking with registry support, care management guidelines, test tracking and follow-up, electronic prescribing, referral tracking, and performance reporting and improvements (NCQA, 2018). With more than 60,000 providers and 12,000 practices recognized by the NCQA, more than 100 payers are supportive of this evaluation program (NCQA, 2018). Through these types of continued commitments from CMS, health plans, and key stakeholders, PCMHs may be a long-term solution to reduce fragmented, highly specialized care to move to prevention and primary care for the individual.

Accountable Care Organizations

Another new model of population-based care designed from prior demonstration projects is the accountable care organizations (ACOs). Through a formal network of healthcare providers, ACOs are designed by agreement to be responsible for the quality of care and accountable to the population that they serve (Shaw, 2014). ACOs are described by CMS as an entity of physicians, hospitals, and other healthcare providers who join together to provide high-quality, coordinated care to a defined population of those on Medicare (CMS, 2017). The organization and structure of ACOs can be multifaceted and intricate depending on the variety of providers joining the entity. Additionally, the funding payer, usually the federal or state government or a private payer such as a health plan, legally binds the ACO for the provision of quality, cost-effective care for a distinct population. With a view to moving toward a highly reliable, safe, reformed healthcare delivery system, ACOs were envisaged to capture the collective spirit of the *Triple Aim* and the early, visionary adopters of prior payment reforms (Dunlap et al., 2017).

As early as 2012, healthcare organizations could apply to the federal government to become ACOs for Medicare enrollees. To increase initial interest, the PPACA created incentives for entities to form ACOs. Once formed, ACOs function with the goal of providing high-quality care and managing healthcare costs. By agreement between the ACO and the CMS as the payer, targets are established for the achievement of health outcomes and for the distribution of any savings achieved in managing the population. When the ACO demonstrates lower costs of care and improved quality metrics per defined baseline targets, the entity would either retain the dollars saved or receive an incentive payment from the funding payer (Gold, 2014). Since the early release of Medicare's Pioneer ACO model in 2012, the ACOs have experienced escalations in the savings at risk. Therefore, the initial shared risk financial model between the ACO and the payer has developed into a comprehensive financial and quality ownership of the population health model (CMS, 2017).

Besides Medicare, Medicaid and commercial health plans such as United Healthcare and Blue Cross Blue Shield have developed ACO models. Whereas the financial arrangements and the structure of the agreement by a payer with an ACO can be comparable, the types of populations they serve and manage are based on the payer's targeted population. Many states use this model to not only drive quality outcomes but also shift the cost burden of care to the providers (Center for Healthcare Strategies, 2016). Lastly, the commercially funded ACOs have seen growth from private and self-insured payers to manage populations such as employer-funded programs and individuals who buy health insurance (Shorter et al., 2014).

The PPACA does not define how an ACO should be managed or structured; however, hospitals and very large physician practices are typically the leaders of an ACO. In addition, ACOs may include skilled nursing centers, long-term acute care facilities, independent physician practices, home care/hospice services, FQHCs, and other outpatient services (CMS, 2017). This structure makes ACOs very unique in the ability to align financial incentives with quality targets across the continuum of care, with a focus on health and wellness rather than on acute care (Casalino, 2015). This model is vastly different from the FFS payment system, which led to an increased volume of tests and procedures along with fragmentation of care. When enrolling in an ACO, individuals identify a primary care provider who will coordinate and manage their care in an integrated manner through a team of healthcare professionals. The aim of ACOs is to move past disjointed, fragmented care delivery systems to one that sees improvement in health outcomes through cost-effective rewards for the providers (Bithoney, 2014).

Alternative Payment Initiatives

Mandated payment models or demonstration projects will continue to be explored to reduce the cost of care, create quality in services rendered, and drive value to the consumer. Hospitals, nursing homes, and home health agencies, along with other providers, will be affected by necessary reforms to their components of the healthcare system. However, to help the nurse develop the required focus and understanding within the ambulatory care setting, payment reform models being currently tested, evaluated, and adapted that affect this environment are explored in what follows.

Quality Payment Program

Through the passage of MACRA of 2015, the physician payment model changed from the sustainable growth rate formula fraught with its weighty payment cuts to providers, huge administrative burden of implementation within practices, and expensive short-range fixes. One payment model, known as the Quality Payment Program (QPP), offers incentive payments for performance in areas such as quality, costs, and the use of the EHR. Implemented through CMMI, two options are offered to eligible physicians through the QPP: Merit-Based Incentive Payment System (MIPS) and Alternative Payment Model (APM) (CMS, 2015; Gruessner, 2016).

The MIPS program combines and coordinates multiple, prior incentive projects that addressed a singular approach to improve clinicians' quality reporting, the use of the EHR, and improvement in value-based metrics. MIPS targets physicians and other clinicians to simultaneously address these improvement strategies, including costs. Besides physicians, other eligible clinicians for MIPS are nurse practitioners, PAs, nurse anesthetists, and clinical nurse specialists. MIPS also promotes the ability of hospital-based physicians to use their facilities' measurements in value-based performance and other quality metrics. Clinicians may be incentivized or could receive penalties of as much as 5% by 2020 with as much as 9% at risk by 2022 based on the collective results of the identified metrics or outcomes (American Hospital Association, 2017).

The APM model under QPP includes demonstration projects, types of ACOs, and certain CMMI models and provides added incentives to providers. APMs must demonstrate that they can improve quality without impacting costs or reduce costs without jeopardizing quality within the overall goal of improving both quality and costs. The difference between MIPS and APMs is that APMs accept financial risk for the care that they provide. Although APMs have increased financial risks, the potential financial rewards are also higher compared with MIPS (CMS, 2015).

Physicians and practitioners who participate in an eligible APM, a more advanced APM, can enjoy bonus payments of up to 5% for cost and quality improvements; likewise, they also carry some level of monetary risks for financial excesses through their delivery of care. An alternative eligibility criterion for APMs can be participation in a CMMI-designated medical home model. Regardless, clinicians within APMs are mandated to use certified technology within their EHR. These providers also receive payments based on quality metrics similarly noted within the MIPS program (CMS, 2015).

Bundled Payments for Care Improvement

Bundled payments for care improvement (BPCI), also known as episode-based payment, is an approach aimed at providing care for a Medicare recipient's condition or treatment tied to a hospitalization and subsequent services for a specific diagnosis. Historically, individual payments were provided to the hospital, the physician, and other services such as laboratory, home healthcare, and skilled nursing homes. The quantity, not the quality, of services rendered was the incentive. Because the payment was not aligned for all services rendered for a condition or treatment, the care was not well coordinated among providers and care settings, leading to fragmentation of care.

BPCI provides a single payment for the entire episode of care to all the different providers. The bundling of payment for services forces hospitals, physicians, and post–acute care settings to collaborate and work collectively together to coordinate care and eliminate services and tests that are wasteful and that offer no value to individual health outcomes. The alignment of the financial incentives among these providers creates an environment that ensures that costs do not exceed the single payment. CMMI initiated work within the bundle of care services within hip and knee replacements and continues to develop and promote different models of BPCI to study and evaluate to enhance care for Medicare beneficiaries (CMS, 2018b; Kurtzman & Johnson, 2014).

Table 2.1 summarizes reform and payment models relevant to ambulatory care settings. These models will continue to be studied and modified and require flexibility in order to

TABLE 2.1 REFORM AND PAYMENT MODELS OF THE 21ST CENTURY

Model	Year Launched	Description
Fee-for-service reimbursement model	1965	Providers (physicians and hospitals) paid by payers for number of services rendered. The incentive is based on volume or quantity of services rather than quality.
P4P demonstration projects	2003	Hospitals that volunteered to receive incentives for improving quality of care through improvement of metrics.
PQRI	2007	Physicians who volunteered to receive incentives for improving quality of care through improvement of metrics.
Medicare PGPD	2005	Group medical practices that volunteered to receive incentives if quality improved and costs were reduced.
VBP	2012	CMS withheld Medicare payments to most hospitals unless they demonstrated improved quality metrics/processes.
PPACA	2010	Signed by President Obama, legislation addressed accessibility of care, reduction of costs, and quality of care, spurring the focus on primary care in ambulatory settings.
PCMHs	2007	Comprises an interdisciplinary care team, including physicians, providing comprehensive, coordinated care throughout all settings for the entire health of an individual.
ACO	2012	Consists of an entity of physicians, hospitals, and other providers responsible for the quality and cost of care for a defined population.
QPP	2015	Provides incentives to physicians for improvement in quality, costs, and use of EHR. Two options exist: (1) MIPS promoting improvement in data reporting, use of EHR, and in quality metrics and (2) APM promotes goals of MIPS and also contains financial risk to the physician practice or organization.
BPCI	2015	An approach to address care for a Medicare recipient's condition or treatment tied to a hospitalization and subsequent services for a specific diagnosis. Provides a single payment for the entire episode of care for all the different providers.

Note. ACO = Accountable Care Organizations; APM = Alternative Payment Model; BPCI = Bundled Payments for Care Improvement; CMS = Centers for Medicare and Medicaid Services; EHR = electronic health record; MIPS = Merit-Based Incentive Payment System; P4P = Pay-For-Performance; PCMHs = Patient-Centered Medical Homes; PGPD = Physician Group Practice Demonstration; PPACA = Patient Protection and Affordable Care Act; PQRI = Physician Quality Reporting Initiative; QPP = Quality Payment Program; VBP = Value-Based Purchasing.

address the charge and mandate for healthcare reform to improve quality and costs for consumers. Even the CMMI, which is tasked with creating, evaluating, and establishing innovative models of care, is being evaluated by the CMS. Policy makers advocate a directional change in its future to one of increased competition among providers for individuals' choice and greater flexibility in payment models. Although continued focus by CMS will be sustained in areas such as APMs, increased interest by CMS is being demonstrated in other areas, including physician specialty models, state and local innovations to include Medicaid and behavioral health, and consumer- or market-directed care (Morse, 2017).

Integrated Care

An area of growing interest is the development and implementation of integrated care through the linking of primary and mental healthcare. The outcomes of behavioral health conditions, including mental health disorders, substance abuse, and lifestyle issues, affect many people, leading to early death. Inappropriate eating behaviors, sedentary lifestyle, smoking, and social isolation have led to obesity, hypertension, diabetes, and cardiovascular disease, resulting in poorer health outcomes, increased mortality rates, and higher healthcare costs. At the same time, the complexity of care delivery systems for these health conditions has become a major obstacle to individuals attempting to access and navigate the process. Key content experts believe that the primary care setting is the gateway to addressing behavioral health conditions and lifestyle choices to improve the health of the whole person (American Psychiatric Association, 2016). The merging of the treatment of medical health conditions and behavioral health into one has developed into the concept and care delivery model known as integrated care. Defined by the Substance Abuse and Mental Health Services Administration (SAMHSA, 2016), integrated care is the systematic coordination of general and behavioral healthcare, producing the best outcomes and the best way to care for people with multiple conditions. Whether integrated care is delivered in primary care settings, behavioral health settings, or PCMHs, the approach is seen as the way to support access to holistic care (Crowley & Kirschner, 2015; Gorman, 2016; SAMHSA, 2016).

In 2013, an estimated 43.8 million U.S. adults, representing 18.5% of the total adult population, had some type of mental health condition that impacted their daily functioning, thoughts, and relationships with others. In addition, mental illnesses that are labeled as being significant, known as serious mental illness, comprise 4.2% of the adult population (Crowley & Kirschner, 2015). On top of these conditions, substance abuse affects 21.6 million U.S. citizens aged 12 or older, according to the National Survey on Drug Use and Health (Crowley & Kirschner, 2015). Therefore, these individuals ultimately die prematurely of chronic medical conditions because of the lack of routine medical care because only 40% of adults with a diagnosable mental health condition receive needed services (Crowley & Kirschner, 2015; Gorman, 2016).

Behavioral health conditions routinely lead to overall mortality and morbidity because of poor nutrition, smoking, lack of physical activity, and social relationships (Blount & Miller, 2009, Crowley & Kirschner, 2015; Gorman, 2016). At least 68% of individuals with a mental illness have at least one medical comorbidity such as obesity, heart disease, or diabetes (Crowley & Kirschner, 2015). The relationship between one's mental health and chronic illness may disrupt the treatment plan, leading to noncompliance by the individual (McGough et al., 2015). Yet the individual receiving only medical care is not receiving the necessary mental or behavioral health treatment to address the total needs of the individual. As an example, only one-third of individuals with diabetes with known mental illness receive care for their mental condition (Crowley & Kirschner, 2015). Less than 20% of individuals with depression and a chronic medical diagnosis receive appropriate intervention by a mental health provider (McGough et al., 2015). Of the seven leading causes of death, five can be associated with unhealthy lifestyle choices that can be addressed by promoting behavioral change for preventative health within the primary care setting (Blount & Miller, 2009; Crowley & Kirschner, 2015). Even without a diagnosis of a mental illness, psychosocial needs can be successfully addressed in primary care with appropriate interventions of using RNs in face-to-face visits (Blount & Miller, 2009). Integrating preventative health changes within primary care supports overall improvement within the health of the community. Many people with mental illness who do access primary care will not access mental healthcare outside of the primary care office, leading primary care to become the "de facto mental health system" (Blount & Miller, 2009).

Future Care Delivery Models

Primary care and ambulatory care are undergoing transformation as more individuals have access to care, aging populations are living longer, and individuals with chronic illnesses have increasingly complex care needs. In addition, the shortage of primary care providers continues to grow. RNs' roles in ambulatory care and primary care are widening in response to expanding demands (Bodenheimer et al., 2015; Needleman, 2015).

Future care delivery models will be driven by healthcare payment models such as VBP and shared savings programs. Many of the quality indicator metrics associated with these financing programs can be achieved by RNs, for example, by developing and implementing programs for individuals to have access to care along with support for self-care management. Additional quality indicator metrics supported by RNs include longitudinal care planning, access to 24-hour care, advanced directives and care planning, activation measures, health information exchange portals, and clinical data registries. Ultimately, RNs will be partners in care with providers to manage panels of individuals in primary, ambulatory, and specialty care settings. A full description and discussion of measures of excellence in the context of future care delivery models can be found in Chapter 5.

Registered Nurse Roles in Ambulatory Care

In addition to the roles discussed in this chapter, a full description and discussion of primary care in the context of the role of RNs is provided in Chapter 10.

RNs are uniquely positioned to impact health outcomes by defining their role in CCTM in ambulatory care settings (AAACN, 2017). CCTM models provide necessary services between community and outpatient settings, hospital to home, and home and subacute settings. ACOs and PCMHs position RNs to coordinate care and manage transitions for individuals in these types of reimbursed care delivery models. In these models, RNs manage care for chronically ill individuals. For example, RNs lead clinics to manage chronic diseases with improved clinical outcomes when compared with a physician-only management model (Bodenheimer & Smith, 2013). As content experts, they save time for providers by spending 30 to 40 minutes on a visit with an individual with diabetes to review education, track labs, discuss exercise and weight management, review medication reconciliation and adherence, and provide counseling and behavior-based goal setting. Improved outcomes lead to an overall lowering of the cost of care, and often there are incentives with pay-for-performance dollars from insurance contracts.

Care Coordination and Transition Management

RNs can initiate the management of chronic disease such as titrating blood pressure medication, adjusting diabetic medication, and managing blood thinners with evidence-based protocols (Bauer & Bodenheimer, 2017). Managing complex care needs for multiple comorbid conditions through care coordination promotes cost reduction and quality improvement, helping to avoid readmissions. Episodic care and preventive care can be accomplished through delegation and use of evidence-based protocols. Using preestablished order sets or protocols in the EHR allows RNs to manage episodic illness and improve health promotion with screening for health maintenance during telephone triage. The clinical assessment of individuals requires critical thinking skills to ensure individuals are moved to a higher level of care if warranted as a result of a health-related concern identified on the call. Including the individual and their family in care planning and education helps optimize adherence to complex care needs using behavioral-based health coaching. Medication reconciliation provides opportunities to ensure the individual has a good understanding of the reason for pharmacologic indication. Using "teach back" technique ensures that the individual and family have a clear understanding of the medication and the importance of adherence and compliance.

New specialized roles are emerging for RNs in ambulatory settings. One example is the role of care manager to follow individuals with complex care needs such as diabetes, mental health disorders, homelessness, care transitions, and home visits. RNs manage medication with protocols, set goals with individuals during counseling for behavioral changes, oversee routine monitoring of diabetes, lead cardiovascular risk reduction visits, and have them set up as "flip visits" with providers. The case study in this chapter describes the role of RNs in managing complex care needs. Chapter 8 contains a full description and discussion of CCTM in the context of the role of RNs.

Leadership

Practice leadership is another role for RNs in overseeing operations. The RN practice leader plays a significant role in analyzing data on in-basket messaging, ensuring individual and family satisfaction, reinforcing infection prevention measures with hand hygiene and compliance with high-level disinfection, and utilizing data to drive process improvement initiatives for positive outcomes. RNs are often responsible for ensuring compliance with the clinical regulatory standards such as The Joint Commission (TJC) and CMS in-office practice settings and oversight of daily operations, including flow, scheduling, and same-day access. Using Lean Six Sigma methodologies, they can lead daily huddles to manage the care team and optimize gaps in care with focused initiatives to improve quality metrics tied to reimbursement with insurance and government standards and contracts.

Technology

Technology is rapidly changing and providing opportunities to use applications known as apps. Applications are software programs, usually on a mobile device, designed to perform a specific function directly for the user. For example, apps can measure individuals' biologic indicators through portals in the EHR. Engagement of the individual to become active in managing their chronic disease is a step in the right direction (Vessey et al., 2015). Other virtual care applications are being developed to download information into the EHR to monitor blood glucose, exercise, pulse oximetry, weights, and other biologic data for assessment of conditions. Practices are offering video visits by RNs for postoperative management under bundled care, rather than return to the clinic within a specific period postprocedure. Doing wound checks over secure platforms can be accomplished and prevents the individual from having a family member take time off work. Success in having individuals return to the clinic for follow-up has improved with gentle reminders through texting prior to appointments. Using technology to remind individuals of important follow-up care has decreased cancellations and no-show rates. RNs can work off platforms, using decision support tools to give care advice and use cost avoidance measures by assessing individuals and avoiding emergency room visits. Measuring cost avoidance is important to capture and helps validate and place value on the role RNs play in producing better outcomes and cost savings.

Institute of Medicine: Future of Nursing

The Future of Nursing: Leading Change, Advancing Health (IOM, 2011) described the future of healthcare and nursing's critical role in safety, quality care, and coverage for all individuals in the healthcare system. The report identified recommendations to prepare nurses for new and vital roles to enhance healthcare delivery for the future. In 2015, the IOM evaluated movement toward its recommendations and released a report titled *Assessing Progress on the Institute of Medicine Report: The Future of Nursing*. Findings reinforced the need to continue developing an RN workforce that (1) practices to the full extent of their education and training; (2) achieves higher levels of education and training through improved education systems that promote seamless academic progression and include nurse residency programs; (3) participates as full partners with physicians and members of the interprofessional healthcare team, partnering in healthcare design and collaborative, team-based care; and (4) utilizes effective workforce planning and policy making that includes better data collection and improved information infrastructure (IOM, 2015).

California Healthcare Foundation: RN Role Reimagined

The California Healthcare Foundation published a report, *RN Role Reimagined: How Empowering Registered Nurses Can Improve Primary Care* (2015). The report identified 12 strategies, aligned with the IOM recommendations, to support the delivery of primary care through enhanced roles for RNs in primary care. These strategies, listed in Box 2.1, are also relevant and applicable to ambulatory care.

Josiah Macy Jr. Foundation Report: Partners in Transforming Care

In 2016, the Josiah Macy Jr. Foundation hosted an invitational conference of thought leaders from academic nursing and medicine, healthcare delivery organizations, professional nursing associations, and healthcare philanthropy to explore the preparation of nurses for enhanced roles in order to meet urgent demands in primary care (Macy, 2016). Facilitators and barriers were examined, and the need for radical change was explored. Actionable recommendations are listed in Box 2.2.

BOX 2.1 Strategies for Enhancing the Role of RNs in Primary Care

1. Provide RNs with additional training in primary care skills, so they can make more clinical decisions.
2. Empower RNs to make more clinical decisions, using standardized procedures.
3. Reduce the triage burden on RNs to free up time for other responsibilities.
4. Include RNs on care teams, allowing them to focus on their team's patients.
5. Implement RN-led new-patient visits to increase patient access to care.
6. Offer patients covisits in which RNs conduct most of the visit, with providers joining in at the end.
7. Deploy RNs as "tactical nurses."
8. Provide patients with RN-led chronic care management visits.
9. Employ RNs' skills to care-manage patients with complex healthcare needs.
10. Train some RNs to take responsibility for specialized functions.
11. Schedule RNs to perform different roles on different days.
12. Preserve the traditional RN role and focus on training medical assistants (MAs) and licensed vocational nurses (LVNs) to take on new responsibilities.

Note. LVN = licensed vocational nurses; MA = medical assistant; RN = registered nurse. Reprinted with permission from the Bodenheimer, T., Bauer, L., Syer, S, & Otaylwola, J. N. (2015). RN role reimagined: How empowering registered nurses can improve primary care. *California Healthcare Foundation.* https://www.chcf.org/publication/rn-role-reimagined-how-empowering-registered-nurses-can-improve-primary-care/

BOX 2.2 Conference Recommendations Josiah Macy Jr. Foundation

1. Leaders of nursing schools, primary care practices, and health systems should actively facilitate culture change that elevates primary care in RN education and practice.
2. Primary care practices should redesign their care models to utilize the skills and expertise of RNs in meeting the healthcare needs of patients—and payers and regulators should facilitate this redesign.
3. Nursing school leaders and faculty should elevate primary care content in the education of prelicensure and RN-to-BSN nursing students.
4. Leaders of primary care practices and health systems should facilitate lifelong education and professional development opportunities in primary care and support practicing RNs in pursuing careers in primary care.
5. Academia and healthcare organizations should partner to support and prepare nursing faculty to educate prelicensure and RN-to-BSN students in primary care knowledge, skills, and perspective.
6. Leaders and faculty in nursing education and continuing education programs should include interprofessional education and teamwork in primary care nursing curricula.

Note. BSN = Bachelor of Science in Nursing; RN = registered nurse. Reprinted with permission from Josiah Macy Jr. Foundation. (2016). *Registered nurses: Partners in transforming primary care.* http://macyfoundation.org/publications/publication/conference-summary-registered-nurses-in-transforming-primary-care

American Academy of Ambulatory Care Nursing: Current and Future Roles

The AAACN's *Position Statement* (2017) highlights current and future roles for all ambulatory care practice settings. In addition, the paper advances a call to action to all ambulatory care RNs, and the activities are described in Box 2.3.

BOX 2.3 Call to Action Activities

1. Communicate the powerful story of professional progress made by ambulatory care nurses and articulate their ability to positively impact patient care and outcomes.
2. Expand the body of knowledge for ambulatory care clinical and telehealth nursing practice by conducting and/or applying the findings of scientific studies that build evidence-based nursing practice.
3. Lead organizational efforts to define and implement professional nursing roles that promote autonomy, enhance collaboration, improve care, and address core competencies in care coordination and transition management.
4. Ensure EHRs include robust documentation tools that support professional ambulatory and telehealth nursing practice.
5. Establish strategic alliances between health systems and academic institutions to develop curricula that prepare students to practice as registered nurses in ambulatory care environments.
6. Pursue partnerships with regulatory and standard setting agencies to identify and measure indicators of patient safety and quality of care in ambulatory nursing practice.
7. Design organizational structures and cultures that spur and reward innovation.
8. Collaborate with professional organizational colleagues to define the duties and responsibilities for each member of the healthcare team.
9. Develop an agenda that informs the nursing community, healthcare professionals, and political stakeholders at the local, state, and federal levels of the value and cost-effectiveness of professional ambulatory care nurses.

Note. EHR = electronic health record. Reprinted with permission from American Academy of Ambulatory Care Nursing. (2017). American Academy of Ambulatory Care Nursing position paper: The role of the registered nurses in ambulatory care. *Nursing Economics, 35*(1), 39–47.

Robert Wood Johnson Foundation: Catalyst for Change

The Robert Wood Johnson Foundation published *Catalysts for Change: Harnessing the Power of Nurses to Build Population Health in the 21st Century* (2017). This work studied the role of RNs in helping to reverse the course of declining health of U.S. citizens and promoting the health of the nation in the 21st century. As value-based care reimbursement models are evolving, specific interventions for targeted populations will need to be addressed with strategies focused on social determinants of health, health equity, healthy behaviors, and access to affordable care.

The report states: "Nurses must develop four key population-focused competencies: 1) a holistic approach considering the physical, mental, social, and spiritual aspects in the context of the environment; 2) coordination of care across providers and sites of care; 3) collaboration with other professionals and community stakeholders; and 4) advocacy for the individual and the community" (p. 4). In addition, the following RN population health and population health management roles were identified: (1) leadership in state and local public health agencies, (2) leadership for population health initiatives for healthcare systems, (3) school nursing, (4) data analytics, (5) chronic disease management, (6) care coordination/management, and (7) leading community benefit and population health initiatives (RWJF, 2017).

Future of Ambulatory Care Nursing

There are approximately 3.7 million RNs who can help transform care in ambulatory care settings (Macy, 2016). With these numbers, RNs are well-positioned to assist in the redesign of care models. Nurses and nurse leaders need to be involved in developing value-based models that include care coordination methodologies to assist meeting metrics for reimbursement in value-based care. Nurses need to be educated differently and empowered to practice to the full scope of their preparation and licensure (IOM, 2011; Macy, 2016).

It is important for the nurse to understand population health and risk stratification as a driver of high cost of care (RWJF, 2017). Using health information and data analytics to build programs and tools helps identify population health variances and outliers early so design changes can be implemented in coordinating care. Nurses with expertise in technology are vital to practice success because they can manage high-risk individuals, as well as rising risk populations (Dunlap et al., 2017).

Ambulatory care nurses are well poised to lead, direct, and support these emerging care delivery and payment reform models. Through acquired knowledge and skills, ambulatory care nurses can manage and use their competencies, focus on the individual and their family, and drive processes for the success of practice redesign and improved access to care. Ambulatory care nurses are critical to the success of healthcare reform in providing care to individuals, communities, and the nation.

Case Study

Helen G is a 74-year-old with a recent history of increased medical problems and complications. Liz, the care coordinator in the primary care provider's office, knows Ms. G well and is responsible for managing Ms. G's ongoing nursing care needs and subsequent follow-up appointments in multiple clinical areas.

Ms. G has a history of hypertension, type 2 diabetes, hypercholesterolemia, and essential tremors and developed a low-grade right-sided astrocytoma near the basal ganglia 1 year ago. She underwent tumor ablation (97% successful), 6 weeks of daily radiation therapy but failed a course of oral chemotherapy because of bone marrow suppression. She subsequently developed multiple deep vein thromboses in the right leg and was started on Lovenox and transitioned to Coumadin over a 3-month period.

Normal pressure hydrocephalus was discovered inadvertently during the brain tumor workup. Symptoms included increasing gait disturbance, urinary incontinence, and mild dementia, which progressed to a complete inability to walk, limited ability to eat, total urinary incontinence, inability to dress and undress, and need for total care. A ventriculoperitoneal shunt was placed about 6 months later. After the shunt surgery, Ms. G was placed in a nursing facility for rehab. Over the next 3 months, Ms. G demonstrated a significant improvement of symptoms. She is walking with a rollator and is able to perform most activities of daily living independently but has developed increased short-term memory loss with poor decision-making, and thus safety is a major concern.

Since Ms. G lives alone and all of her family members live in different states, her friend Mary is her power of attorney for healthcare and primary caregiver who assists Ms. G in making healthcare decisions. Ms. G wants to return home or to a local assisted living facility.

1. What actions will the CCTM-RN take to assist Ms. G in accomplishing the identified goals?
2. What interventions will be performed in collaboration with providers or other care team members?

Key Points for Review

- Ambulatory care nurses have the ability to impact the health of individuals they care for in any of the settings that comprise ambulatory care. Partnering with individuals and other members of the healthcare team, care delivery in the ambulatory setting has evolved from the basic care provided in homes and schools in the 19th century to the highly technical and sophisticated care provided in ambulatory settings today, in the 21st century.
- Care payment models relevant to ambulatory care settings have been reformed from paying for volume to paying for value. Care models continue to be studied, change, and require flexibility in order to address the charge and mandate for healthcare reform to improve quality and costs for consumers. Policy makers suggest a directional change in its future to one of increased competition among providers for individuals' choice and greater flexibility in payment models.
- RNs are uniquely positioned to impact health outcomes by defining the enhanced and emerging roles for RNs in ambulatory care, including care coordination, managing transitions, chronic disease management, telehealth practice, nurse-led specialty care, community-based primary care, health promotion, wellness, disease prevention models, and home care. In addition, ambulatory RNs are employed in ACOs and PCMHs to manage care for chronically ill individuals.
- National reports will continue to guide the evolution of roles for ambulatory care nurses.

REFERENCES

American Academy of Ambulatory Care Nursing. (2017). American Academy of Ambulatory Care Nursing position paper: The role of the registered nurses in ambulatory care. *Nursing Economics$, 35*(1), 39–47. PMID: 29984958.

American Hospital Association. (2017). *CMS finalizes key physician quality payment program policies for 2020 [Press release]*. https://www.aha.org/system/files/advocacy-issues/bulletin/2017/171103-bulletin-qpp.pdf

American Psychiatric Association. (2016). *Dissemination of integrated care within adult primary care settings: The collaborative model*. American Psychiatric Association/Academy of Psychosomatic Medicine. https://www.integration.samhsa.gov/integrated-care-models/APA-APM-Dissemination-Integrated-Care-Report.pdf

Arend, J., Tsang-Quinn, J., Levine, C., & Thomas, D. (2012). The patient-centered medical home: History, components, and review of the evidence. *Mount Sinai Journal of Medicine: A Journal of Transnational and Personalized Medicine, 79*(4), 423–523. https://doi.org/10.1002/msj.21326

Bauer, L., & Bodenheimer, T. (2017). Expanding roles of registered nurses in primary care delivery of the future. *Nursing Outlook, 65*(5), 624–632. https://doi.org/10.1016/j.outlook.2017.03.011

Berwick, D., Nolan, T., & Whittington, J. (2008). The triple aim: Care, health, and cost. *Health Affairs, 27*(3), 759–769. https://doi.org/10.1377/hlthaff.27.3.759

Bithoney, W. (2014). 6 necessary guidelines to create and manage a successful ACO. Becker's Hospital Review. https://www.beckershospitalreview.com/accountable-care-organizations/6-necessary-guidelines-to-create-and-manage-a-successful-aco.html

Blount, F., & Miller, B. (2009). Addressing the workforce crisis in integrated primary health. *Journal of Clinical Psychology in Medical Settings, 16*, 113–119. https://doi.org/10.1007/s10880-008-9142-7

Blumenthal, D., Abrams, M., & Nuzum, R. (2015). *The Affordable Care Act at 5 years*. http://www.nejm.org/doi/full/10.1056/NEJMhpr1503614

Bodenheimer, T., & Sinsky, C. (2014). From triple to quadruple aim: Care of the patient requires care of the provider. *Annals of Family Medicine, 12*(6), 573–576. https://doi.org/10.1370/afm.1713

Bodenheimer, T., Bauer, L., Syer, S, & Otaylwola, J. N. (2015). RN role reimagined: How empowering registered nurses can improve primary care. *California Healthcare Foundation.* https://www.chcf.org/publication/rn-role-reimagined-how-empowering-registered-nurses-can-improve-primary-care/

Bodenheimer, T. S., & Smith, M. D. (2013). Primary Care: Proposed solutions to the physician shortage without training more physicians. *Health Affairs,* (32), 1881–1886. https://doi.org/10.1377/hlthaff.2013.0234

Casalino, L. (2015). Pioneer accountable care organizations: Traversing rough country. *Journal of the American Medical Association, 313*(21), 2126–2127. https://doi.org/10.1001/jama.2015.5086

Center for Healthcare Strategies. (2016). *Medicaid accountable care organization learning collaborative*. http://www.chcs.org/project/medicaid-accountable-care-organization-learning-collaborative-phase-iii/

Centers for Disease Control and Prevention. (2018). *Progress reviews for health people 2020.* https://www.cdc.gov/nchs/healthy_people/hp2020/hp2020_progress_reviews.htm

Centers for Medicare and Medicaid Services. (2009). *Roadmap for implementing value driven healthcare in the traditional Medicare fee-for-service program.* https://www.cms.gov/Medicare/Quality-Initiatives-Patient-Assessment-Instruments/QualityInitiativesGenInfo/Downloads/VBPRoadmap_OEA_1-16_508.pdf

Centers for Medicare and Medicaid Services. (2015). *The Medicare Access & CHIP Reauthorization Act of 2015: Path to value*. https://www.cms.gov/Medicare/Quality-Initiatives-Patient-Assessment-Instruments/Value-Based-Programs/MACRA-MIPS-and-APMs/MACRA-LAN-PPT.pdf

Centers for Medicare and Medicaid Services. (2017). *Accountable care organizations: Overview.* http://www.cms.gov/ACO

Centers for Medicare and Medicaid Services. (2018a). *About the CMS innovation center.* https://innovation.cms.gov/About

Centers for Medicare and Medicaid Services. (2018b). *Bundled Payment for Care Improvement (BPCI) Initiative: General information*. https://innovation.cms.gov/initiatives/bundled-payments

Colla, C., Wennberg, D., Meara, E., Skinner, J., Gottlieb, D., Lewis, V., Snyder, C. M., Fisher, E. (2012). Spending differences associated with the Medicare Physician Group Practice Demonstration. *Journal of American Medical Association, 308*(10), 1015–1023. https://doi.org/10.1001/2012.jama.10812

Crowley, R., & Kirschner, N. (2015). The integration of care for mental health, substance abuse, and other behavioral health conditions into primary care: Executive summary of an American College of Physicians position paper. *Annals of Internal Medicine, 163*(4), 298–299. https://doi.org/10.7326/M15-0510

David, G., Saynisch, P. A., & Smith-McLallen, A. (2018)., The economics of patient centered care. *Journal of Health Economic,* (59), 60–77. https://doi.org/10.1016/j.jhealeco.2018.02.012

Davis, K., Abrams, M., & Stremikis, K. (2011). How the affordable care act will strengthen the nation's primary care foundation. *Journal of General Internal Medicine, 26*(10), 1201–1203. https://doi.org/10.1007/s11606-011-1720-y

de Bruin, S. R., Baan, C. A., & Struijs, J. N. (2011). Pay-for-performance in disease management: A systematic review of the literature. *BMC Health Services Research, 11*(1), 272. https://doi.org/10.1186/1472-6963-11-272

Dunlap, C., Green, A., Cropley, S., & Estes, L. (2017). Making sense of ACOs: A guide for nurse leaders. *Nurse Leader, 15*(3), 193–198. https://doi.org/10.1016/j.mnl.2017.03.001

Federman, A. D., & Keyhani, S. (2011). Physicians' participation in the Physicians' Quality Reporting Initiative and their perceptions of its impact on quality of care. *Health Policy, 102*(2–3), 229–234. https://doi.org/10.1016/j.healthpol.2011.05.003

Fillmore, H., DuBard, C. A., Ritter, G. A., & Jackson, C. T. (2014). Health care savings with the patient-centered medical home: Community Care of North Carolina's experience. *Population Health Management, 17*(3), 141–148. https://doi.org/10.1089/pop.2013.0055

Gold, J. (2014). *FAQs on ACOs: Accountable care organizations explained.* http://www.kaiserhealthnews.org/

stories/2011/january/13/aco-accountable-care-organization-faq.aspx

Goodson, J. (2010). Patient Protection and Affordable Care Act: Promise and peril for primary care. *Annals of Internal Medicine, 152*, 742–744. https://doi.org/10.7326/0003-4819-152-11-201006010-00249

Gorman, A. (2016). *Bridging the gap between medical and mental health care. California Healthline*, 1–6. http://californiahealthline.org/news/bridging-the-gap-between-medical-and-mental-health-care

Gruessner, V. (2016). *How MACRA resolves sustainable growth rate formula challenges. HealthPayer Intelligence.* https://healthpayerintelligence.com/news/how-macra-solves-challenges-of-sustainable-growth-rate-formula

Guterman, S., Davis, K., Stremikis, K., & Drake, H. (2010). Innovation in Medicare and Medicaid will be central to health reform's success. *Health Affairs, 29*(6), 1188–1193. https://doi.org/10.1377/hlthaff.2010.0442

Hadley, J. (2003). Sicker and poorer—The consequences of being uninsured: A review of the research on the relationship between health insurance, medical care use, health, work, and income. *Medical Care Research and Review, 60*(2), 3S–75S. https://doi.org/10.1177/1077558703254101

Hoffman, C. (2014). The uninsured and underinsured-On the cusp of health reform. In D. Mason, J. Leavitt, & M. Chaffee (Eds.), *Policy and politics in nursing and health care* (6th ed., pp. 187–197). Elsevier.

Institute of Medicine. (1978). *A manpower policy for primary health care: Report of a study.* The National Academies Press.

Institute of Medicine. (2011). *The future of nursing leading change, advancing health.* The National Academies Press.

Institute of Medicine. (2015). *Assessing progress on the Institute of Medicine Report The Future of Nursing.* The National Academies Press.

Josiah Macy Jr. Foundation. (2016). *Registered nurses: Partners in transforming primary care.* http://macyfoundation.org/publications/publication/conference-summary-registered-nurses-in-transforming-primary-care

Kilo, C., & Wasson, J. (2010). Practice redesign and the patient-centered medical home: History, promises, and challenges. *Health Affairs, 29*(5), 773–778. https://doi.org/10/1377/hlthaff.2010.0012

Kurtzman, E., & Johnson, J. (2014). Quality and safety in health care: Policy issues. In D. Mason, J. Leavitt, & M. Chaffee (Eds.), *Policy and politics in nursing and health care* (6th ed., pp. 366–374). Elsevier.

McClellan, M., Feinberg, D., Bach, P., Chew, P., Conway, P., Leschly, N., Marchand, G., Mussallem, M., & Teeter, D. (2017). *Payment reform for better value and medical innovation A vital direction for health and health care.* National Academy of Medicine.

McGough, P., Bauer, A., Collins, L., & Dugdale, D. (2015). Integrating behavioral health into primary care. *Population Health Management*, *0*(0), 1–7. https://doi.org/10.1089/pop.2015.0039

Morse, S. (2017). *CMS says it will change direction of CMMI, wants providers to have greater flexibility in payment model. Health Care Finance News.* http://www.healthcarefinancenews.com/news/cms-says-it-will-change-direction-cmmi-wants-providers-have-greater-flexibility-payment-model

National Committee for Quality Assurance. (2018). *NCQA PCMH recognition: Better quality. Lower costs.* https://www.ncqa.org/programs/recognition/practices/patient-centered-medical-home-pcmh

Needleman, J. (2015). *Expanding the role of the registered nurses in primary care: A business case.* Prepared for the Josiah Macy Jr. Foundation.

Nichols, L., Cuellar, A., Helmchen, L., Gimm, G., & Want, J. (2017). *What should we conclude from "mixed" results in payment reform evaluations?.* https://www.healthaffairs.org/do/10.1377/hblog20170814.061537/full/

Nightingale, F. (1859). *Notes on nursing: What it is, what it is not.* Harrison.

Public Broadcasting Service. (2012). *Health costs: How the U.S. compares with other countries.* https://www.pbs.org/newshour/health/health-costs-how-the-us-compares-with-other-countries

Pulcini, J., & Hart, M. (2014). Financing health care in the United States. In D. Mason, J. Leavitt, & M. Chaffee (Eds.), *Policy and politics in nursing and health care* (6th ed., pp. 135–146). Elsevier. https://www.cms.gov/Research-Statistics-Data-and-Systems/Statistics-Trends-and-Reports/NationalHealthExpendData/NationalHealthAccountsProjected

Reinhardt, U. (1997). Wanted: A clearly articulated social ethic for American health care. *Journal of American Medical Association, 278*(17), 1446–1447. https://doi.org/10.1001/jama.1997.03550170076036

Rhodes, D. C. (1988). The impact of DRGs on the cost and quality of healthcare in the United States. *Health Policy, 9*(2), 117–131. https://doi.org/10.1016/0168-8510(88)90029-2

Robert Wood Johnson Foundation. (2017). *Catalysts for change: harnessing the power of nursing to build population health in the 21st century.* https://www.rwjf.org/en/library/research/2017/09/catalysts-for-change--harnessing-the-power-of-nurses-to-build-population-health.html

Shaw, J. (2014). *Accountable care organizations: What is the evidence*? http://www.vtlegalaid.org/sites/default/files/Accountable Care Organizations - What is the Evidence.pdf

Shorter, T., Bartlett, P., & Kirsner, J. (2014). In P. Pavarini, C. McGinty, & M. Schaffi (Eds.), *The ACO handbook: A guide to accountable care organizations* (2nd ed.). American Healthcare Lawyers Association.

Shrank, W. (2013). The Center for Medicare and Medicaid Innovation's blueprint for rapid-cycle evaluation of new care and payment models. *Health Affairs, 32*(4), 807–812. https://doi.org/10.1377/hlthaff.2013.0216

Sikka, R., Morath, J., & Leape, L. (2015). The quadruple aim: care, health, cost and meaning in work. *BMJ Quality & Safety, 0*, 1–3. https://doi.org/10.1136/bmjqs-2015-004160

Stulberg, J. (2008). The physician quality reporting initiative—A gateway to pay for performance: What every health care professional should know. *Quality Management in Healthcare, 17*(1), 2–8. https://doi.org/10.1097/01.QMH.0000308632.74355.93

Substance Abuse & Mental Health Services Administration. (2016). *What is integrated care?* http://www.integration.samhsa.gov/about-us/what-is-integrated-care

Vessey, J., Mc Crave, J., Curro-Harrington, C., & Di Fazio, R. (2015). Enhancing care coordination through patient-and family-initiated telephone encounters: A quality improvement project. *Journal of Pediatric Nursing,* (30), 915–923. https://doi.org/10.1016/j.pedn.2015.05.012

Werner, R., Kelsted, J., Stuart, E., & Polsky, D. (2011). The effect of pay-for-performance in hospitals: Lessons for quality improvement. *Health Affairs, 30*(4), 690–698. https://doi.org/10.1377/hlthaff:2010.1277

3

Social, Economic, and Policy Influences on Ambulatory Care

Karen Alexander

PERSPECTIVES

"Researchers and policy makers have known for decades that access to health care is not sufficient for addressing health disparities because of the socially situated roots of the disparities. We argue that the lack of progress in alleviating health disparities is the result of a lack of overarching framework to guide both policy makers and researchers in their efforts."

Thurman & Harrison (2017), p. 26

LEARNING OBJECTIVES

Upon completion of this chapter, the reader will be able to:

1. Describe the national and global movement toward understanding social determinants of health as important predictors of health outcomes.
2. Understand the health disparities that exist racially, economically, and in terms of place and gender.
3. Understand the role of public health and public health nursing efforts to monitor and ensure health outcomes.
4. Explain the role of the ambulatory care nurse in distinct population health roles.
5. Compare and contrast the types of policy that may influence health in the future.

KEY TERMS

Health policy
Population health
Public health system
Social determinants of health
Vulnerable populations

Social Determinants of Health

Increasingly, social and environmental context has been influential in predicting long-term health outcomes, health risk, and health quality (Adler et al., 2016). The study of **social determinants of health** has developed in order to explore the context in which individuals live and is a focus in current **health policy** and practice. Healthcare governing bodies in the United States have embraced the term and have used social determinants of health to guide their policy and practice recommendations. The Centers for Disease Control and Prevention (CDC) and Healthy People 2020 define social determinants of health as the "conditions in the environments in which people are born, live, work, learn, play, worship and age that affect a wide range of health, functioning and quality of life outcomes and risks" (United States Department of Health and Human Services, 2017). The National Academies of Health have convened a task force to shape policy based on the latest evidence regarding social determinants of health (Adler et al., 2016). Globally, the World Health Organization (WHO) also recognizes the need to account for the environmental and social context when addressing policy and directing interventions (Magnan, 2017). The health policies that these organizations target "refer to decisions, plans, and actions that are undertaken to achieve specific health care goals within a society" (World Health Organization, 2018). As a result, these contextual influences on health are now paramount to incorporate in clinical practice for nursing and other healthcare professions.

Although the last century highlighted many medical interventions and technologic advancements, modifiable factors in the surrounding environment that influence individual behavior have emerged in the 21st century as the most important component of health outcomes. Approximately 80% to 90% of modifiable contributors to healthy outcomes are related to social determinants of health and the remaining 10% to 20% to medical treatment (Hood et al., 2016). Preventable disease is still the highest risk factor in mortality worldwide. The modifiable risk factors that influence mortality risk, in such conditions as cardiovascular disease, are more strongly correlated with social determinants of health than access to medical intervention (Mahony & Jones, 2013). With the overall shift in payment to a value-based system focused on outcomes in the United States, interventions and systems that take into account social determinants of health are increasingly emerging (Magnan, 2017).

Social determinants of health help explain differences between groups of people based on upstream and downstream factors. The emphasis on social determinants of health acknowledges that health outcomes occur as a result of the convergence of a complex set of factors. Often, the individual sees only the immediate downstream choices (smoking or not smoking, eating healthy choices or not)—but these choices exist as the result of a bigger picture. A perspective that takes into account social determinants of a health model encompasses larger, upstream factors as well. Upstream factors include the environmental context and the greater policy and societal factors that influence the choices available to the population. Both downstream and upstream factors contribute to overall health outcomes, which in turn affect both life expectancy and quality of life.

Public Health and Social Determinants of Health

The **public health system** ensures that everyone in society can be healthy through a well-established process comprised of screening, monitoring, and evaluation activities. Public health is not a new concept but one that does not receive adequate credit for the overall wellness and health of our modern society. In the first half of the 20th century, large leaps in life expectancy occurred as a result of public reforms worldwide. These reforms included sanitary reform, food and water safety, vaccinations, and antibiotic treatment.

As important as quality medical care is for a person's health, it has been insufficient to ensure better health outcomes in the population. Medical advancements are necessary and life giving but are ultimately individually focused and come at a great economic cost. Public health intervention can extend to every arena of life that could affect health, including air pollution, motor vehicle safety, and food safety. With governmental regulation and oversight, these environmental and behavioral factors have improved steadily to keep society as a whole healthier (Adler et al., 2016; Braveman & Gottlieb, 2014). Yet despite the public health efforts that have controlled many diseases such as cholera, tuberculosis, and measles, application of the same public health principles to diseases with large behavioral components (ie, substance use) has been slower (Levy & Sidel, 2013; Thurman & Harrison, 2017).

In addition, health disparities among distinct groups of our society prevail despite marked improvements in the overall health of the population. For example, most racial minority populations in the United States experience a lower life expectancy, higher incidence of major causes of morbidity, and a higher infant mortality rate (Chetty et al., 2016; David & Collins, 2007). Economically, income status remains a leading indicator of a person's life expectancy and overall health quality despite overall decreases in poverty rates in the last 50 years (Galea et al., 2011). Finally, gender disparities exist, with women experiencing differences in health outcomes compared with men, and this certainly extends to those individuals who define their gender as nonbinary or transgendered (*Millennial Development Goal 3: Promote Gender Equality and Empower Women*, 2015). Health access and delivery falls short in all these groups of individuals, but it is not the only factor in such disparities. Income differences, differences in food access, and racial and gender differences are all pivotal in determining the health equity of all of these groups.

With the exploration of the connection between social determinants and health disparities, investigation into the distinct health needs of populations has emerged within public health movements. **Population health** is defined as the study of the health outcomes for discrete groups of people (Adler et al., 2016). The implementation of strategies to improve the health of the population falls under the purview of public health, and the overall public health system is therefore crucial for the success of all populations.

Public Health Efforts for Populations in the 21st Century

In response to the need for a better public health effort to influence social determinants of health and health disparities for distinct populations, the CDC and Healthy People 2020 have developed a framework in relation to social determinants of health that integrates three key areas of prevention (DeSalvo et al., 2016). Figure 3.1 illustrates the crossover of care that occurs as traditional clinical prevention and population prevention occur through innovative services that can be provided outside the clinical setting (Auerbach, 2016). There are vital public health services offered by nursing and other healthcare professionals in acute and ambulatory settings in the traditional clinical prevention bucket, including vaccinations and routine screenings. Innovative clinical prevention can include home-based and technology-based interventions provided in response to the needs of populations, such as asthma home environmental evaluations (Auerbach, 2016; Schroeder et al., 2018). Population prevention occurs at the community level and involves policy change, structural change, and financial incentive restructuring for providers.

As preventative interventions that influence social determinants of health emerge, Healthy People 2020 identified five key areas for targeted intervention: the neighborhood and built environment, health and healthcare, social and community context, education, and economic stability. Tool kits have been developed and are publicly available on the Department of Health

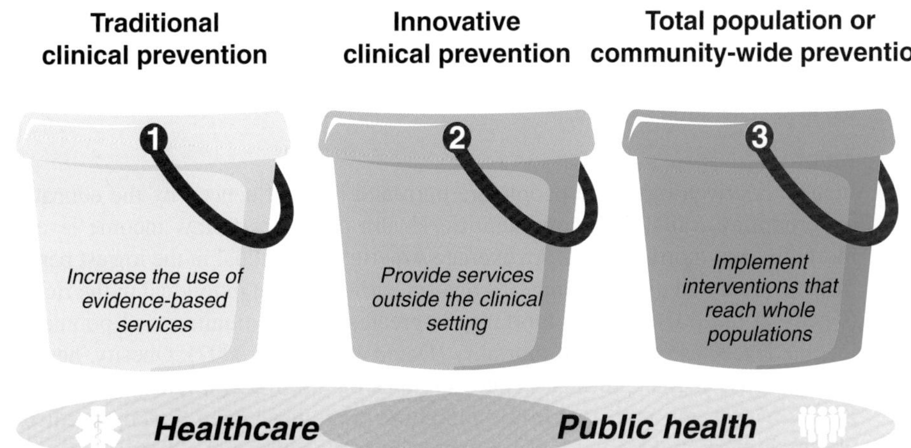

FIGURE 3.1 Centers for Disease Control and Prevention: three buckets of prevention. (Auerbach, J. [2016]. The 3 buckets of prevention. *Journal of Public Health Management and Practice, 22*[3], 215–218. https://doi.org/10.1097/phh.0000000000000381)

and Human Services (DHHS) website. Public health campaigns with advertising targeted at specific populations have a far reach and effect on behaviors such as safe sleep, smoking and alcohol use, and texting while driving (DeSalvo et al., 2016).

Even with the resources of governmental agencies, nurses and other healthcare professionals may feel that affecting social determinants of health is outside the domain of their practice and influence. Yet it is important for nurses and all healthcare professionals to survey the evidence in distinct areas of environmental and social context in relation to health outcomes and learn from existing, effective interventions. Nursing has a legacy of advocating and partnering with the community in public health efforts (Braveman & Gottlieb, 2014). Just as patients are now considered a part of the healthcare team, community members need to be a part of public health initiatives. A shared vision can promote long-term sustainability through multiple funding sources and provide a unique structure tailored to that population's needs (Braveman & Gottlieb, 2014). Addressing the following social determinants of health is crucial to health policy, not just social policy.

Place of Residence

Recent published research indicates that zip code of birth may be the leading indicator of health outcomes in the United States, emphasizing the importance of beginnings and residence (Adler et al., 2016; Johnson et al., 2011). Place of residence is linked to housing quality, food security, income potential, access to quality education, and access to quality healthcare (Galea et al., 2011). Rural residents in the United States are disproportionately disadvantaged when accessing the primary and acute care they need (Bryant-Moore et al., 2018). Outcomes for those seeking substance use treatment are poorer in rural states than in states with urban centers (Hand et al., 2017).

Most clearly, place of birth is linked most directly to life expectancy in recent studies (Woolf, 2017). For example, within the city of Philadelphia there are many zip codes that encompass small geographic areas. Life expectancy can be as disparate as 20 years between one zip code and another that are both within the city limits but a mile or two apart (Chetty et al., 2016). Researchers have, in fact, tried moving individuals out of a low-poverty neighborhood to improve life expectancy, and although those who moved experienced better mental health, morbidity and mortality remained the same (Galea et al., 2011).

Communities that have experienced affordable housing shortages and insecurity for decades are more vulnerable to poor health outcomes. Therefore, it is the systems that can improve whole neighborhoods, caught in cycles of poverty, which will have an influence on the next generation's health.

Income

Income is driven by where people are born and live, influenced by the educational and job opportunities available to communities. Health outcomes follow income levels, as seen in morbidity and mortality data. An average American individual in the lowest percentiles of the income strata will die on average 14.6 years earlier than an individual in the richest percentile (Chetty et al., 2016). Infant mortality is greatest in communities and populations at lower income levels, as is maternal mortality (David & Collins, 2007). Obesity, heart disease, and diabetes have higher prevalence rates in areas of lower socioeconomic status (Galea et al., 2011). In fact, the increases in the minimum wage have been directly predicted to reduce obesity in the population of low-income workers (Conklin et al., 2016).

Food Insecurity

Millions of children nationwide (and globally) spend days without adequate food supply for their caloric needs (United States Department of Health and Human Services, 2017).

Children are the most vulnerable to inadequate food supplies, but food insecurity touches all populations, including older people. In modern society, environments where food is not consistently provided are directly related to the consumption of calorie-rich but nutritionally deficient foods. The result is weight gain and obesity epidemics in food-insecure populations, especially those experiencing poverty (Nguyen et al., 2017).

Programs such as Supplemental Nutrition Assistance Programs (SNAPs) have been directly able to increase children's consumption of fresh fruits and vegetables. Participation in the mother and child program, Women, Infants and Children (WIC), has been associated with better birth outcomes and child immunization rates (Nguyen et al., 2017).

Race

Although place of residence, income, and food security can largely explain the health disparities in the United States, race is still an important independent, social determinant of health that needs to be highlighted. Controlling for socioeconomic status, minority racial groups still experience dissimilar maternal mortality rates, infant mortality rates, and rates of disease compared with the White majority population in the United States (Thurman & Harrison, 2017). For example, among women who did not finish high school, the infant mortality rate of children born to African American women is twice that of children born to White women (Williams, 2012). In addition, African Americans have a 30% higher overall mortality rate than White individuals living in the United States (Williams, 2012). Racial disparities exist among groups of veterans, as well, who, theoretically, have similar access to outpatient and inpatient care (Thurman & Harrison, 2017). Other racial groups, such as Hispanics and Asians, tend to be disparate in their health outcomes based on years spent in the United States. The longer the time spent in the United States, the worse these racial minority groups' health outcomes become (Singh & Hiatt, 2006).

Ambulatory Care for Specific Vulnerable Populations: Applications of Population Health

Ambulatory care nurses work with a view of both populations and individuals. The day-to-day practice of an ambulatory care nurse telescopes in between both worlds, confronting both downstream choices and upstream influences. The practice of care coordination addresses population health by bringing the population and individual aspects of nursing care together. Population-focused nursing practice occurs when nurses are addressing key aspects of overall health management for a group of people who share a common characteristic, such as children with asthma or older people with mental illnesses. The individual aspect of nursing care occurs when one-on-one care is being performed for an individual, such as when one needs a refill on a prescription or a referral to a community service. Care coordination is occurring at each of these levels and is a vital function of the ambulatory care nurse.

It should be noted that when discussing the **vulnerable populations** that follow in this chapter, person-first language is used. No longer are nurses to see the diagnosis first, but, rather, the person behind the diagnosis should be brought to the forefront. A child with asthma or a mother with a substance use disorder integrates context into the language of healthcare. Instead of seeing individuals as their illness, the change in our language reflects a transformation in posture toward the population and the individual. It is culturally sensitive and socially responsible to alter terminology when caring for vulnerable populations. Individual care needs and population care needs differ in relation to specific vulnerable populations.

Children

Disparities related to child health that are predominantly linked to social determinants of health are most clearly seen in the management of asthma and prevalence of infant mortality (Oliva et al., 2010; Schroeder et al., 2018). Infants born to African American women are smaller and experience more adverse health events in the first year of life compared with White infants (Johnson et al., 2011). Immigrant children also see disparate birth weight figures, with small for gestational age babies occurring more frequently as years spent in the United States increase (David & Collins, 2007). Asthma, a disease managed primarily in an ambulatory care setting, is markedly affected by social determinants of health, with Black and Hispanic children much more likely to die as a result of the disease than White children (Schroeder et al., 2018). Emergency room and urgent care visits related to asthma are four times more likely among African American children than among White children (Schroeder et al., 2018).

Yet intervention in the ambulatory care setting aimed at addressing these social determinants is possible. A randomized controlled trial of primary care assessment and referral to resources for mothers and children successfully enrolled families in more than one new resource annually (Garg et al., 2015). The families who received the intervention also had a greater likelihood of being employed, having a child in child care, receiving fuel assistance, and lower odds of experiencing homelessness (Garg et al., 2015). In addition, school nurses can promote and accomplish community-based interventions that reduce environmental triggers and increase asthma safety plan usage (Schroeder et al., 2018).

People Experiencing Incarceration

Women and men who have been incarcerated are a marginalized people within our society. Housing, employment, and healthcare access are all disrupted by their time in jail or prison and also prove difficult to access once released from incarceration. Incarceration has demonstrated effects on the transmission of infectious diseases, which then become communicated to family members on release (Adler et al., 2016). Racial disparities exist in incarceration rates and are widely documented (Fox et al., 2014). Substance use disorders are almost universal among prison inmates, although inmates have limited access to treatment during and postincarceration (Binswanger et al., 2012; Davis et al., 2003). Social isolation and financial constraints make transition into home life difficult. Shelters and transitional group housing postincarceration are often marked by violence, detachment from family support, and full of opportunities to obtain drugs (Binswanger et al., 2012).

Ambulatory care nurses interact with individuals experiencing incarceration transitions frequently, and a particular concern for engagement and coordination on release is important. This is especially a concern for women who are often transitioning to the care of their children or managing a pregnancy. Nonjudgmental care of individuals with incarceration history is paramount to improved quality of care and referral to resources for this population (Colbert et al., 2013).

People With a Substance Use Disorder

Substance use is most often initiated in the teenage and young adult years, before the age of 25 (Borelli et al., 2010). It is during this formative time, when development is still unfolding, that the brain and the body are most susceptible to the ill effects of substance abuse. Currently the leading cause of accidental death, opioid overdose often occurs in younger, newer opioid users (Huang et al., 2018). Public health interventions, in traditional clinical settings as well as in community settings, can influence attitudes and behaviors toward early initiation of substance use. School nurses and pediatric ambulatory care nurses are instrumental in preventative education and early screening and referral to treatment for adolescent substance users. Larger, upstream factors can also change the behaviors of youth through neighborhood stability and job availability (Cattell, 2001).

In addition, substance use during pregnancy affects not only the mother but also her child in the immediate and long term. Home visiting programs, especially ones that partner nurses with mothers, are effective in lowering substance use rates, increasing adherence to substance use treatment programs, and decreasing child maltreatment rates (Wu et al., 2017). Early referral to treatment improves outcomes for mother and child and increases breastfeeding rates and decreases referrals to child protective services (Earnshaw et al., 2013; Ordean et al., 2013).

Implications of Social Determinants of Health on Ambulatory Care Nursing Practice

In this overview of social determinants of health and correlated health disparities, the direction of governmental organizations has been highlighted as a guiding force. Healthy People 2030 goals are now emerging, and the future perspective will be to shape practice and policy with a large-scale community approach to intervention. Health policy that monitors our practice comes along slower and with more political discourse. Nevertheless, nurses should advocate for environmental and social policies that lead to better health outcomes for all populations. Schools are an important place where health outcomes can be improved by maintaining a safe environment, free of contaminants and pollutants, where good nutritional practices and safe exercise are encouraged. Ambulatory care practices can promote preventative education, screening, and early referral to treatment, all of which maintains and improves public health universally.

It can be difficult for a practicing nurse to see the connection between policy and their daily work. Yet, just as it is difficult to see how upstream social factors connect to downstream individual choices in health behaviors, policies affect nursing practice as well. A number of nursing organizations have crafted position statements addressing the need to incorporate social and economic context when practicing in the community. Policies have allowed funding to be made available, which in turn has provided resources for nurses in primary and ambulatory care practice. It is important that nurses access the healthcare technology, tool kits, and continuing education that are available in multiple formats from governing health organizations and professional nursing organizations. For example, the CDC produces tool kits that are specific to disease prevention and management, from infectious diseases to chronic heart disease.

Ambulatory care nurses can utilize the developed individual-specific information, fact sheets, and data to better serve their target populations. Statistics on the regional spread of disease are updated often, and social media messaging is included that can be conveyed to the desired audience. These tools can guide nurses in focusing not only on the individual's care but also on the care of the population.

National survey data are widely available and can help nurses understand the distribution of disease and illness in their communities of practice. Demonstration projects, such as state innovation models and accountable health communities, are linking population health and clinic care in the community. Finally, policies that now place an emphasis on value-based payment models require the coordination of care at the population level. Nurses are at the front line of this coordination of care, especially in the unique populations emphasized in this chapter.

Summary

Most of the work of nurses was outside of an acute care setting until modern times, and ambulatory care nursing has recently been seeing increasing prominence. Nurses have focused for centuries on large-scale, population-level interventions stemming from the sanitary reforms and epidemiologic research of Florence Nightingale. Nurses continue to be at the front line of prevention and maintenance of wellness in vulnerable populations. An awareness of the relationship between social determinants of health and health disparities for key populations is essential to provide excellent nursing care in this century. Policy development and advocacy for all groups of people will transform health for populations despite their background and context.

Case Study

Jeannette is a nurse working in a medication-assisted treatment clinic serving a population of mothers diagnosed with an opioid use disorder. Her role is to triage illnesses when individuals present at the clinic, in addition to coordinating appointments and resources for the mothers. She frequently has mothers bring their children in for evaluation.

A mother walks into the clinic with her 6-month-old child. The infant is crying and irritable, and the mother comes into the nurse's office for an evaluation of the child because she feels the child is ill. Jeannette performs a physical assessment of the infant and asks about formula or breastfeeding intake. The infant's vital signs are normal. The mother reports that she has been breastfeeding and supplementing with formula. Jeannette asks if the child has been to a pediatrician recently, and the mother tells her she was able to make the 3-month appointment but has not been recently.

Critical Thinking:

1. What is the next piece of physical assessment information that Jeannette needs today?
2. What are some reasons the mother has not been adherent to the expected well-child visits at her pediatrician?
3. How could Jeannette intervene to connect this mother to a pediatrician more regularly?

Key Points for Review

- Although public health organizations have made efforts to address social disparities to improve health, much remains to be done.
- Healthcare workers can have a positive impact on social determinants of health both through practice and public policy.
- Vulnerable populations such as children, the incarcerated, and those with substance use disorders are especially affected by socioeconomic factors.

REFERENCES

Adler, N. E., Cutler, D. M., Fielding, J. E., Galea, S., Glymour, M. M., Koh, H. K., and Satcher, D. (2016). Addressing social determinants of health and health Disparities: A vital direction for health and health care. *NAM Perspectives*. Discussion Paper, National Academy of Medicine, Washington, DC. https://doi.org/10.31478/201609t

Auerbach, J. (2016). The 3 buckets of prevention. *Journal of Public Health Management and Practice, 22*(3), 215–218. https://doi.org/10.1097/phh.0000000000000381

Binswanger, I. A., Nowels, C., Corsi, K. F., Glanz, J., Long, J., Booth, R. E., & Steiner, J. F. (2012). Return to drug use and overdose after release from prison: A qualitative study of risk and protective factors. *Addiction Science & Clinical Practice, 7*, 3. https://doi.org/10.1186/1940-0640-7-3

Borelli, J. L., Luthar, S. S., & Suchman, N. E. (2010). Discrepancies in perceptions of maternal aggression: Implications for children of methadone-maintained mothers. *American Journal of Orthopsychiatry, 80*(3), 412–421. https://doi.org/10.1111/j.1939-0025.2010.01044.x

Braveman, P., & Gottlieb, L. (2014). The social determinants of health: It's time to consider the causes of the causes. *Public Health Reports, 129*(1_suppl2), 19–31. https://doi.org/10.1177/00333549141291S206

Bryant-Moore, K., Bachelder, A., Rainey, L., Hayman, K., Bessette, A., & Williams, C. (2018). Use of service learning to increase master's-level nursing students' understanding of social determinants of health and health disparities. *Journal of Transcultural Nursing, 29*, 473–479. https://doi.org/10.1177/1043659617753043

Cattell, V. (2001). Poor people, poor places, and poor health: the mediating role of social networks and social capital. *Social Science and Medicine, 52*(10), 1501–1516. https://doi.org/10.1016/S0277-9536(00)00259-8

Chetty, R., Stepner, M., Abraham, S., Lin, S., Scuderi, B., Turner, N., Bergeron, A., & Cutler, D. (2016). The association between income and life expectancy in the United States, 2001–2014. *JAMA, 315*(16), 1750–1766. https://doi.org/10.1001/jama.2016.4226

Colbert, A. M., Sekula, L. K., Zoucha, R., & Cohen, S. M. (2013). Health care needs of women immediately post-incarceration: A mixed methods study. *Public Health Nursing, 30*(5), 409–419. https://doi.org/10.1111/phn.12034

Conklin, A. I., Ponce, N. A., Frank, J., Nandi, A., & Heymann, J. (2016). Minimum wage and overweight and obesity in adult women: A multilevel analysis of low and middle income countries. *PLoS One, 11*(3), e0150736. https://doi.org/10.1371/journal.pone.0150736

David, R., & Collins, J., Jr. (2007). Disparities in infant mortality: What's genetics got to do with it? *American Journal of Public Health, 97*(7), 1191–1197. https://doi.org/10.2105/ajph.2005.068387

Davis, T. M., Baer, J. S., Saxon, A. J., & Kivlahan, D. R. (2003). Brief motivational feedback improves post-incarceration treatment contact among veterans with substance use disorders. *Drug and Alcohol Dependence, 69*(2), 197–203. https://doi.org/10.1016/S0376-8716(02)00317-4

DeSalvo, K. B., O'Carroll, P. W., Koo, D., Auerbach, J. M., & Monroe, J. A. (2016). Public health 3.0: Time for an upgrade. *American Journal of Public Health, 106*(4), 621. https://doi.org/10.2105/AJPH.2016.303063

Earnshaw, V., Smith, L., & Copenhaver, M. (2013). Drug addiction stigma in the context of methadone maintenance therapy: An investigation into understudied sources of stigma. *International Journal of Mental Health and Addiction, 11*(1), 110–122. https://doi.org/10.1007/s11469-012-9402-5

Fox, A. D., Anderson, M. R., Bartlett, G., Valverde, J., Starrels, J. L., & Cunningham, C. O. (2014). Health outcomes and retention in care following release from prison for patients of an urban post-incarceration transitions clinic. *Journal of Health Care for the Poor and Underserved, 25*(3), 1139–1152. https://doi.org/10.1353/hpu.2014.0139

Galea, S., Tracy, M., Hoggatt, K. J., Dimaggio, C., & Karpati, A. (2011). Estimated deaths attributable to social factors in the United States. *American Journal of Public Health, 101*(8), 1456–1465. https://doi.org/10.2105/ajph.2010.300086

Garg, A., Toy, S., Tripodis, Y., Silverstein, M., & Freeman, E. (2015). Addressing social determinants of health at well child care visits: A cluster RCT. *Pediatrics, 135*(2), e296–e304. https://doi.org/10.1542/peds.2014-2888

Hand, D. J., Short, V. L., & Abatemarco, D. J. (2017). Substance use, treatment, and demographic characteristics of pregnant women entering treatment for opioid use disorder differ by United States census region. *Journal of Substance Abuse Treatment, 76*, 58–63. https://doi.org/10.1016/j.jsat.2017.01.011

Hood, C. M., Gennuso, K. P., Swain, G. R., & Catlin, B. B. (2016). County health rankings: Relationships between determinant factors and health outcomes. *American Journal of Preventive Medicine, 50*(2), 129–135. https://doi.org/10.1016/j.amepre.2015.08.024

Huang, X., Keyes, K. M., & Li, G. (2018). Increasing prescription opioid and heroin overdose mortality in the United States, 1999–2014: An age-period-cohort analysis. *American Journal of Public Health, 108*(1), 131–136. https://doi.org/10.2105/ajph.2017.304142

Johnson, T. S., Malnory, M. E., Nowak, E. W., & Kelber, S. (2011). Using fetal and infant mortality reviews to improve birth outcomes in an urban community. *Journal of Obstetric, Gynecologic, and Neonatal Nursing, 40*(1), 86–97. https://doi.org/10.1111/j.1552-6909.2010.01201.x

Levy, B. S., & Sidel, V. W. (Eds.). (2013). *Social injustice and public health* (2nd ed.). Oxford University Press.

Magnan, S. (2017). *Social determinants of health 101 for health care: Five plus five*. https://nam.edu/social-determinants-of-health-101-for-health-care-five-plus-five/

Mahony, D., & Jones, E. J. (2013). Social determinants of health in nursing education, research, and health policy. *Nursing Science Quarterly, 26*(3), 280–284. https://doi.org/10.1177/0894318413489186

Millennial development goal 3: Promote gender equality and empower women. (2015). http://www.un.org/millenniumgoals/gender.shtml

Nguyen, B. T., Ford, C. N., Yaroch, A. L., Shuval, K., & Drope, J. (2017). Food security and weight status in children: Interactions with food assistance programs. *American Journal of Preventive Medicine, 52*(2s2), S138–s144. https://doi.org/10.1016/j.amepre.2016.09.009

Oliva, G., Rienks, J., & Smyly, V. (2010). African American's awareness of disparities in infant mortality rates and sudden infant death syndrome risks. *Journal of Health Care for the Poor and Underserved, 21*(3), 946–960. https://doi.org/10.1353/hpu.0.0341

Ordean, A., Kahan, M., Graves, L., Abrahams, R., & Boyajian, T. (2013). Integrated care for pregnant women on methadone maintenance treatment: Canadian primary care cohort study. *Canadian Family Physician, 59*(10), e462–e469.

Schroeder, K., Malone, S. K., McCabe, E., & Lipman, T. (2018). Addressing the social determinants of health: A call to action for school nurses. *Journal of School Nursing, 34*, 182–191. https://doi.org/10.1177/1059840517750733

Singh, G. K., & Hiatt, R. A. (2006). Trends and disparities in socioeconomic and behavioural characteristics, life expectancy, and cause-specific mortality of native-born and foreign-born populations in the United States, 1979–2003. *International Journal of Epidemiology, 35*(4), 903–919. https://doi.org/10.1093/ije/dyl089

Thurman, W. A., & Harrison, T. (2017). Social context and value-based care: A capabilities approach for addressing health disparities. *Policy, Politics & Nursing Practice, 18*(1), 26–35. https://doi.org/10.1177/1527154417698145

United States Department of Health and Human Services. (2017). *Social determinants of health: Know what affects health*. https://www.cdc.gov/socialdeterminants/

Williams, D. R. (2012). Miles to go before we sleep: Racial inequities in health. *Journal of Health and Social Behavior, 53*(3), 279–295. https://doi.org/10.1177/0022146512455804

Woolf, S. H. (2017). Progress in achieving health equity requires attention to root causes. *Health Affairs, 36*(6), 984–991. https://doi.org/10.1377/hlthaff.2017.0197

World Health Organization. (2018). *Health policy*. http://www.who.int/topics/health_policy/en/

Wu, J., Dean, K. S., Rosen, Z., & Muennig, P. A. (2017). The cost-effectiveness analysis of nurse-family partnership in the United States. *Journal of Health Care for the Poor and Underserved, 28*(4), 1578–1597. https://doi.org/10.1353/hpu.2017.0134.

UNIT 2

Measuring Impact

4

Nursing Practice: Regulation and Advocacy

Barbara E. Trehearne and Mary Hines Vinson

PERSPECTIVES

"As a community, as a patient, as an individual trying to maintain wellness or seeking different levels of care, it is reassuring to know that a professional group defines what might be expected. This is communicated through standards and criteria and assured through regulation and certification. Also welcome is role clarification of the various members of a group and the commitment to working with teams of health givers in today's world."

Norma M. Lang, RN, PhD, FAAN, Professor and Dean Emerita, University of Pennsylvania School of Nursing and University of Wisconsin Milwaukee College of Nursing.

LEARNING OBJECTIVES

Upon completion of this chapter, the reader will be able to:

1. Describe the purpose of regulating nursing practice.
2. Define scope of practice.
3. Identify key regulatory agencies that impact scope of practice.
4. Describe how standards of practice defined by professional organizations influence scope of practice.
5. Understand how the employer defines scope of practice.
6. Explain how the setting of care impacts scope of practice.
7. Recognize micro- and macrosocial levels of advocacy.
8. Define the role of the registered nurse as patient advocate.

KEY TERMS

Board of Nursing
Nurse practice act
Nursing licensure
Nursing regulation
Professional Nursing Organization

Regulation of Nursing

From the end of the 19th century onward, nursing recognized the need for regulation of nursing practice. North Carolina became the first state, in 1903, to pass laws to regulate the practice of nurses by registering nurses and issuing licenses (Lambert & Lambert, 2005). **Nursing regulation** is government oversight of the practice of nursing in each of the 50 states and

U.S. territories. The regulatory process gives states the authority to determine qualifications needed for individuals to engage in nursing practice (Lambert & Lambert, 2005). State boards of nursing (BON) are the governmental agencies that determine the rules and processes by which a nurse (a) has a license in their state; (b) may practice in other states, both physically and electronically; and (c) may be subject to the state's practice law and regulation (Lambert & Lambert, 2005).

Initially, practice acts were written for a few healthcare professions. Currently, however, there may be as many as 30 practice acts within a state. Changes in technology and education as well as increasing complexity in healthcare have increased the need for regulation as well as changes in scope of practice.

Purpose and Elements of Regulation

The primary purpose of regulation in healthcare is to ensure protection of the public and assurance that regulated individuals are competent to provide certain services in a safe and effective manner (Schmitt, 2015). Regulation also:

- Provides a means to manage individuals who fail to comply with standards set forth by the profession.
- Is the authority of each state.
- Grants licenses that become the property right of the individual.
- Establishes standards that determine who can practice, what they must know, and what it takes to qualify for the licenses.
- Includes three mechanisms: registration, certification, and licensure (Schmitt, 2015).

Nursing regulation exists to protect the health, safety, and welfare of the public in their receipt of nursing services, and much more (National Council of State Boards of Nursing [NCSBN], n.d.). Box 4.1 summarizes the guiding principles for nursing regulation as identified by the NCSBN.

State Boards of Nursing

Through these guiding principles, the BON develop administrative rules or regulations to make the laws governing nursing practice more specific (Russell, 2012). Although specifics may vary, each practice act within a state includes the following elements:

- Definitions
- Authority, power, and composition of the BON
- Educational program standards
- Standards and scope of nursing practice
- Types of titles and licenses
- Protection of titles
- Requirements for licensure
- Grounds for disciplinary action, other violations, and possible remedies (Russell, 2012)

The BON rules define the responsibility of the registered nurse (RN) to supervise and oversee the practice of nursing when care is delivered by others (Russell, 2012). Membership of a BON generally consists of registered and licensed practical/vocational nurses, advanced practice nurses, and public representatives. However, membership varies by state and depends on state statutes.

The BON sets standards for prelicensure nursing education programs and clinical experience. Additionally, the BON establishes standards and scope of practice to direct and measure nursing practice. Each state has a **nurse practice act** (NPA) which is defined by the NCSBN

BOX 4.1 Guiding Principles of Nursing Regulation

Protection of the public

- Nursing regulation exists to protect the health, safety, and welfare of the public in their receipt of nursing services.
- Involvement of nurses in nursing regulation is critical to public protection.

Competence of all practitioners regulated by the board of nursing

- Nursing regulation is responsible for upholding licensure requirements for competence of the various levels of nursing practice.
- Competence is assessed at initial licensure/entry and during the career life of all practitioners.

Due process and ethical decision-making

- Nursing regulation ensures due process rights for practitioners.
- Boards of nursing hold practitioners accountable for conduct based on legal, ethical, and professional standards.

Shared accountability

- Nursing regulation requires shared accountability for enhancing safe patient care.

Strategic collaboration

- Nursing regulation requires collaboration with individuals and agencies in the interest of public protection, patient safety, and the education of nurses.

Evidence-based regulation

- Nursing regulation uses evidence-based standards of practice, advances in technology, and demographic and social research in its mission to protect the public.

Response to the marketplace and healthcare environment

- Nursing regulation requires timely and thoughtful responsiveness to the evolving marketplace.
- Scope of practice clarity and congruence with the community needs for nursing care are essential.

Globalization of nursing

- Nursing regulation occurs at the state level and concurrently works to standardize regulations and access to licensure.
- Nursing regulation requires fair and ethical practices and policies to address the social, political, and fiscal challenges of globalization.

Note. Adopted from 2007 National Council of State Boards of Nursing Delegate Assembly.
From National Council of State Boards of Nursing. (2007). *Guiding principles of nursing regulation*. https://www.ncsbn.org/3933.htm

as "All states and territories legislated a nurse practice act (NPA) which establishes a **board of nursing** (BON) with the authority to develop administrative rules or regulations to clarify or make the law more specific" (NCSBN n.d.). The standards defined in the nurse practice acts often include nursing assessment, collaboration with the healthcare team, patient-centered healthcare plans, decision-making, critical thinking, provision of care as ordered by authorized healthcare providers, evaluation of interventions, development of teaching plans, delegation of nursing care, and advocacy for the patient (Russell, 2012).

Levels of Regulation: Registration, Certification, Licensure

Registration is the simplest form of regulation and usually requires only name, address, and some relevant background information. Certification in a specific specialty area provides title protection and may require specified education, training, or experience (Schmitt, 2015). Licensure is the most restrictive regulatory process and applies to both RNs and licensed practical/vocational nurses (LP/VNs).

The use of the words certification and certificate can be confusing. Certification often involves a process in which individuals achieve and then demonstrate a level of knowledge and skill to perform their roles within the profession (Schmitt, 2015). In nursing, certification may be a voluntary or mandatory process and may depend on employer requirements for various roles. The certification itself is awarded by a third party such as the American Nurses Credentialing Center (ANCC) and allows the recipient to identify the certification with the initials BC (Board Certified) or C (Certified) after their licensure (eg, RN-C).

Certification involves a set of standards established by the professional group and typically has ongoing requirements to maintain the certification and use of a title after one's professional title (Schmitt, 2015). Examinations and recertification based on continuing education are processes to support certification.

On the other hand, a certificate program is generally a training program established by employers or educational institutions that is a course of study not dependent on previous experience or skill level (Schmitt, 2015). A certificate may be issued by an employer or a third party but generally does not rise to the same rigor as certification.

Licensure is the most rigorous level of regulation. Licensure in nursing is held by the RN, Advanced Practice RN (APRN), and Licensed Practical or Vocational Nurse (LPN/LVN). Examples of licensure and certification may be found in Table 4.1.

Scope of Practice

Scope of practice is integral to the role of nurses and nursing staff across the continuum of care. In order to practice safely, nurses must know and understand how scope of practice is determined and defined. In ambulatory practice settings, this knowledge and understanding is paramount owing to the added complexity of multiple clinical positions and roles. While scope of practice is derived from legal statutes, it is also informed by regulatory and professional groups as well as employers of nurses.

It is important to remember that the Board of Nursing for each state is responsible for establishing the scope or practice for RNs and APRNs, as well as LVN/LPNs. Changes in healthcare technology, workforce, practice settings, and demand are driving the need to reconsider scope of practice for many healthcare professions, nursing included.

Definition

The American Nurses Association (ANA) defines scope of practice as "the description of services that a qualified health professional is deemed competent to perform, and permitted to undertake, in keeping with the terms of their professional license" (American Nurses Association, n.d.). Licensing laws establish the scope of practice and include specific activities only licensees may perform (Schmitt, 2015). These licensing laws are referred to as practice acts. Although these laws are designed to protect the public, they also provide guidance for nursing practice (Russell, 2012). They become the basis for determining scope of

TABLE 4.1 NURSING EDUCATION AND CERTIFICATIONS

Registration or Designation	Education	Additional Qualifications	Designation[a]
RN	AD or ADN or BSN	Optional national certification in specialties such as: Palliative Care Case Management Ambulatory Care, Care Coordination and Transition Management	RN-C (certified) or RN-BC (board certified)
APRN	**Master's level:** MSN or MN or MS with nursing major. **Doctoral level:** DNP (RNs with a PhD are at the doctoral level but not licensed as an APRN).	National certification such as: FNP, CRNA, CNM	Specialty designation may be followed by C or BC Example: FNP-BC
LPN or LVN	Vocational or technical school with diploma or longer program with Associate Degree	Variety of specialty topics offering additional certificates or certification in areas such as wound care or long-term care	Designation by certifying body such as National Association of Practical Nurse Education and Service
UAP Examples: MA, Nursing Assistant, Home Healthcare Assistant	No specific national requirement; may have state-specific requirements	May obtain certification such as CMA, or CNA	

Note. AD or AND = Associate Degree Nurse; APRN = Advanced Practice RN; BSN = Bachelor of Science in Nursing; CMA = Certified Medical Assistant; CNA = Certified Nursing Assistant/Aide; CNM = Certified Nurse Midwife; CRNA = Certified Registered Nurse Anesthetist; DNP = Doctor of Nursing Practice; FNP = Family Nurse Practitioner; LPN = Licensed Practical Nurse; LVN = Licensed Vocational Nurse; MA = Medical Assistant; MN = Master of Nursing; MS = Master of Science; MSN = Master of Science in Nursing; PhD = Doctor of Philosophy degree; RN = registered nurse; UAP = Unlicensed Assistive Personnel.
[a]C or BC is applied to the credentials depending on the specific certifying organization.

practice. The ANA uses the "who," "what," "when," "where," "why," and "how" to illustrate nursing scope of practice:

- Who: RNs and Advanced Practice Registered Nurses (APRNs) comprise the "who" constituency and have been educated, titled, and maintain active licensure to practice nursing.
- What: Nursing is the protection, promotion, and optimization of health and abilities; prevention of illness and injury; facilitation of healing; alleviation of suffering through the diagnosis and treatment of human response; and advocacy in the care of individuals, families, groups, communities, and populations.
- Where: Wherever there is a patient in need of care.
- When: Whenever there is a need for nursing knowledge, compassion, and expertise.
- Why: The profession exists to achieve the most positive patient outcomes in keeping with nursing's social contract and obligation to society (American Nurses Association, n.d.).

A Federation of State Medical Boards (2005) report defined scope of practice as "the activities that an individual health care practitioner is permitted to perform within a specific profession. Those activities should be based on appropriate education, training, and experience.

Scope of practice is established by the practice act of the specific practitioner's board, and the rules adopted pursuant to that act" (Federation of State Medical Boards, 2005, p. 8). Thus, the nursing boards through the establishment of standards and rules establish the legal scope of practice for licensed nurses. Not all states require continuing education for relicensure, but all specify the educational requirements for nurses.

Registered Nurses

RN practice generally includes independent and dependent functions. RN scope of practice includes independent accountability for execution of nursing interventions, which may include assessment, goals of care, evaluation of care, development of a plan of care, and delegation (Russell, 2012). Dependent functions are the execution of orders for the provision of care as prescribed by authorized providers such as medical doctors (Russell, 2012). Rules for delegating care require the RN to organize, manage, and supervise the practice of nursing when delivered by others such as unlicensed healthcare workers.

The BONs also provide rules to assure safe care. Complaints may be initiated by an employer, a patient, or another healthcare worker. Through investigation, a board may determine a need to take formal action, including, but not limited to, suspension or revocation of the nursing license (Russell, 2012). **Nursing licensure** is defined by the NCSBN as "the process by which boards of nursing grant permission to an individual to engage in nursing practice after determining that the applicant has attained the competency necessary to perform a unique scope of practice" (NCSBN n.d.). Disciplinary cases may be in one or more of the following areas: practice, drugs, boundary violations, sexual misconduct, abuse, fraud, or positive criminal background check (Russell, 2012).

Questions about scope of practice for RNs emerge in a variety of ways. New technologies, new healthcare workers, changes in practice settings, and overlapping roles often serve as the basis for scope of practice issues. It is important for RNs to know their practice acts and how decisions are made to determine whether a given task or responsibility is within their scope.

Four major nursing organizations convened to develop a scope of practice decision tree developed by an expert panel (Ballard et al., 2016). The decision-making framework is applicable to licensed nurses in all practice settings in all roles, illustrated in Figure 4.1. Its purpose supports safety, accountability, communication with other healthcare professionals and employing organizations, and education of students and practicing nurses (Ballard et al., 2016).

Regardless of the role, nurses are accountable for their actions and adhering to both state, organizational, and professional standards of practice. The decision-making framework provides guidance to determine the scope of practice.

Advanced Practice Registered Nurses

APRNs generally include four groups: certified nurse practitioners (CNP), clinical nurse specialist (CNS), nurse anesthetists (CRNA), and certified nurse midwives (CNM). They are prepared at the master's or post master's education level. APRNs are also under the authority of the BON in each state, and all states regulate advanced practice nurses in some way (NCSBN, n.d.). Authority to practice may be through licensure, certification, registration, or similar means. Each of the four groups of APRNs has a unique history and context but shares the commonality of being APRNs.

While education, accreditation, and certification are necessary components of an overall approach to preparing an APRN for practice, the licensing boards, governed by state regulations and statutes, are the final arbiters of who is recognized to practice within a given state (Federation of State Medical Boards, 2005). Currently, there is no uniform model of regulation of APRNs across the states. Each state independently determines the APRN legal scope of practice, the roles that are recognized, the criteria for entry into advanced practice, and the certification examinations accepted for entry-level competence assessment. This has created

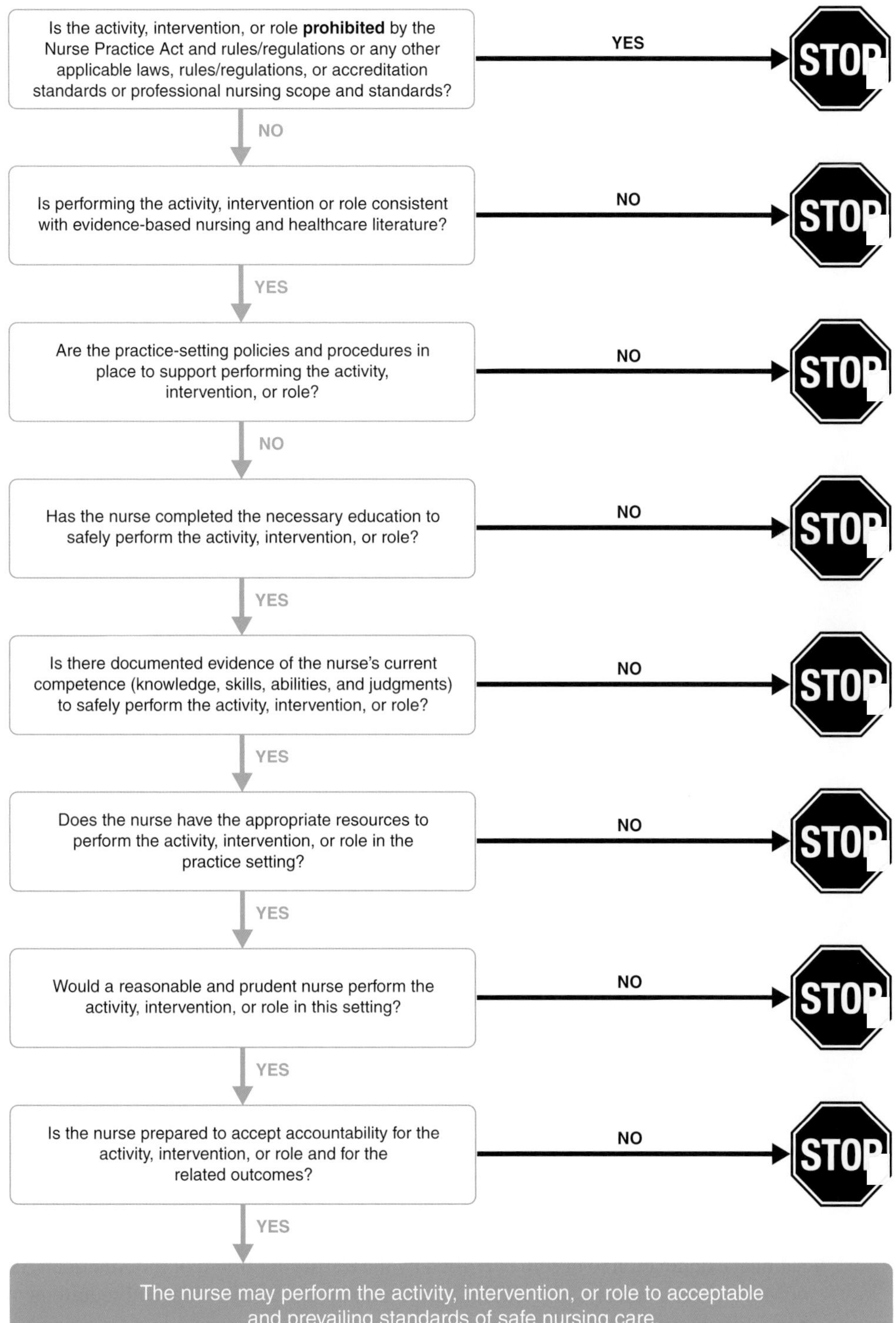

FIGURE 4.1 Scope of practice decision-making framework. (Ballard, K., Haagenson, D., Christiansen, L., Damgaard, G., Halstead, J. A., Jason, R. R., Joyner, J. C., O'Sullivan, A. M., Silvestre, J., Cahill, M., Radtke, B., & Alexander, M. [2016]. Scope of nursing practice decision-making framework. *Journal of Nursing Regulation*, 7[3], 19–21. https://doi.org/10.1016/S2155-8256(16)32316-X)

a challenge for APRNs to easily move from state to state and has decreased access to care for patients (NCSBN, 2008).

BON require certification by a national professional body to practice as an APRN and are thus subject to the standards for registered nursing as well as additional regulation. In addition to the RN scope of practice within the state, the APRN role generally includes:

1. Conducting an advanced assessment
2. Ordering and interpreting diagnostic procedures
3. Establishing primary and differential diagnoses
4. Prescribing, ordering, administering, dispensing, and furnishing therapeutic measures
5. Delegating and assigning therapeutic measures to assistive personnel (American Association of Nurse Practitioners, n.d.).

Frequently, Physician Assistants (PAs) are also part of the healthcare team and generally work at the same level as the APRN. They are collaborative members in healthcare delivery but have a different licensure process.

Licensed Practical/Vocational Nurses

LPN/LVNs are usually educated in technical or vocational programs that award a certificate or diploma but not a degree, although some programs may offer an associate degree with additional time. Programs vary in length from 12 to 18 months. LPN/LVNs provide basic or routine nursing services under the direction of an RN, Doctor of Medicine (MD), or an advanced practice provider. Most are employed in long-term care facilities or community and ambulatory care settings. Although LPN/LVNs usually function under the direction of an RN or MD, in long-term care facilities they may have greater administrative responsibility.

Similar to RNs, the type of care provided by LPN/LVNs is regulated by the state practice acts. These acts vary in regard to how LPN/LVNs contribute to assessment, care planning, delegation, and supervision. The practice acts regulate the way in which RNs direct LPN/LVN practice (National League of Nursing, 2014). However, most functions of the LPN/LVN are assistive in nature to the RN or based on delegated functions by the RN.

Unlicensed Assistive Personnel

There is increasing use of unlicensed assistive personnel (UAP) in healthcare. "The term 'unlicensed assistive personnel' refers to those health care workers who are not licensed to perform nursing tasks; it also refers to those health care workers who may be trained and certified, but are not licensed. Examples of UAPs include (but are not limited to) certified nursing assistants, home health aides, and patient care technicians" (Department of Consumer Affairs, n.d.). Tasks are generally assigned or delegated by an RN and include routine tasks and activities for patients who are stable and not acutely ill. Such tasks may include basic hygiene, bathing, feeding, ambulation, vital signs, and maintaining a safe environment.

The medical assistant (MA) is one type of UAP and may or may not be regulated by the state. One distinction between MAs and most other UAP is that the MA may also take a national examination to become certified by the Certifying Board of the American Association of Medical Assistants (AAMA). This certification is not a state or federal requirement but may be required by employers.

In some states, MAs, as well as other UAP, may function at the direction of the MD as well as the RN. Although a UAP may work at the direction of the physician or medical provider, they must adhere to state and employer policies/guidelines that define the provider's scope of practice. Their roles may be clinical as well as administrative and, depending on the clinical setting, they may support specialized procedures as well.

When working with a UAP, the RN must oversee, monitor, and delegate functions and tasks. The NCSBN defines delegation as "transferring to a competent individual the authority to perform a selected nursing task in a selected situation. Responsibility for the performance of an activity is transferred to the delegate while the delegator retains accountability for the outcome. The RN uses professional judgment to determine appropriate activities to delegate" (Academy of Medical-Surgical Nurses, 2012).

Healthcare shortages and increased demand for healthcare and nursing services will continue to require unlicensed staff, and the RN must be able to assess the risk and potential harm to patients when determining whether a task can be performed by a UAP. Tasks that require substantial knowledge or professional judgment are generally not delegated. Specific delegation rules are established by each state in the practice acts, but most states recognize aspects of the nursing process that should be performed only by RNs:

1. performance of a comprehensive assessment;
2. validation of the assessment data;
3. formulation of the nursing diagnosis for the individual;
4. identification of goals derived from nursing diagnosis;
5. determination of the nursing plan of care, including appropriate nursing interventions derived from the nursing diagnosis; and
6. evaluation of the effectiveness of the nursing care provided (Department of Consumer Affairs, n.d.).

Regardless of the practice setting, clear job descriptions and employer policies are necessary to ensure clarity about roles, supervision, and delegation. It is also incumbent on the RN or APRN to be familiar with the scope of practice requirements for their state.

Scope of Practice Considerations

Increasingly, care is delivered virtually, via the telephone, text, video, and electronic messaging. Sites of care are no longer the traditional clinic or office setting where patients are seen face to face with readily available equipment and technology. Nurses must navigate this increasingly complex environment in which scope of practice may be further blurred. Because scope of practice is state based, practicing "across state lines" by delivering care telephonically may require licensure in another state. The introduction of the Nurse Licensure Compact, which allows RNs to practice seamlessly between specified states, has helped to address this challenge. However, more information is needed to understand implications for scope of practice when care is delivered via video or other non-face-to-face methods.

Scope of practice is statutorily established by each state through nurse practice acts, and each state legislature has the authority to make changes in a particular scope. This often raises concerns from professions about "encroachment" or economic impact (Changes in Healthcare Professions Scope of Practice, 2012). An example of encroachment might include the ability of medical assistants to prepare and administer medications when allowed by the employer or state regulation. There are some who believe this encroaches on the role of the RN who has historically held the responsibility for medication administration. Owing to lower wages for the MA, employers might make decisions to hire MA staff rather than RNs, which may cause concerns about level of care as well as potentially impact the economic status of RNs.

In an ambulatory setting, scope of practice may also be a factor, because the RN is normally accountable for ensuring complete assessment, intervention, and evaluation of care. In settings with lower numbers of licensed nursing staff, safety and quality of care must be monitored.

Regulatory Agencies

In addition to the regulatory functions of the State BON discussed earlier, there are a number of other agencies that may impact nursing practice. Healthcare regulatory agencies monitor healthcare practitioners and facilities, provide information about industry changes, promote safety, and ensure legal compliance and quality services. These agencies at the federal, state, and local levels establish rules and regulations for the healthcare industry. The rules and regulations are mandatory, but some agencies such as those that accredit healthcare organizations/facilities may require voluntary participation. Nonetheless, participation is often needed to meet other requirements such as reimbursement (What Are Health Care Regulatory Agencies, 2017).

Role of the Federal Government

In addition to the state laws covered earlier, federal laws, other regulatory requirements, and government-sponsored programs such as Medicare and Medicaid also impact nursing practice. The Centers for Medicare and Medicaid Services (CMS) specify requirements for privacy, reimbursement, and security, among other areas that impact nursing practice. The CMS establishes conditions of participation and coverage that apply to any organization that provides care to those over 65 years, those under 65 years with disabilities, and those with end-stage renal disease (What Are Health Care Regulatory Agencies, 2017).

The health and safety standards are designed to protect the safety and improve quality for beneficiaries. The Drug Enforcement Agency enforces controlled substance laws and regulation in the United States. The Department of Health and Human Services Office for Civil Rights (OCR) is in charge of HIPAA enforcement, by auditing healthcare providers (Field, 2008). The Occupational Safety and Health Administration (OSHA) is an agency of the U.S. Department of Labor. Its role is to promote the safety and health of America's workforce, including healthcare workers, by setting and enforcing standards; providing training, outreach and education; establishing partnerships; and encouraging continual process improvement in workplace safety and health (What Are Health Care Regulatory Agencies, 2017).

Other Regulatory and Accrediting Bodies

Agencies at the state and federal levels, along with a host of private organizations, are involved in regulation of healthcare functions, facilities, personnel, and processes. Accrediting agencies such as The Joint Commission accredit hospitals and other healthcare-related functions such as laboratories. The National Commission for Quality Assurance is another example of an agency that ensures quality of managed care plans.

The agencies and regulations are designed to provide additional safety and standards for healthcare organizations and personnel. Nurses must be familiar with the rules and regulations of the agencies that are relevant in their employment settings. They should know and understand the nature of the regulations and impact on their day-to-day practice and overall scope of practice.

Professional Organizations

There are numerous nursing organizations that students and practicing nurses can join. They are focused on specialties, roles, practice settings, or nursing as a professional group. The important feature of many of these **professional nursing organizations** is the ability to provide education, professional development, and certification for their members. Those organizations that provide certification also establish standards of practice for nurses within the specialty area, which become a reference point for nurses in that practice setting. Professional standards determine and define the competent level of care as well as desirable levels of performance.

Specialty Organizations

Standards for care are critically important in nursing owing to increasing complexity, the variety of specialty areas of practice, and the growing need to ensure ongoing competence of nurses. Many standards are developed by specialty areas and serve the following functions:

- Outline what the profession expects of its members.
- Promote, guide, and direct professional nursing practice—important for self-assessment and evaluation of practice by employers, individuals, and other stakeholders.
- Provide nurses with a framework for developing competencies (Current Nursing, n.d.).

Standards set by professional organizations can be used to set clinical and educational expectations for practice within an organization. At the very least, they are one means of measuring performance, establishing expectations for care, and determining the qualifications needed for staff. The standards become relevant in determining scope of practice, education needed for specialty practice, and ongoing competency. There are multiple examples of organizations that establish standards of practice used by educational institutions and employers to ensure safe practice, many of which apply to specialty areas such as oncology, cardiology, or perioperative nursing.

Ambulatory Care Organizations

The American Academy of Ambulatory Nursing is one organization that provides extensive resources and a large network to practicing nurses, managers, and educators in ambulatory care. Additionally, the Case Management Society of Nursing provides resources for professional case managers across the continuum of care. There are a growing number of organizations focused on ambulatory care settings.

In addition to professional organizations focused on specialty areas, there are also organizations such as the ANA, which is a full-service organization. The purpose of the ANA is to advance the profession of nursing by setting standards of practice and to provide a code of ethics and leadership in policy initiatives (Lambert & Lambert, 2015). These ANA standards of practice serve as a foundation for practice for all RNs regardless of specialty or practice setting.

In addition to standards set by professional organizations, employers of nurses also establish standards of practice through policies, procedures, protocols, and guidelines for nursing staff. These processes are usually informed by expert nurses, such as CNSs, current evidence, community practice, and best practices. Along with job descriptions, they form an additional basis for defining scope of practice within the employment setting.

Many employers of nurses use employer-based credentialing processes to further define scope and standards of practice. These may include credentialing in IVs, wound care, chemotherapy, and other procedures or processes. The purpose is to ensure a consistent practice level and a method for evaluating practice. Internal credentialing also serves to reduce the likelihood of error and harm by ensuring clear expectations, especially for processes that bear higher risk, such as chemotherapy administration.

Shared Responsibility

In today's complex healthcare environment, most professions share some skills or procedures with other professions. Given the increasing number of roles within healthcare, it is not reasonable to expect that any given profession has a unique scope of practice that is exclusive (Changes in Healthcare Professions Scope of Practice, 2012). Care is delivered in teams in most settings. In ambulatory settings, there may be a higher percentage of unlicensed staff whose practice is not regulated. This requires employers, regulatory agencies, and individual professionals to be informed and educated about all roles within their practice environments.

As demand for healthcare services increases, demand for healthcare personnel also increases. In order to meet the needs of the population, healthcare workers must ensure that the various skills and knowledge possessed by any one professional group become part of the larger whole of care delivery. It is the combined efforts of the RN, APRN, PA, MD, social worker, and medical/nursing assistant, working in collaboration, that results in a better outcome for the patient. On the first page of his article, Wagner (2000) defines a patient care team as "a group of diverse clinicians who communicate with each other regularly about the care of a defined group of patients and participate in that care." Each of these clinicians brings a set of skills and a knowledge base that contribute to the care. Some of the clinicians will share some skills such as starting an IV or conducting an assessment, but it is the combination of these skills and knowledge that lends itself to the ability to provide a higher level of care.

The current healthcare environment is changing rapidly. Demand for healthcare services is increasing as the population ages. Many people have limited access to healthcare, and there are those that believe scope of practice can be a limiting factor in promoting access to care (Reforming Scope of Practice, 2010). Ongoing debates suggest scope of practice laws need to be regularly reviewed and reformed in order to keep pace with the changes in healthcare.

Advocacy

Advocacy is the foundation of nursing practice in care coordination roles and the key to success in meeting the goals of the Quadruple Aim and the National Quality Strategy (NQS). At the patient and family level, advocacy is best described as a process that involves a series of strategies and actions for preserving, representing, and safeguarding the best interests and values of individuals, families, and populations within the healthcare system. At this level, there is agreement that humanistic relationships between the nurse and the patient are the foundation for integrating advocacy into practice (Water et al., 2016).

The practice of advocacy has its theoretical roots in nursing ethics. The Code of Ethics for Nursing (American Nurses Association, 2015) delineates the role of advocacy in professional nursing practice at the individual, organizational, and system levels. This important document outlines the values, moral norms, and ideals that guide nurses and nursing organizations. The Code of Ethics clearly speaks to nursing's primary commitment to the patient, whether an individual, family, group, community, or population. The Code also speaks directly to the responsibility of the RN to respect the individual's right to determine what will be done with and to their own person, known as the right to self-determination.

All RNs are expected to embrace these ethical standards in every nursing action. To practice effectively, ambulatory nurses in care coordination and transitional care settings require an understanding of the meaning and importance of advocacy in professional nursing practice. Milliken and Grace (2017) describe ethical nursing care as those actions taken by nurses to address needs that are in accordance with the profession's goals and perspectives. Nurses should be aware of the areas of their practice that are central to ethical standards.

The early work of Bu and Jezewski (2007) describes three core attributes of nursing advocacy. These include ensuring patient autonomy and self-determination, acting on behalf of patients, and championing social justice in healthcare. Advocacy interventions are described by the context (level) of care in which they occur (Bu & Jezewski, 2007; Tahan, 2016). These levels are described as microsocial and macrosocial.

Advocacy at the *microsocial level* refers to nursing interventions directed toward individuals, families, or groups. *Macrosocial level advocacy* refers to advocacy directed toward a population, organization, or society in general (Tahan, 2016). Figure 4.2 depicts the levels of advocacy.

Microsocial-level Advocacy

Acting in the role of patient advocate at the microsocial level includes actions taken by ambulatory care nurses to ensure that the patient has a voice in all matters related to the provision of healthcare services. Ambulatory care nurses establish a plan of care that addresses the

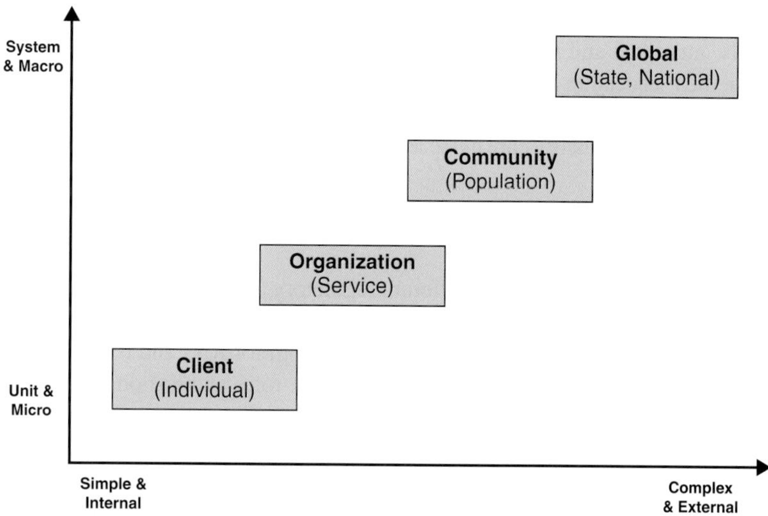

FIGURE 4.2 Types of advocacy. (NCSBN guiding principles: https://www.ncsbn.org/1325.htm)

patient's culture, value systems, spiritual beliefs, social support systems, gender and sexual orientation considerations, and language preferences.

As advocates, nurses are expected to recognize that self-determination is dependent on awareness of the decision and that it can be impacted by cognitive ability, literacy, language proficiency, educational level, visual or hearing impairment, anxiety, or fear. Therefore, information is provided accurately, completely, and in a manner that facilitates informed decision-making. At the individual level, the nurse practices ethical sensitivity by promoting; advocating for; and protecting the rights, health, and safety of individuals and families by respecting privacy and confidentiality (American Nurses Association, 2015).

Macrosocial-level Advocacy

At the macrosocial level, nurses understand the importance of acquiring and maintaining appropriate practice competencies to support professional practice, as well as participating in the development, implementation, review, and adherence to organizational and professional policies that promote patient health and safety, reduce errors and waste, and sustain a culture of safety. Also at the macrosocial level, nurses integrate social justice into nursing and health policy by collaborating with other health professionals and the public to protect human rights, promote health diplomacy, and reduce health disparities (American Nurses Association, 2015).

The call for nurses to engage in health policy leadership has been growing, not only within the ranks of the nursing profession, but also from governmental and healthcare organizational leaders. Involvement in policy decisions may be seen as an important aspect of patient advocacy and can ensure that the importance of activities by ambulatory care nurses is inherently reflected in public policy.

Nursing Advocacy

Nurse leaders, acting as advocates, are responsible for the quality of care and services in their organizations. These leaders are positioned to use their professional knowledge base to lead care coordination initiatives and oversee models of care that manage services longitudinally across the healthcare continuum, as well as vertically among a variety of complex care delivery systems. Ambulatory care nurse leaders act as advocates at both the microsocial and macrosocial levels when they respect the dignity, worth, and contributions of others, proactively anticipate and recognize the needs of others, and advocate for safe environments.

In their leadership roles, nurses promote safe and healthy workplace and professional practice environments (American Academy of Ambulatory Care Nursing, 2016). By recognizing their role as advocates, ambulatory care nurse leaders ultimately contribute to achieving the goals of the NQS.

Summary

This chapter has discussed the different regulatory and ethical forces that have an impact on professional nursing. Scope of practice laws, determined by individual states, are essential in determining the parameters of practice in nursing, both for RNs and for APRNs. An essential part of nursing practice also includes understanding the roles and responsibilities of all team members, especially LPNs and unlicensed personnel, who come under the responsibility of the RN.

Advocacy is part of ethical nursing care and may be initiated at different levels: individual, family, group, population, or societal. In applying these and other competencies, nurses must be accountable for knowing and understanding how laws, regulatory agencies, professional organization standards, and employer policies impact their optimal practice of nursing.

Case Study

The RN in a primary care clinic directs the MA to call a patient with the results of their laboratory tests for cholesterol, which are within normal range. The clinic has developed a set of routine instructions for these types of calls. However, the RN overhears the MA giving information to the individual about diet, exercise, and why they should be cautious about certain foods. These instructions are not part of the routine information.

1. Is the MA governed by scope of practice? If not, who develops the parameters for the MA's response?
2. At what point should the RN intervene? What would be an appropriate way for the RN to intervene without undermining another team member?
3. Following the call, what should the RN discuss with the MA regarding limitations on the information the MA can provide and appropriate referral?

Key Points for Review

- The purpose of regulating practice is to ensure the protection of the public and the competence of individuals to provide services in a safe and effective manner.
- Scope of practice is the activities that an individual healthcare practitioner is permitted to perform within a specific profession and is based on appropriate education, training, and experience.
- Regulatory agencies impact scope of practice and include State BON, CMS, The Joint Commission, and more.
- Standards of practice are defined by both professional organizations and the employer of nurses and are affected by the practice setting.
- Advocacy is an essential part of nursing responsibility and is applied both on the individual or family level (micro) and on the population or societal level (macro).

REFERENCES

Academy of Medical-Surgical Nurses. (2012). *Unlicensed assistive personnel*. https://www.amsn.org/practice-resources/position-statements/archive/unlicensed-assistive-personnel-uap

American Academy of Ambulatory Care Nursing. (2016). *Scope and standards of practice for registered nurses in care coordination and transition management* (1st ed.). Author.

American Association of Nurse Practitioners. (n.d.). *What's an NP?* https://www.aanp.org/all-about-nps/what-is-an-np#services

American Nurses Association. (2015). *Code of ethics for nurses with interpretative statements*. Nursebooks.org

American Nurses Association. (n.d.). *Scope of practice*. https://www.nursingworld.org/practice-policy/scope-of-practice/

Association of Perioperative Nurses. (n.d.). *Guidelines and clinical resources*. https://www.aorn.org/guidelines

Ballard, K., Haagenson, D., Christiansen, L., Damgaard, G., Halstead, J. A., Jason, R. R., Joyner, J. C., O'Sullivan, A. M., Silvestre, J., Cahill, M., Radtke, B., & Alexander, M. (2016). Scope of nursing practice decision-making framework. *Journal of Nursing Regulation, 7*(3), 19–21. https://doi.org/10.1016/S2155-8256(16)32316-X

Bu, X., & Jezewski, M. A. (2007). Developing a mid-range theory of patient advocacy through concept analysis. *J Adv Nurs., 57*(1), 101-10. doi: 10.1111/j.1365-2648.2006.04096.x. PMID: 17184379.

Changes in Healthcare Professions' Scope of Practice. (2012). *Legislative considerations*. https://www.ncsbn.org/cps/rde/xchg/SID-34C40F62-16D608C6/ncsbn/hs.xsl/4625.htm

Current Nursing. (n.d.). *Nursing management and nursing standards*. http://currentnursing.com/nursing_management/nursing_standards.html

Department of Consumer Affairs. (n.d.). *Unlicensed assistive personnel*. https://www.nationalnursesunited.org/sites/default/files/nnu/files/pdf/nursing-practice/advisories/uap.pdf

Federation of State Medical Boards. (2005). *Assessing scope of practice in health care delivery: Critical questions in assuring public access and safety*. http://www.fsmb.org/globalassets/advocacy/policies/assessing-scope-of-practice-in-health-care-delivery.pdf

Field, R. I. (2008). Why is health care regulation so complex? *Pharmacy and Therapeutics, 33*(10), 607–608. https://www.ncbi.nlm.nih.gov/pmc/articles/PMC2730786/

Lambert, V. A., & Lambert, C. E. (2005). Professionalism: The role of regulatory bodies and nursing organizations. In J. Daly, et al. (Ed.), *Professional nursing concepts, issues, and challenges*. Springer Publishing Co.

Milliken, A., & Grace, P. (2017). Nurse ethical awareness: Understanding the nature of everyday practice. *Nursing Ethics, 24*(5), 517–524. https://doi.org/10.1177/0969733015615172

National Council of State Boards of Nursing. (2008). *Consensus model for APRN regulation: Licensure, accreditation, certification & education*. https://www.ncsbn.org/aprn-consensus.htm

National Council of State Boards of Nursing. (2016). National guidelines for nursing delegation. *Journal of Nursing Regulation, 7*(1), 5–14. https://www.ncsbn.org/1625.htm

National Council of State Boards of Nursing. (n.d.). *Guiding principles of nursing regulation*. https://www.ncsbn.org/1325.htm

National League of Nursing. (2014). *Board of Governors on a vision for recognition of the role of licensed practical/vocational nurses in advancing the nation's health*. http://www.nln.org/docs/default-source/about/nln-vision-series-

Reforming Scope of Practice. (2010). https://www.ncsbn.org/739.htm

Russell, K. A. (2012). Nurse practice: Acts guide and govern nursing practice. *Journal of Nursing Regulation, 3*(3), 36–42. https://doi.org/10.1016/S2155-8256(15)30197-6

Schmitt, K. (2015). *Demystifying occupational and professional regulation*. Professional Testing Inc.

Tahan, H. M. (2016). Essentials of advocacy in case management: Part 1: Ethical underpinnings of advocacy-theories, principles, and concepts. *Professional Case Management, 21*(4), 163–179. https://doi.org/10.1097/NCM.0000000000000162

Wagner, E. (2000). The role of patient care teams in chronic disease management. *BMJ, 320*(7234), 569–572. https://doi.org/10.1136/bmj.320.7234.569

Water, T., Ford, K., Spence, D., & Rasmussen, S. (2016). Patient advocacy by nurses—Past, present and future. *Contemporary Nurse, 52*(6), 696–709. https://doi.org/10.1080/10376178.2016.1235981

What are health care regulatory agencies? (2017). *pocketsense.com*. https://pocketsense.com/what-are-health-care-regulatory-agencies-12196961.html

5

Measurement and Value

Rachel E. Start, Diane Brown, Harriet Udin Aronow, and Ann Marie Matlock

PERSPECTIVES

"As healthcare reform and reimbursement models are reshaping care delivery, the demand for ambulatory care nurses will be growing in exponential rates. Nurses providing care for primary and complex chronic diseases are needed to develop and innovate care models that provide access to healthcare, preventative health services, management of costly diseases, and to define and improve quality outcomes. Ambulatory nurses can support the healthcare delivery system by creating value through quality and costs in care."

Nancy May, DNP, RN-BC, NEA-BC, Chief Nursing Officer for Ambulatory Care and the University of Michigan Medical Group, University of Michigan Health System

LEARNING OBJECTIVES

Upon completion of this chapter, the reader will be able to:

1. Describe the history of evaluating quality in healthcare and nursing.
2. Discuss the Centers for Medicare and Medicaid Services' (CMS) leadership and the importance of value and measures of excellence in today's healthcare landscape related to ambulatory care nursing.
3. Discuss quality measurement in healthcare, including individual satisfaction.
4. Understand nursing measurement and benchmarking in ambulatory care.
5. Define measuring structure, process, and outcomes of current and emerging ambulatory care nursing models and roles.

KEY TERMS

Endorsed measures
Individual satisfaction
Nurse-sensitive indicators (NSIs)
Quality measurement

Introduction

Nursing has a long tradition of earning the public's trust (Gallup Organization, 2017). With that trust comes the professional obligation to understand the performance of the healthcare delivery systems where nurses practice to ensure quality and value for the public. Without meaningful measurement, value cannot be assessed, improved, or utilized as a tool to create useful care delivery. Measuring value can be challenging. Porter (2010) has defined the value equation as quality divided by cost. Ownership of the value equation is a mandate that engages nurses in the examination of clinical practice and performance outcomes, as well as cost and the potential for revision of payment structures to improve affordability (Porter-O'Grady & Malloch, 2006). Meaningful measurement of nurses' contributions to transformative healthcare change as a catalyst for improved value is a mandate that cannot be ignored in this dynamic industry.

Pursuit of value in healthcare in the United States is the solution to some of the most complex challenges facing the populations that most need care continuity and health promotion (Schneider et al., 2016). The United States spends far more on healthcare than other countries, only to have poor access to primary care, inadequate prevention and management of chronic disease, delayed diagnoses, incomplete adherence to treatments, wasteful overuse of drugs and technology, higher infant mortality, and lower healthy life expectancy (Schneider et al., 2017). Perhaps most sobering is the lack of equitable healthcare delivery where financial barriers create poor performance for lower income individuals (Berwick et al., 2008; Schneider et al., 2016).

Three national strategies, described as the Triple Aim, were developed to address the need for improved value: improvement of the individual experience of care, improvement in the health of populations, and reduction of the per capita costs of care for populations (Berwick et al., 2008). This Triple Aim was later broadened into the Quadruple Aim with an added element of improvement to the life of clinicians and staff (Bodenheimer & Sinsky, 2014). These strategies were followed by authoritative policies found in the Patient Protection and Affordable Care Act (PPACA, 2010) and in reports by the Institute of Medicine (IOM, 2001, 2010, 2015) supporting quality, as well as the engagement and leadership of nurses at all points in the care continuum.

Nursing has been called on throughout these strategies to lead the transformation of healthcare (IOM, 2010; Macy, 2016). Specifically, "the nursing professional has the potential to affect wide-reaching changes in the healthcare system ... to lead in the improvement and redesign of its many practice environments ... to bridge the gap between coverage and access ... to coordinate increasingly complex care for a wide range of patients and to fulfill their potential as primary care providers to the full extent of their education and training and to enable the full economic value of their contributions across practice settings to be realized" (pp. 2–4) (IOM, 2010).

With the pursuit of high-value healthcare, there has been a shift in the locations in which individuals receive care (AHA, 2015; Paschke et al., 2017; Roski & Gregory, 2001; Start et al., 2016). Ambulatory care has become the focus of policy related to healthcare transformation, seen for its potential for increased prevention, important care coordination as well as decreased cost. As a result, ambulatory registered nurses (RNs) are uniquely positioned to assume expanded roles in the design and delivery of high-quality affordable care (Bodenheimer et al., 2015; Paschke et al., 2017; Roski & Gregory, 2001; Start et al., 2018; Swan et al., 2006).

Measurement of nurse-sensitive contributions to the value equation in the ambulatory setting has been a strategy pursued by ambulatory care nurses in recent years (Brown & Aronow, 2017; Martinez et al., 2015; Matlock et al., 2016; Start et al., 2016, 2018). Ambulatory nursing practice has not always been professionally socialized, structurally empowered, supported to be autonomous, or involved in leadership of interprofessional processes (Start et al., 2016). Quantifying the value of the role of the ambulatory RN empowers nurses to be better equipped to meet the growing healthcare needs in this setting, supporting growth as an autonomous, leadership-based specialty (American Academy of Ambulatory Care Nursing [AAACN], 2017; Paschke et al., 2017; Start et al., 2016).

This chapter will educate the reader on healthcare industry trends related to measurement and value in the ambulatory setting, highlighting **nurse-sensitive indicator (NSI)** development, measurement, and benchmarking opportunities.

History of Evaluating Quality in Healthcare and Nursing

One of our first nursing leaders, Florence Nightingale, famously initiated nursing's scientific ownership of data to impact public policy through her work during the Crimean War (Montalvo, 2007). She conducted studies of hospital and public health reports, making her own statistical analyses (Calabria & Macrae, 1994; Dossey et al., 2005; Montalvo, 2007; Nightingale, 1860). Avedis Donabedian introduced the medical community to a framework to evaluate healthcare using a foundational conceptual model that segments quality into structure, process, and outcomes of care (Donabedian, 1966). He described the outcomes of care as the most obvious measures of quality, while stating that it may be necessary to measure the process or the structure behind any given outcome in order to impact overall quality. This seminal work has shaped quality assessment and measurement across healthcare disciplines with measures delineated into structure, process, and outcome categories.

Nurse-Sensitive Indicators

In the 1970s, the American Nurses Association (ANA) began nursing practice **quality measurement** utilizing the Quality Assurance Model (Rantz, 1995) and the Donabedian framework (1988). **Nurse-sensitive indicators (NSIs)** continue to be delineated as measures that relate to the structure, processes, or outcomes of care delivery (Montalvo, 2007). By the 1990s, there was a national nursing movement to evaluate staffing and its linkage with quality and patient outcomes (Montalvo, 2007). The ANA funded six pilot studies to develop NSIs in the inpatient setting (Brown & Wolosin, 2013; Brown et al., 2010; Montalvo, 2007; Start et al., 2016).

The Collaborative Alliance for Nursing Outcomes (CALNOC) and the National Database of Nursing Quality Indicators (NDNQI) emerged as the two prominent acute care NSI databases for benchmarking nursing care quality. An initial set of 15 NSI standardized evidence-based measures for acute care were endorsed by the National Quality Forum (NQF) in 2004 (NQF, 2004). Using these measures, researchers began the journey to quantify the extent to which nurses contribute to individual safety, quality, and the professional work environment. The literature from this work is extensive, and these measures are now the gold standard for communicating the value of nursing care in the inpatient setting (Aiken et al., 2003; Buerhaus et al., 2006; Needleman et al., 2006). This early work allowed for the development of care models, revision of staffing models to support high-quality care, and the promotion of a value argument for inpatient nurses to support their contributions (Aiken et al., 2003; Curtin, 2003).

Magnet Recognition Program

The latter part of the 20th century saw the beginning of the American Nurses Credentialing Center (ANCC) Magnet Recognition Program. In 1983, the American Academy of Nursing Task Force on Nursing Practice in Hospitals conducted a study to identify work environments that attracted and retained well-qualified nurses while also obtaining excellent outcomes (ANCC, n.d.). Forty-one of those 163 (25%) institutions were able to attract and retain well-qualified nurses in the midst of a national nursing shortage. Those institutions, mostly representing inpatient nursing care, had common themes of structure, process, or outcome that are now called the "forces of magnetism" (ANCC, 2013).

As of 2011, about 7% of registered hospitals had achieved Magnet Recognition and are known for excellence in outcomes relative to nursing staff satisfaction, patient care quality, and excellent interprofessional collaboration (ANCC, n.d.). Throughout this time, organizations pursuing Magnet Recognition have had to demonstrate NSIs that outperformed national benchmarks along with compliance with other program-specific requirements, which supported widespread advancement and empowerment of autonomous practice in any organization pursuing Magnet Recognition.

Guidelines From Organizations

In 2001, the IOM published a landmark report highlighting the impact of medical errors in hospitals and the need for a culture of safety. In 2006, the NQF introduced physician-focused ambulatory care measures and the Physicians Quality Reporting System (PQRS) for the Centers for Medicare and Medicaid Services (CMS) (NQF, 2006; Swan, 2008). In 2008, NQF released a broad set of ambulatory measures focusing primarily on the provider's performance (Swan, 2008). This came on the heels of the National Committee on Quality Assurance (NCQA), a private healthcare quality organization, releasing Healthcare Effectiveness Data and Information Set (HEDIS) measures for primarily ambulatory settings in the 1990s (Roski & Gregory, 2001).

HEDIS measures provide standardized information on the quality of care provided by managed care organizations (MCOs) primarily in ambulatory environments. They are related to measurement of the effectiveness of care, access and availability of care, utilization of services, and satisfaction with the experience of care (Roski & Gregory, 2001). Most recently, the multiple organizations have initiated specialty certification programs for patient-centered medical homes (PCMH), a team-based model of care delivery with an emphasis on improved value, efficiency, and care coordination (AHRQ, n.d.; NCQA, n.d.-a). Table 5.1 summarizes the important national measure creation entities, measurement drivers, and measurement databases driving practice in the ambulatory care arena.

The IOM report on the *Future of Nursing: Leading Change, Advancing Health* (2010) challenged nurses to lead healthcare reform and transformation. This report issued mandates for nurses to practice to the full extent of their education and training, achieve higher levels of education and training, be full partners in redesigning healthcare, and perform effective workforce planning that relies on better data collection and improved information infrastructure to achieve key elements of much needed transformation in healthcare. The AAACN took the lead in responding to this call for ambulatory nursing. A series of supportive documents were produced that would advance the ambulatory nurse to top-of-scope in role, education, leadership, and research, as well as track the value contribution through the development of NSIs specific to ambulatory nursing (AAACN, 2011a, 2011b, 2016, 2017; Paschke et al., 2017; Start et al., 2016).

AAACN and other professional organizations began to formally propose measurement of NSIs in the ambulatory setting (ANCC, 2013; Lewis, 2014; Start et al., 2016). The ANA convened an ambulatory summit where multiple organizations provided input on ideas for ambulatory nurse-sensitive measurement topics (Lewis, 2014; Start et al., 2016). NDNQI published early measures for ambulatory measurement relative to pending diagnostic tests and medication reconciliation (Start et al., 2016), whereas CALNOC published measures for the ambulatory surgery arena that were coupled with important volume, staffing, and stratification structures to aid in meaningful benchmarking (Brown & Aronow, 2017; Start et al., 2016). Additionally, much of the literature emerging during this push for measurement discussed the role of the nurse in care coordination and the strategic position that the ambulatory nurse had for improved coordination along the continuum (AAACN, 2016; Haas & Swan, 2014; Lamb, 2014). Other national organizations were issuing documents on the importance of care coordination with many of the required

TABLE 5.1 **NATIONAL MEASURE CREATION ENTITIES, DRIVERS, AND DATABASES**

	NQF	CMS Macra 2018 Measures	AHRQ	HEDIS	PCORI PROMIS Measures	CEDR/ACEP	ASC-Q
About	NQF is a not-for-profit, nonpartisan membership-based organization that works to catalyze improvements in healthcare.	Medicare Access and CHIP Reauthorization Act (2015). Quality payment program. Streamlines quality programs under MIPS and gives bonus payments for participation in APMs.	Federal agency. 1 of 12 agencies within the Department of Health and Human Services that support the quality of health in America.	HEDIS. Developed by the NCQA to measure health plan performance. NQF endorsed measures.	PCORI funds development of PROMIS about physical, mental, and social health.	The ACEP CEDR. Reports healthcare quality and outcomes specific to emergency medicine.	Formed in 2006 to focus on healthcare quality and safety.
Work	Consensus-based organization. Endorsement process takes measures from organizations throughout the country for others to use.	Quality measures for processes, outcomes, and patient care experiences. Organizations submit at least six measures (one must be outcome related).	Develops tools to improve the healthcare system and help Americans, healthcare professionals, and policy makers make informed health decisions	A tool used by more than 90% of America's health plans to measure performance on dimensions of care and service.	Largest public research funder focusing primarily on clinical effectiveness research.	First Emergency Medicine specialty-wide registry at the national level, designed to measure and report healthcare quality and outcomes.	Measure development, public reporting of quality data, advancing ASC quality and advocacy.
Impact	Approx. 300 NQF endorsed measures used in federal public reporting and pay for performance programs as well as private and state programs.	With a focus on Value = Quality/Cost, rather than volume, CMS hopes to hold partners accountable to transforming healthcare quality while decreasing cost.	Conducts and supports health services research, both within AHRQ and in academic institutions, hospitals, physicians' offices, healthcare system.	Comprise a majority of the ambulatory quality improvement measures.	PCORI is an independent, nonprofit, nongovernmental organization authorized by Congress in 2010.	Collects and provides data on patients from all payers, including CMS, as well as benchmarks from national and regional cohorts.	

Link to NSI	AAACN/CALNOC utilize NQF as the gold standard to align with national quality priorities	https://qpp.cms.gov/mips/quality-measures	Multiple tools are available on the AHRQ website to assist with practice and quality.	AAACN/CALNOC reflected on HEDIS measures to guide care coordination, telehealth, population health NSI measurement	AAACN/CALNOC reflected on PROMIS measures to guide development of NSIs that would be inclusive of a patient-centered focus.	CALNOC ambulatory measures reflect similar quality and when aligned with staffing and nurse demographics provide quality insights.	AAACN/CALNOC adopted measures endorsed by NQF and created by ASC-QC as its first set of quality outcomes for nurses in ambulatory.
Other	NQF published reports on care coordination and telehealth measures	Also for ACOs and PCMHs		HEDIS measures used in NCQA certification and PCMH accreditation program		Approved as a CMS qualified clinical data registry to meet CMS requirements.	
Website	qualityforum.org	https://cms.gov/Medicare/Quality-Initiatives-Patient-Assessment-Instruments/Value-Based-Programs/MACRA-MIPS-and-APMs/MACRA-MIPS-and-APMs.html	ahrq.gov	http://ncqa.org/hedis-quality-measurement	https://pcori.org http://healthmeasures.net/explore-measurement-systems/promis/intro-to-promis	Acep.org https://acep.org/administration/quality/cedr/cedr-home/#sm.001epl3ll1cxpflwsqu12euxf16ov	http://ascquality.org

Note. AAACN = American Academy of Ambulatory Care Nursing; ACEP = American College of Emergency Physicians; ACO, Accountable Care Organizations; AHRQ = Agency for Healthcare Research and Quality; APM = alternative payment model; ASC-Q = Ambulatory Surgical Quality Collaboration; CALNOC = Collaborative Alliance for Nursing Outcomes; CEDR = Clinical Emergency Data Registry; CHIP = Children's Health Insurance Program; CMS = Centers for Medicare and Medicaid Services; HEDIS = Healthcare Effectiveness Data and Information Set; MIPS = Merit-based Incentive Payment System; NCQA = National Committee for Quality Assurance; NQF = National Quality Forum; PCORI = Patient-Centered Outcomes Research Institute; PCMH, Patient-Centered Medical Home; PROMIS = Patient Reported Outcomes Measures. Start, R., Brown, D., Matlock, A. M., Soban, L., and Aronow, H. (2019).

activities in line with nursing strengths (AHRQ, 2014; CMS, 2014, 2015, 2018a, 2018i; Craig et al., 2011; Macy, 2016; NQF, 2014a, 2014b, 2017; NTOCC, 2008).

Accreditation and Certification

Accreditation and certification emerged in the latter part of the 20th century as important tools for both consumers and payers to identify organizations that met minimum thresholds for industry standards and to receive payment from CMS. Accreditation is earned by an entire healthcare organization such as a hospital, nursing home, or ambulatory organization (The Joint Commission [TJC], 2018), whereas certification is earned by programs or services within an organization, for example, an organization's diabetes program or heart disease program.

TJC is one body that both accredits organizations and certifies programs. Healthcare organizations must be in compliance with health and safety requirements in federal regulations in order to receive federal payment from Medicare or Medicaid programs (TJC, 2018). This compliance is assessed and documented through certification and/or accreditation by CMS-approved national accrediting organizations. For example, TJC accredits ambulatory surgical centers, clinical laboratories, critical access hospitals, home health agencies, hospice agencies, hospitals, and psychiatric hospitals. TJC also certifies programs that relate to cardiac care, disease-specific care, staffing, integration, palliative care, perinatal care, and primary care medical homes (TJC, 2018).

CMS provides a full list of organizations that it supports as accreditation bodies (CMS, 2018b). One of those organizations, the National Committee for Quality Assurance (NCQA), accredits health plans, case management programs, wellness and health promotion plans, accountable care organizations (ACOs), and managed behavioral healthcare organizations (NCQA, n.d.-b). NCQA also certifies different programs within those organizations that meet standards for specific populations or programs.

Multiple agencies may offer the same accreditation or certification services. For example, PCMH certification is offered by NCQA, the Utilization Management Accreditation Commission (URAC), TJC, and the Accreditation Association for Ambulatory HealthCare (AAAHC). PCMH accreditation or certification is tied to increased reimbursement from health plans as it demonstrates the organization's willingness to improve quality and affordability (Medical Economics, 2015).

Centers for Medicare and Medicaid Services Leadership of Measurement and Value

There are multiple drivers to measure healthcare improvement in the United States. Key healthcare stakeholders include the recipients of healthcare, providers and care teams, and insurers. Each stakeholder is vested in achieving the Triple Aim in different ways—improving the care experience, improving the health of populations, and reducing the cost of healthcare (Berwick et al., 2008; Institute for Healthcare Improvement [IHI], 2018a).

Improving quality and affordability in the healthcare system is a critical strategic priority in the United States. Healthcare spending reached $3.3 trillion, or $10,348 per person, in 2016, representing almost 18% of the gross domestic product (GDP) (CMS, National Health Expenditures 2016 Highlights, 2018i). Hospital services and physician/clinical services reflected the highest proportion of costs, while CMS was the largest single payer source. National healthcare spending projections are staggering. Between 2017 and 2026, costs are expected to reach $5.7 trillion, growing 1% faster per year than GDP to 19.7% by 2026 (CMS, National Health Expenditure Projections 2017–2026, 2018j). This growth is driven by increased prices for goods and services but also by enrollment shifts from private health insurance to Medicare related to the aging of the population, as depicted in Figure 5.1 A and B.

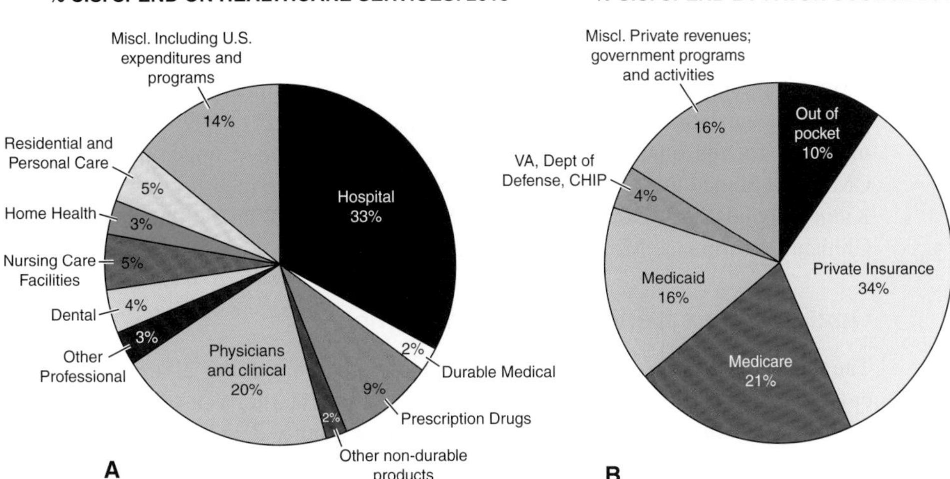

FIGURE 5.1 **A.** Percent U.S. spend on healthcare services 2016. **B.** Percent U.S. spend by payer source. (Created by D. Brown and adapted from Centers for Medicare and Medicaid Services. [2018]. *National health expenditures 2016 highlights*. https://www.cms.gov/Research-Statistics-Data-and-Systems/Statistics-Trends-and-Reports/NationalHealthExpendData/Downloads/highlights.pdf)

CMS Funding

It is important for nurses to understand healthcare funding, because reimbursement models for the healthcare organizations that employ nurses and provide care are increasingly tied to specific healthcare funding sources and the populations that organizations serve. CMS, a division of the U.S. Department of Health and Human Services, administers healthcare insurance for two major programs, Medicare and Medicaid, each supporting distinct populations.

In 1965, President Johnson signed into law the bill that led to the creation of the CMS, which has evolved over the years with additional benefits and eligibility (CMS, CMS' Program History, 2018c). Medicaid is health insurance funded by the federal government in partnership with states for families experiencing low income, pregnant women, people of all ages with disabilities, and people who need long-term care. States are not obligated to participate in Medicaid. Each state tailors its Medicaid program with respect to eligibility standards and the specific services provided. As a result, there is a wide variation in the Medicaid program from state to state.

Medicare is a federal government entitlement program—most citizens earn the right to enroll by working and paying taxes (eHealth, Medicare, 2018a). Coverage is provided for citizens aged 65 and older, those under 65 receiving Social Security Disability Insurance, or those with severe progressive disease such as end-stage renal disease (ESRD). Medicare can be confusing for nurses and consumers because there are four different parts to the program. Parts A and B are often referred to as *Original Medicare*. Part A covers inpatient hospital care, some skilled nursing care facility, limited home healthcare services, and hospice care. Part B benefits cover nonhospital medical expenses like doctors' office visits, blood tests, X-rays, diabetic screenings and supplies, and outpatient hospital care. Medicare Part C, or *Medicare Advantage*, is offered by private insurance companies to provide a benefits package as an alternative to Original Medicare through CMS contracts. Medicare Advantage plans may cover additional benefits like eye exams, hearing aids, dental care, or drug plans. Part D is optional prescription drug coverage, available as a stand-alone drug plan through private insurance companies. "Dual-eligibles" are individuals with both Medicare and Medicaid.

Over the years, additional legislation has been passed to further improve our national healthcare system. For example, in 1997, the Children's Health Insurance Program (CHIP) was created to give health insurance and preventive care to uninsured American children (CMS, CMS' Program History, 2018c). All 50 states and the District of Columbia have CHIP plans that cover many children who are victims of the working poor disparities—uninsured families earning more than Medicaid eligibility requirements. Healthcare quality became apparent as a priority in legislation. For example, the Balanced Budget Act of 1997 required CMS to develop measures for the quality of renal dialysis services provided under the Medicare program. CMS then funded the development of clinical performance measures on the basis of National Kidney Foundation's Dialysis Outcome Quality Initiative Clinical Practice Guidelines (CMS, Clinical Performance Measure Project, 2018a).

Quality Transparency for the Consumer

The consumer's perspective of quality gained momentum in the 21st century, leveraging the emerging availability of the World Wide Web and the Internet as a vehicle for transparency in healthcare quality assessment. Public reporting of quality data began and continued to grow exponentially in the decades that followed. In order to assist consumers, CMS developed a Star Rating process to summarize public information to make it easier to review using a Star Rating (one star to represent poor care and five stars to represent excellent care) (eHealth, Star Ratings, 2018b).

In 2002, CMS began a national Nursing Home Quality Initiative (NHQI) (CMS, Nursing Home Compare, 2018k). Quality measures from resident assessment data that nursing homes routinely collected were converted to quality measures to give consumers information on how well nursing homes were caring for their residents' physical and clinical needs and preferences and life care wishes. The site now allows comparison of more than 15,000 nursing homes around the country certified by Medicare and Medicaid (www.medicare.gov/nursinghomecompare).

Also in 2002, Hospital Compare was created by Medicare and the Hospital Quality Alliance, a public–private collaboration to promote quality reporting (CMS, Hospital Compare, 2018f). The intention was to make it easier to inform consumers for hospital healthcare decision-making. This began in 2005 with the first set of 10 core process of care measures focused on heart attack, heart failure, pneumonia, and surgical care. The site has continued to grow, making quality transparent to consumers seeking hospital care (www.medicare.gov/hospitalcompare).

Beginning in 2003, CMS began posting home health data, a subset of OASIS (Outcome and Assessment Information Set)-based quality performance information, on Home Health Compare (CMS, Home Health Compare, 2018e). These publicly reported measures include outcome measures that indicate how well home health agencies assist their patients in regaining or maintaining their function and process measures to evaluate the home health agency use of evidence-based processes of care (www.medicare.gov/homehealthcompare).

Experimenting with different ways to incentivize quality, CMS initiated a Physician Quality Reporting System (PQRS) in 2006 to provide financial incentives to voluntarily report healthcare quality data—pay for performance (CMS, PQRS, 2018n). The Tax Relief and HealthCare Act (TRHCA) included a provision for a 1.5% incentive payment to eligible providers who successfully submitted quality data to CMS. By 2015, CMS identified 254 quality measures to choose from, but by 2016 PQRS was sunset and transitioned to the Merit-based Incentive Payment System (MIPS) under the Quality Payment Program.

Innovative Models

The PPACA intended to make affordable health insurance available to more people, to expand Medicaid income criteria to those below 138% of the federal poverty level, and to lower costs of healthcare by supporting innovative delivery methods. Since then, healthcare reform has seen a flurry of approaches to achieve the Triple Aim of improving the care experience, health, and affordability. As the largest single payer for healthcare services, CMS became a major driver for healthcare reform and transformation of the nation's healthcare system. In addition to those described, numerous other organizations have a role in national healthcare quality. These organizations have in many instances worked in tandem with the Triple Aim, CMS, PPACA, and other national initiatives to further advance the quality and efficiency of healthcare. Table 5.1 gives a synopsis of these organizations and the measures adopted.

Center for Medicare and Medicaid Innovation

Medicare has taken the lead in testing care models with financial incentives for providers to collaborate in lowering costs and improving care (CMS, CMS Innovation Center, 2018m; Kaiser Family Foundation, 2018). The Center for Medicare and Medicaid Innovation (CMMI) was established by the PPACA, which authorized an appropriation of $10 billion for CMMI through 2019 (and for each subsequent decade) to test innovative payment and delivery models across Medicare, Medicaid, and CHIP. Three such Medicare payment models are as follows:

1. Accountable Care Organizations (ACOs): Groups of healthcare providers (doctors, hospitals, and other providers) form partnerships to share accountability for quality and cost and receive financial incentives for lowering cost and improving quality.
2. Medical Home Models: Team-based primary care practices that coordinate the majority of their individuals' care, for monthly care management fees, to improve quality and streamline care delivery. Different models are the Federally Qualified Health Center (FQHC), Advanced Primary Care Practice (APCP), Multi-Payer Advanced Primary Care Practice (MAPCP), Comprehensive Primary Care (CPC) Initiative, Independence at Home, and Comprehensive Primary Care Plus (CPC+).
3. Bundled Payment Models: For a given episode of care, a total Medicare budget is established for all services provided. Providers assume the risk of sharing savings below the budget or incur losses that exceed the budget.

Medicare Access and CHIP Reauthorization Act

The Medicare Access and CHIP Reauthorization Act of 2015 (MACRA) is another example of legislation to improve quality incentives in the ambulatory environment and transform healthcare delivery models (CMS, MACRA, 2018g). This Quality Payment Program changed the way clinicians were rewarded, shifting from volume-based to value-based practices. It also streamlined multiple quality programs under MIPS in addition to bonus payments for participation in eligible alternative payment models (APMs).

Meaningful Measures

In an effort to organize all of these quality improvement (QI) measurement models, CMS, in 2017, announced a Meaningful Measures framework (CMS, Meaningful Measures, 2018h). This framework intends to prioritize quality measurement and improvement by assessing core issues most critical to high-quality care and improving outcomes. Quality measures are defined as tools to quantify healthcare processes, outcomes, patient perceptions, and organizational structures or systems associated with high-quality healthcare and relate to one or more quality goals, including effective, safe, efficient, individual-centered, equitable, and timely care.

Using a collaborative approach with stakeholders, the framework was developed drawing on prior work of the NQF and the National Academies of Medicine (NAM), and it includes the perspective of individuals, clinicians, and providers. The framework contains 19 areas, organized into specific, overarching quality priorities. The goals of the initiative are as follows:

- Promote alignment across quality initiatives and programs to minimize provider burden.
- Promote focused measure development toward meaningful outcomes.
- Identify quality issues that are the highest priority in improving health and healthcare.
- Communicate how CMS programs and measures improve individuals' health and meet the needs of those individuals.

Individual Satisfaction Measurement

Individual satisfaction is often used as a metric for determining the quality of care in a healthcare setting (Al-Abri & Al-Balushi, 2014; Rama & Kanagaluru, 2011; Tonio et al., 2011). It has been used in the inpatient setting for the past two decades through the use of valid and reliable tools. These data can be benchmarked and used to make financial decisions both in performance metrics for leaders and in reimbursement for services. In many instances, the data are available for healthcare consumers to use for decision-making about where to go for care and treatment. As part of the recommended performance measures for ambulatory care, the National Academy of Science in 2006 recommended ambulatory care surveys to evaluate aspects of patient satisfaction, including receiving appropriate care and communication of healthcare providers and office staff (IOM, 2006).

Surveys

The Agency for Healthcare Research and Quality (AHRQ) and CMS have numerous data sources for surveys administered to individuals asking about their experiences with ambulatory care providers, including physicians' offices, and health plans (CMS, 2018d). In 1997, the AHRQ released the Consumer Assessment of Health Plan Survey (CAHPS) to assess care received by individuals. The use of this survey tool is required by many health plans for accreditation. The CAHPS survey domains include communication, coordination of care, and customer service. The majority of CAHPS data collection is done using the mail system. Newer methodologies have been attempted via web surveys, but this method did not improve response rates (Tesler & Sorra, 2017).

A variety of CAHPS surveys focus on different aspects of care, including clinician and groups, ACOs, outpatient and ambulatory, and home health. Other tools focus on individual disease processes such as the patient satisfaction survey for HIV care in ambulatory (IHI, 2018b) or behavioral healthcare (IOM, 2006). The CAHPS survey tools do not include questions directly regarding the role of the RN. Specific areas address office staff and how well providers communicate. Organizations may choose to add additional questions to the surveys specific to their services or populations served, which provides an opportunity to insert questions related to nursing practice. If standardized questions are available, benchmarking performance would be possible in the future. According to CMS, CAHPS surveys are an integral part of efforts to make improvements in the healthcare provided in the United States (CMS, 2018d). Some of the CAHPS surveys are used for financial incentives and are a part of value-based purchasing/pay for performance initiatives (CMS, 2018d). This change moves from strictly paying for the number of services rendered to reimbursing for high-quality services.

Numerous other tools assist caregivers in obtaining individual feedback about their experience and satisfaction with care. As care coordination continues to be an important focus within healthcare, the AHRQ suggests obtaining feedback via surveys from a multitude of perspectives in order to ensure all points within the continuum, including the individual and family, are adding to the overall improvement of care and experience. Box 5.1 contains a sample of surveys that assist caregivers in obtaining feedback for performance improvement from individuals and families (AHRQ, 2014).

Nursing Measurement and Benchmarking in Ambulatory Care

Learning from the acute care NSI journey, there has been a need for research to generate evidence comparing quality outcomes with structure and process measures important to the nursing profession and practice. Acute care measures supporting performance

BOX 5.1 Healthcare Consumer Feedback Surveys

- Coleman Measures of Care Coordination
- CAHPS and CAHPS PCMH Survey
- Individual Perception of Coordination Questionnaire
- Care Transitions Measure
- Individual Assessment of Chronic Illness Care
- Family-Centered Care Self-Assessment Tool
- Primary Care Assessment Survey
- National Survey of Children with Special Health Care Needs
- Medical Home Family Index and Survey
- Resources and Support for Self-Management
- Care Evaluation Scale for End-of-Life Care
- Oncology Patients' Perceptions of the Quality of Nursing Care

Note. CAHPS = Consumer Assessment of Health Plan Survey; PCMH = patient-centered medical homes.

improvement have historically included structural measures around the provision of nursing care, including staffing and demographics describing the nursing workforce (education, certification turnover), as well as volume descriptors to understand the size of practices and individual populations served (Brown & Wolosin, 2013; Brown et al., 2010; Montalvo, 2007; Start et al., 2016). Process measures have focused on the nursing assessment of individuals to identify the plan of care to improve outcomes and interventions based on those assessments, for example, risk mitigation for falls or pressure injuries or adverse events.

Individual outcomes related to these processes of care can then be evaluated for variation. These measures become the basis of comparisons between organizations, known as benchmarking, and the variation helps nurses identify best practices or improvement opportunities. Nursing unit rates of adverse outcomes, such as inpatient falls or hospital-acquired pressure injuries, have been shown to be related to staff mix of RNs and unlicensed assistive personnel and the education and certification level of the nurses working on nursing units personnel (Aydin et al., 2015; Boyle et al., 2016; Butler et al., 2011).

In 2013, the AAACN commissioned a task force to address NSIs specific to ambulatory nursing (Start et al., 2016). The AAACN NSI task force began this journey by conducting literature reviews on best practices and industry trends, compared with published statements on the ambulatory RN role (AAACN, 2010; AAACN, 2011) and care coordination and transition management (Haas & Swan, 2014). The result of this effort was a published report outlining existing measures for ambulatory NSI benchmarking and proposed priorities for measure development (Start et al., 2016).

AAACN/CALNOC Collaborative

In the fall of 2015, AAACN and CALNOC formalized a collaboration to move the priorities proposed by the NSI task force forward (Brown & Aronow, 2017). A core group from both organizations created a framework for ambulatory measure development. The initial NSIs launched were for Ambulatory Surgery and Procedure units, followed by measures sets for urgent care, primary care, specialty care, and birthing centers. The research leaders of CALNOC were able to translate learnings from acute care NSI development into ambulatory NSI development.

The CALNOC registry already included a full set of NSIs reflecting nursing practice in emergency care and outpatient observation units, ambulatory care settings that have traditionally been included in inpatient nursing performance measurement. Like emergency departments and observation units, ambulatory surgery centers and procedure units have more standardized nurse staffing patterns and nursing practices and are often under the auspices of, or outgrowths of, inpatient facilities. With advice and consultation from experts in ambulatory care, the first set of measures was introduced in 2016. The work of the ASC Quality Collaboration (2018) with their experience in standardized quality measure since 2006 was built on to reflect measures sensitive to nursing practice.

Engaging nurses nationally in the measure development process has been critical to reaching a tipping point for NSI ambulatory quality measurement and benchmarking. The core group leveraged the networks of both the AAACN and CALNOC to enlist interested nurses to serve on virtual Technical Expert Panels (TEPs). A TEP is a group of stakeholders and experts convened as part of the measure development process to provide input and direction to measure development teams (CMS, 2017). The TEP engaged more than 200 individual nurses—including leaders, clinical practice specialists, researchers, and staff nurses—representing large and small systems, specialty practice areas, and hospital-based and free-standing organizations. These nurses advised the core group in reviewing national **endorsed measures**, refining measures to represent ambulatory nursing practice, pilot testing them for feasibility and clarity, and charting the direction for further development.

The AAACN/CALNOC Collaborative development of measures for NSI benchmarking followed a well-defined process based on decades of inpatient measure development. The Donabedian (1976) quality framework has been used to frame the performance of discrete ambulatory care units across varied settings. The full set of ambulatory measures in the CALNOC registry as of 2018 is shown in Table 5.2. This table represents the comprehensive work of more than 150 participant organizations from across the country with TEP participants under the leadership of the AAACN/CALNOC Collaborative. Ambulatory nursing is on the journey to benchmark quality. As more ambulatory organizations participate in the use of these measures, performance improvement conclusions and meaningful benchmarks will emerge and drive value.

Benchmarking

Developing standard measures across the industry for use in individual organizations is the first step toward understanding the impact of the RN in the ambulatory setting. However, understanding performance in comparison with other organizations more broadly influences organizations' approach to improving healthcare delivery and the health of the nation. Repeated measurement over time helps nurses understand whether structure and processes are improving outcomes. Without reference to the performance of other organizations, it is impossible to know whether performance is a best practice in the industry, failing, or somewhere in between. Benchmarking performance to compare across organizations is a critical step in the NSI QI journey.

Collection of structure, process, and outcome measures within an organization is a critical step toward understanding improvement opportunities and monitoring the improvement of initiatives. These become more powerful when compared with other organizations—the process of benchmarking. The first step on the benchmarking journey is to develop "like" practices for comparison. For example, in the hospital setting, comparisons are made between like units such as age groups (ie, adult or pediatrics), types of units (ie, critical care, step down, medical surgical, trauma ED, newborn, postpartum), and size of the organization (ie, number of ED encounters or procedures or deliveries, or average daily census).

Ambulatory nursing must also develop a taxonomy to define like units, in addition to stratifications to reflect key differentiating characteristics of like unit types for meaningful comparisons. As an example, in the CALNOC benchmarking repository, ambulatory programs classifying individual care units by their setting type (ie, surgery/procedure unit, specialty care, primary care, urgent care, etc.), unit type (ie, cardiac, oncology, medical home, etc.), in addition to other structural features (ie, practice size, hospital affiliation) allow comparison with similar unit types. When enough units are submitting measures to mask identity, organizations can monitor trends on and compare performance with other similar participating units (the benchmark).

TABLE 5.2 **AAACN/CALNOC EXISTENT AMBULATORY NURSING MEASURES**

Measures	Ambulatory Care Setting					
	Primary Care	Specialty Care	Surgery/ Procedure Centers	Birthing Centers	Urgent Care	Emergency Care
Structure of Care						
Hours of direct care	X	X	X	X	X	X
Nursing staff skill mix	X	X	X	X	X	X
Nurse turnover	X	X	X	X	X	X
RN education/certification	X	X	X	X	X	X
Process of Care						
Pain assessment and follow-up	X	X	X			
Risk assessment and follow-up: hypertension, community falls, body mass index, depression	X	X				
No shows/cancellations	X	X	X	X		
Median encounter time					X	X
ED encounters admitted to hospital						X
Pts left: Without being seen; before treatment complete; against medical advice					X	X
Number of boarded patients						X
Outcomes of Care						
Unplanned transfers to hospital			X	X	X	
Falls and falls with injury	X	X	X	X	X	X
Number of visits with any wrongs (site, side, implant, etc.)			X			
Number of visits with burns			X			

Note. AAACN = American Academy of Ambulatory Care Nursing; CALNOC = Collaborative Alliance for Nursing Outcomes; RN = registered nurse. Start, R., Matlock, A. M., Brown, D., Aronow, H., & Soban, L. (2018). Realizing momentum and synergy: Benchmarking meaningful ambulatory care nurse sensitive indicators. *Nursing Economics*, 36(5), 246–251.

Future Phases of NSI

The next phase of the NSI journey will focus on measures that reflect care coordination, transitional care, chronic disease management, advanced care planning, and opioid management while incorporating PCMH and telehealth (virtual care) delivery models. Involvement of TEPs will be critical to the success of this development process, just as national benchmarking through registry participation is critical to the production of valid benchmark measures by which nursing leaders can improve and demonstrate the roles and value of nurses in ambulatory care.

Ambulatory organizations are beginning to provide dedicated performance improvement resources. As certification or accreditation of programs such as PCMHs gain momentum as required elements for reimbursement, organizations are beginning to provide the infrastructure for quality measurement much like acute care has done. Ambulatory RNs must engage in performance improvement methodologies, gain access to administrative data for measurement, and provide support to develop the infrastructure to compare quality across departments, sites or branches, or outside organizations.

RNs have the potential to positively impact individuals' outcomes and make changes in the care delivery models to improve care and decrease cost. As healthcare resources are precious, nurses must provide evidence to support care delivery model changes to improve care. Without ongoing performance improvement measurement, it is difficult to provide evidence beyond independent research studies that record results from a static point in time.

As the AAACN continued its mission to advance nursing practice in the ambulatory environment, a strategy evolved to advocate for more comprehensive inclusion of ambulatory nursing practice into the ANCC Magnet Recognition process. Given that the Magnet Recognition program has been a catalyst for positive change in inpatient settings, it has been strategic to the same in ambulatory practices. In the 2014 Magnet Recognition Manual (ANCC, 2013), ambulatory NSIs and settings were included, although measures and structural supports were in their infancy. The ANA had just convened a task force focused on ambulatory (Lewis, 2014), and the AAACN had previously convened a task force to develop NSIs (Start et al., 2016). This initiated focus on the ambulatory nursing environment, and the capability of performance to Magnet standards (Start et al., 2016). In the spring of 2016, a delegation of AAACN members approached the ANCC Magnet Commission advocating for a more comprehensive formalized appraisal of ambulatory nursing excellence throughout the Magnet Recognition program.

In the 2019 ANCC Magnet Manual (2017), all areas of nursing practice are accountable to the same sources of evidence for the Magnet Recognition process. Demographics displaying levels of education, certification, turnover, and vacancy are required for all nurses, including ambulatory. For example, professional governance, performance evaluation, peer evaluation, and leadership with a minimum educational preparation of a Bachelor of Science in Nursing (BSN) apply to all areas of nursing practice within an applicant organization.

Performance expectations are high. For example, in eight quarters organizations must outperform in four of seven nurse satisfaction or engagement domains (including ambulatory areas) and in four of seven patient satisfaction domains. Nurse-sensitive clinical indicators must also be provided for eight quarters, outperforming national benchmarks in at least two of the suggested measures (falls with injury; ambulatory surgical center patient burns; adverse outcomes of care: wrong site, side, individual, procedure, implant or device; return to acute care; HbA_{1c} target levels; extravasation rate; door-to-balloon time; antibiotic stewardship; delay in treatment; and telehealth appropriate disposition).

Summary

Society is looking to nursing for the vital transformation of healthcare. Leadership of value through meaningful measurement is imperative for the development of new care delivery models, insightful outreach to individuals in the community, and improving access for all populations. Luther Christman (1976) timelessly stated, "It is possible for nurses to move in as many levels of the profession and bring about innovation and change ... Nurses are caught up in the seething excitement of revamping the profession ... If this new vigor can spark new forms of organization and new leadership models, then the future of the professional can be viewed with great optimism." The American public trusts the nursing profession to ignite the transformation needed to achieve access to quality and affordable healthcare. Nursing is arguably the most prepared profession to transform healthcare for diverse populations that struggle with chronic illness, social disparities, and care continuity in a predominately ambulatory delivery environment (IOM, 2010, 2015).

With great need, there is great opportunity. Nursing ownership to improve healthcare quality and service to the society that relies on it requires measurement of nursing's unique contribution to generate the evidence needed for healthcare transformation. Amid a sobering landscape, the opportunity for nursing to lead important change for individuals and their families is vital. Nurses are on the front line of care delivery, building relationships with individuals and their families and earning the trust of the American public. The measurement mandate for nursing practice has never been stronger, and nurses are well positioned to lead the future of healthcare.

Case Study

As the staff RN for an ambulatory surgery center, you would like to initiate a QI project; however, you are not sure how to proceed. Your nurse manager supports your idea, partly because the center is in the process of applying for Magnet designation. The manager has provided you with some questions to help you focus your project on the basis of current NSIs.

1. What organizations could provide resources for implementing this project?
2. What are the current NSIs for ambulatory surgery centers?
3. Choosing one NSI, what would be some key questions for you to frame your QI project?
4. How might your project fit with requirements for Magnet designation?

Key Points for Review

- With the pursuit of high-value healthcare, there has been a shift in evaluating quality and a shift in the locations in which individuals receive care, with ambulatory care becoming the focus of policy related to healthcare transformation. As a result, ambulatory RNs are uniquely positioned to assume expanded roles in the design and delivery of high-quality affordable care.
- Public reporting of quality data has grown exponentially. It is important for nurses to understand healthcare funding, because reimbursement models for the healthcare organizations that employ nurses and provide care are increasingly tied to specific healthcare funding sources and the populations organizations serve. In order to assist consumers, CMS developed a Star Rating process to summarize public information so as to make it easier to review quality.
- Individual satisfaction is often used as a metric for determining the quality of care in healthcare settings. It has been employed in acute care settings for the past 20 years using valid and reliable tools. These data can be benchmarked and used to make financial decisions—both in performance metrics for leaders and in reimbursement for services. In many instances, the data are available to healthcare consumers to use for decision-making about where to go for care and treatment. As part of the recommended performance measures for ambulatory care, the National Academy of Science, in 2006, recommended that ambulatory care surveys evaluate aspects of patient satisfaction including receiving appropriate care and communication of healthcare providers and office staff.
- The AAACN/CALNOC Collaborative's development of measures for NSI benchmarking followed a well-defined process based on decades of inpatient measure development. The Donabedian quality framework has been used to frame the performance of discrete ambulatory care units across varied settings. A full set of ambulatory measures in the CALNOC registry represents the comprehensive work of more than 150 participant organizations from across the country with TEP participants under the leadership of the AAACN/CALNOC Collaborative. Ambulatory nursing is on the journey to benchmark quality. As more ambulatory organizations participate in the use of these measures, performance improvement conclusions and meaningful benchmarks will emerge and drive value.

REFERENCES

Agency for Healthcare Research and Quality. (2014). *Care coordination measures atlas*. Author.

Agency for Healthcare Research and Quality. (n.d.). *Defining the PCMH. AHRQ Website*. https://pcmh.ahrq.gov/page/defining-pcmh

Aiken, L. H., Clarke, S. P., Silber, J. H., & Sloane, D. (2003). Educational levels of hospital nurses and surgical patient mortality. *JAMA, 290*(12), 1617–1623. https://doi.org/10.1001/jama.290.12.1617

Al-Abri, R., & Al-Balushi, A. (2014). Patient satisfaction survey as a tool towards quality improvement. *Oman Medical Journal, 29*(1), 3–7. https://doi.org/10.5001/omj.2014.02

American Academy of Ambulatory Care Nursing. (2010). *Scope and standards of practice for professional telehealth nursing*. Author.

American Academy of Ambulatory Care Nursing. (2011). *What is ambulatory care nursing*? Author. https://www.aaacn.org/what-ambulatory-care-nursing

American Academy of Ambulatory Care Nursing. (2016). *Scope and standards of practice for registered nurses in care coordination and transition management*. Author.

American Academy of Ambulatory Care Nursing. (2017). *The role of the registered nurse in ambulatory care position statement*. https://www.aaacn.org/sites/default/files/documents/PositionStatementRN.pdf

American Hospital Association. (2015). Utilization and volume. In *Trend watch chart book 2015: Trends affecting hospitals and health systems*. Author. http://aha.org/research/reports/tw/chartbook/2014/chapter3.pdf

American Nurses Credentialing Center. (2013). *2014 Magnet application manual: American nurses credentialing center*. Author.

American Nurses Credentialing Center. (n.d.). *History of the Magnet Program. ANCC Website*. https://www.nursingworld.org/organizational-programs/magnet/about-magnet/

ASC Quality Collaboration. (2018). *ASC quality collaboration measures*. http://ascquality.org

Aydin, C., Donaldson, N., Aronow, H., Fridman, M., & Brown, D. (2015). Improving hospital patient falls: Leveraging staffing characteristics and processes of care. *JONA, 45*(5), 254–262. https://doi.org/10.1097/NNA.0000000000000195

Berwick, D. M., Nolan, T. W., & Whittington, J. (2008). The triple aim: Care, health, and cost. *Health Affairs, 27*(3), 759–769. https://doi.org/10.1377/hlthaff.27.3.759

Bodenheimer, T., & Sinsky, C. (2014). From triple to quadruple aim: Care of the patient requires care of the provider. *Annals of Family Medicine, 12*(6), 573–576. https://doi.org/10.1370/afm.1713

Bodenheimer, T., Bauer, L., Syer, S., & Olayiwola, J. N. (2015). *RN role reimagined: How empowering registered nurses can improve primary care*. California HealthCare Foundation. http://www.chcf.org/~/media/MEDIA%20LIBRARY%20Files/PDF/PDF%20R/PDF%20RNRoleReimagined.pdf

Boyle, D. K., Jayawardhana, A., Burman, M. E., Dunton, N. E., Staggs, V. S., Bergquist-Beringer, S., & Gajewski, B. J. (2016). A pressure ulcer and fall rate quality composite index for acute care units: A measure development study. *International Journal of Nursing Studies, 63*, 73–81. https://doi.org/10.1016/j.ijnurstu.2016.08.020

Brown, D. S., & Aronow, H. U. (2017). Ambulatory care nurse-sensitive indicators series: Reaching for the tipping point in measuring nurse-sensitive quality in the ambulatory surgical and procedure environments. *Nursing Economic$, 34*(3), 147–151.

Brown, D. S., & Woolosin, R. (2013). Safety culture relationships with hospital nursing-sensitive metrics. *Journal for Healthcare Quality, 35*(4), 61–74. https://doi.org/10.1111/jhq.12016

Brown, D. S., Donaldson, N. E., Burnes Bolton, L., & Aydin, C. (2010). Nursing sensitive benchmarks for hospitals to gauge high reliability performance. *Journal of Healthcare Quality, 32*, 9–17. https://doi.org/10.1111/j.1945-1474.2010.00083.x

Buerhaus, P. I., Donelan, K., Ulrich, B. T., Norman, L., & Dittus, R. (2006). State of the registered nurse workforce in the United States. *Nursing Economic$, 24*(1), 6–12.

Butler, M., Collins, R., Drennan, J., Halligan, P., O-Mathuna, D. P., Schultz, T. J., Sheridan, A., & Visis, E. (2011). Hospital nurse staffing models and patient and staff-related outcomes. *Cochrane Database of Systematic Reviews, (7)*. https://doi.org/10.1002/14651858.CD007019.pub2

Calabria, M., & Macrae, J. (Eds.) (1994). *Suggestions for thoughts by Florence Nightingale: Selections and commentaries*. University of Pennsylvania Press.

Center for Medicare and Medicaid Innovation. (2014). *Comprehensive primary care initiative: eCQM user manual*. Version 3.0. https://innovation.cms.gov/files/x/cpci-ecqm-manual2014.pdf

Centers for Medicare and Medicaid Services. (2015). *How does the Medicare Access and CHIP Reauthorization Act, 2015 (MACRA) reform Medicare payment*. https://www.cms.gov/Medicare/Quality-Initiatives-Patient-Assessment-Instruments/Value-Based-Programs/MACRA-MIPS-and-APMs/MACRA-MIPS-and-APMs.html

Centers for Medicare and Medicaid Services. (2017). *Technical expert panels*. https://www.cms.gov/Medicare/Quality-Initiatives-Patient-Assessment-Instruments/MMS/Technical-Expert-Panels.html

Centers for Medicare and Medicaid Services. (2018a). *Clinical performance measure project*. https://www.cms.gov/Medicare/End-Stage-Renal-Disease/CPMProject/index.html

Centers for Medicare and Medicaid Services. (2018b). *CMS-approved accrediting organization contacts for prospective clients*.https://cms.gov/Medicare/Provider-Enrollment-and-Certification/SurveyCertificationGenInfo/Downloads/Accrediting-Organization-Contacts-for-Prospective-Clients-.pdf

Centers for Medicare and Medicaid Services. (2018c). *CMS' program history: Medicare & Medicaid*. https://www.cms.gov/About-CMS/Agency-Information/History/index.html

Centers for Medicare and Medicaid Services. (2018d). *Consumer assessment of healthcare providers and systems (CAHPS)*. https://cms.gov/Research-Statistics-Data-and-Systems/Research/CAHPS/

Centers for Medicare and Medicaid Services. (2018e). *Home health compare*. https://www.cms.gov/Medicare/Quality-Initiatives-Patient-Assessment-Instruments/HomeHealthQualityInits/index.html

Centers for Medicare and Medicaid Services. (2018f). *Hospital compare*. https://www.cms.gov/medicare/quality-initiatives-patient-assessment-instruments/hospitalqualityinits/hospitalcompare.html

Centers for Medicare and Medicaid Services. (2018g). *MACRA: What's MACRA?* https://www.cms.gov/Medicare/Quality-Initiatives-Patient-Assessment-Instruments/Value-Based-Programs/MACRA-MIPS-and-APMs/MACRA-MIPS-and-APMs.html

Centers for Medicare and Medicaid Services. (2018h). *Meaningful measures initiative.* https://www.cms.gov/Medicare/Quality-Initiatives-Patient-Assessment-Instruments/QualityMeasures/index.html

Centers for Medicare and Medicaid Services. (2018i). *National health expenditures 2016 highlights.* https://www.cms.gov/Research-Statistics-Data-and-Systems/Statistics-Trends-and-Reports/NationalHealthExpendData/Downloads/highlights.pdf

Centers for Medicare and Medicaid Services. (2018j). *National health expenditure projections 2017-2026.* https://www.cms.gov/Research-Statistics-Data-and-Systems/Statistics-Trends-and-Reports/NationalHealthExpendData/Downloads/ForecastSummary.pdf

Centers for Medicare and Medicaid Services. (2018k). *Nursing home compare.* https://www.medicare.gov/nursinghomecompare

Centers for Medicare and Medicaid Services. (2018l). *Quality measures list. CMS Quality Payment Program.* https://qpp.cms.gov/mips/quality-measures, https://qpp.cms.gov/mips/explore-measures/quality-measures?py=2018#measures

Centers for Medicare and Medicaid Services. (2018m). *The CMS innovation center.* https://innovation.cms.gov

Centers for Medicare and Medicaid Services. (2018n). https://www.cms.gov/Medicare/Quality-Initiatives-Patient-Assessment-Instruments/PQRS

Craig, C., Eby, D., & Whittington, J. (2011). *Care coordination model: Better care at lower cost for people with multiple health and social needs.* IHI Innovation Series white paper. Institute for Healthcare Improvement. www.IHI.org

Curtin, L. L. (2003). An integrated analysis of nurse staffing and related variables: Effects on patient outcomes. *Online Journal of Issues in Nursing, 8*(3), 5.

Donabedian, A. (1966). Evaluating the quality of medical care. *Milbank Quarterly, 83*(4), 691–729. https://doi.org/10.1111/j.1468-0009.2005.00397.x

Donabedian, A. (1976). Foreword. In M. Phaneuf. *The nursing audit: Self-regulation in nursing practice* (2nd ed.). Appleton-Century-Crofts.

Donabedian, A. (1988). The quality of care: How can it be assessed? *Journal of the American Medical Association, 260*(12), 1743–1748. https://doi.org/10.1001/jama.260.12.1743

Dossey, B., Selanders, L., Beck, D., & Attewell, A. (2005). *Florence Nightingale today: Healing, leadership, global action* (1st ed.). American Nurses Association.

eHealth. (2018a). *Facts about Medicare.* https://www.ehealthmedicare.com/about-medicare-articles/facts-about-medicare/

eHealth. (2018b). *What are the Medicare plan star ratings and how are they measured?* https://www.ehealthmedicare.com/faq/what-are-medicare-plan-star-ratings

Gallup Organization. (2017). *Nurses keep healthy lead as most honest, ethical profession. Economy.* https://news.gallup.com/poll/224639/nurses-keep-healthy-lead-honest-ethical-profession.aspx

Haas, S., & Swan, B. A. (2014). Developing the value proposition for the role of the Registered Nurse in care coordination and transition management in ambulatory care settings. *Nursing Economic$, 32*(2), 70–79.

Institute for Healthcare Improvement. (2018a). *A primer on defining the triple aim.* http://www.ihi.org/communities/blogs/a-primer-on-defining-the-triple-aim

Institute for Healthcare Improvement. (2018b). *Patient satisfaction survey for HIV ambulatory care.* New York Stated Department of Health AIDS Institute. http://ihi.org/resources/Pages/Tools/PatientSatisfactionSurveyforAmbulatoryCare.aspx

Institute of Medicine of the National Academies. (2006). *Performance measurement: Accelerating improvement.* The National Academies Press.

Institute of Medicine. (2001). *Crossing the quality chasm: A new heath system for the 21st century.* National Academy Press.

Institute of Medicine. (2010). *The future of nursing leading change, advancing health.* The National Academies Press.

Institute of Medicine. (2015). *Assessing progress on the Institute of Medicine Report* The Future of Nursing. The National Academies Press.

Kaiser Family Foundation. (2018). *Medicare delivery system reform: The evidence link.* https://www.kff.org/medicare-delivery-system-reform-the-evidence-link

Lamb, G. (2014). *Care coordination: The game changer. How nursing is revolutionizing quality care.* American Nurses Association.

Lewis, L. (2014). Charting a new course: Advancing the next generation of nursing-sensitive indicators. *The Journal of Nursing Administration, 44*(5), 247–249. https://doi.org/10.1097/NNA.0000000000000061

Macy, J., Jr. (2016). Registered nurses: Partners in transforming primary care. Presented at the Macy Foundation conference on preparing nurses for enhanced roles in primary care. Josiah Macy Jr. Foundation.

Martinez, K., Battaglia, R., Start, R., Mastal, M. F., & Matlock, A. M. (2015). Nursing-sensitive indicators in ambulatory care. *Nursing Economic$*, 33(1), 59–66.

Matlock, A., Start, R., Aronow, H., & Brown, D. (2016). Ambulatory care nursing-sensitive indicators. *Nursing Management, 47*(6), 16–18. https://doi.org/10.1097/01.NUMA.0000483126.48107.cf

Medical Economics. (2015). *PCMH accreditation: Is it worth it?* http://medicaleconomics.com/health-law-policy/pcmh-accreditation-it-worth-it

Montalvo, I. (2007). The National Database of Nursing Quality Indicators (NDNQI). *OJIN: The Online Journal of Issues in Nursing, 12*(3), Manuscript 2. https://doi.org/10.3912/OJIN.Vol12No03Man02

National Committee for Quality Assurance. (n.d.-a). *Patient-centered medical home (PCMH) recognition. NCQA Website.* http://ncqa.org/programs/recognition/practices/patient-centered-medical-home-pcmh

National Committee for Quality Assurance. (n.d.-b). *NCQA certification programs. NCQA Website.* http://ncqa.org/programs/certification

National Quality Forum. (2004). *National voluntary consensus standards for nursing-sensitive care: An initial performance set, a consensus report.* www.qualityforum.org

National Quality Forum. (2006). *National voluntary consensus standards for ambulatory care: An initial performance measure set.* http://www.qualityforum.org/docs/ambulatory_care/tbAMB3%201APPAspecifications05-26-06.pdf

National Quality Forum. (2014a). *NQF-Endorsed measures for care coordination: Phase 3, 2014*. Technical Report. ISBN 978-1-933875-78-1.

National Quality Forum. (2014b). *Care coordination table of endorsed measures*. www.qualityforum.org

National Quality Forum. (2017). *Creating a framework to support measure development for telehealth*. Author.

Needleman, J., Buerhaus, P. I., Stewart, M., Zelevinsky, K., & Matke, S. (2006). Nurse staffing in hospitals: Is there a business case for quality? *Health Affairs (Project Hope), 25*(1), 204–211. https://doi.org/10.1377/hlthaff.25.1.204

Nightingale, F. (1860). *Suggestions for Thought to the searchers after Truth among the Artizans of England*. F. Nightingale.

Paschke, S. M., Witwer, S., Richards, W. C., Jessie, A., Harden, L., Martinez, K., & Vinson, M. H. (2017). American Academy of Ambulatory Care Nursing position paper: The role of the registered nurse in ambulatory care. *Nursing Economic$, 35*(1), 39–47.

Patient Protection and Affordable Care Act. (2010). Pub L. NO. 111-148, Sec. 3026.

Porter, M. (2010). What is value in healthcare? *New England Journal of Medicine, 363*(26), 2477–2481. https://doi.org/10.1056/NEJMp1011024

Porter-O'Grady, T., & Malloch, K. (2006). Partnership economics: Creating value through evidence-based workload management. In K. Malloch & T. Porter-O'Grady (Eds.), *Introduction to evidence-based practice in nursing and healthcare* (1st ed., pp. 183–220). Jones and Bartlett Publishers.

Rama, M., & Kanagaluru, S. K. (2011) A study on the satisfaction of patients with reference to hospital services. *International Journal of Business Economics & Management Research, 1*(3). http://zenithresearch.org.in/

Rantz, M. (1995). *Nursing quality measurement: A review of nursing studies*. American Nurses Publishing. http://www.worldcat.org/title/nursing-quality-measurement-a-review-of-nursingstudies/oclc/32384295

Roski, J., & Gregory, R. (2001) Performance measurement for ambulatory care: Moving towards a new agenda. *International Journal for Quality in Health Care, 13*(6), 447–453. https://doi.org/10.1093/intqhc/13.6.447

Schneider, E. C., Sarnak, D. O., Squires, D., Shah, A., & Doty, M. M. (2016). *Mirror, mirror 2017: International comparison reflects flaws and opportunities for better U.S. HealthCare*. http://www.commonwealthfund.org/publications/fund-reports/2017/jul/mirror-mirror-international-comparisons-2017

Start, R., Matlock, A. M., & Mastal, P. (2016). *Ambulatory care nurse-sensitive indicator industry report: Meaningful measurement of nursing in the ambulatory patient care environment*. American Academy of Ambulatory Care Nursing.

Start, R., Matlock, A. M., Brown, D., Aronow, H., & Soban, L. (2018). Realizing momentum and synergy: Benchmarking meaningful ambulatory care nurse sensitive indicators. *Nursing Economics, 36*(5), 246–251.

Swan, B. A. (2008). Making nursing-sensitive quality indicators real in ambulatory care. *Nursing Economic$, 26*(3), 195–205.

Swan, B. A., Conway-Phillips, R., & Griffin, K. F. (2006). Demonstrating the value of the RN in ambulatory care. *Nursing Economic$, 24*(6), 315–322.

Tesler, R., & Sorra, J. (2017). *CAHPS survey administration: What we know and potential research questions*. https://www.ahrq.gov/sites/default/files/wysiwyg/cahps/about-cahps/research/survey-administration-literature-review.pdf

The Joint Commission. (2018) *What is accreditation? The Joint Commission Website*. https://jointcommission.org/accreditation/accreditation_main.aspx

Tonio, S., Joerg, K., & Joachim, K. (2011). Determinants of patient satisfaction: A study among 39 hospitals in an in-patient setting in Germany. *International Journal for Quality in HealthCare, 23*(5), 503–509. https://doi.org/10.1093/intqhc/mzr038

6

Research, Evidence-Based Practice, and Quality Improvement

Sharon Tucker, Cindy J. Dawson, Lynda R. Hardy, and Michele Farrington

PERSPECTIVES

"Research, quality, and evidence help us to see what cannot always be seen through the lens of daily practice. We investigate with curiosity to produce high quality data, to focus the lens and align practice with evidence."

Roy L. Simpson, DNP, RN, DPNAP, FAAN, FACMI Emory University School of Nursing

LEARNING OBJECTIVES

Upon completion of this chapter, the reader will be able to:

1. Describe the difference between research, evidence-based practice, and quality improvement in the ambulatory care setting.
2. Explain the use and importance of data collection as it relates to research.
3. Describe the uses of big data and the electronic health record to support improvement in health outcomes.
4. Understand the role of the registered nurses and the nurse leader in participating in and leading health improvement projects and research.

KEY TERMS

Big data
Evidence-based practice
Informatics
Nursing research
Quality improvement

Introduction

The vast majority of healthcare takes place in the ambulatory care setting (Agency for Healthcare Research and Quality, 2017). Yet the efforts to improve safety and quality have focused predominantly on the inpatient setting, where the stakes and costs are higher. With the continued push for healthcare in outpatient settings along with pay-for-performance and meaningful use requirements that include electronic health record (EHR) standards (HealthIT.gov, 2015), ambulatory care teams are recognizing the importance of methods and models to promote safe, high-quality care that optimizes individuals' outcomes. As healthcare costs continue to drive change and as models of care are implemented, ambulatory care nurses need to be equipped to lead change and systematically guide discovery, innovation, and process improvement. Knowledge and skills in the models and processes of research, **evidence-based practice (EBP)**, and **quality improvement (QI)** will be essential to leading change.

This chapter differentiates research, EBP, and QI and then discusses each area's relevance to ambulatory nursing care. The current state of ambulatory nursing models, practices, and supporting evidence is reviewed along with evidence-based competencies that should be implemented and studied. Health **informatics** and nursing's role in data use in guiding change and improving individuals' outcomes in the ambulatory setting is discussed. The chapter weaves in opportunities for ambulatory nurses to maximize role competencies and improve care through research, EBP, and QI methods.

This chapter is not intended to provide an in-depth description of research, QI, and EBP; any of these topics could justify an entire chapter, or even an entire book. Rather, the goal of this chapter is to offer an overview of practice improvement principles, the tools that support those initiatives, and the application to ambulatory care nursing.

Comparison: Research, EBP, and QI

There is considerable confusion in healthcare as to definitions and differences between research, EBP, and QI models to improve individuals' care. Although all these models share systematic steps (such as identifying a purpose and question, building on existing knowledge or data, implementing a practice or intervention, and evaluating outcomes), they are differentiated by their intentions (Table 6.1). The research method aims to generate new knowledge, advance the

TABLE 6.1 RESEARCH, EVIDENCE-BASED PRACTICE, AND QUALITY IMPROVEMENT COMPARISON

	Research	Evidence-Based Practice	Quality Improvement
Intent	Discover and disseminate knowledge that can be generalized	Improve quality and safety by implementing best evidence in ambulatory decision-making	Improve local ambulatory setting system (processes) quality, safety, and efficiencies
Expected outcomes	Advance science and generalize to other ambulatory systems and patients	Promote best ambulatory healthcare quality and safety for optimal patient, provider, and cost outcomes	Improve ambulatory system performance for best patient, provider, and cost outcomes
Tools	Formal research plan with a priori defined question/hypotheses, design, conceptual and operational variables; valid and reliable tools; procedures; statistical analyses	EBP model to guide PICO question, review literature, collect baseline and postimplementation data; implementation strategies; basic statistics and tracking of existing health metric data	Quality improvement models (Lean Six Sigma, PDSA, continuous improvement); use of system data; locally focused
Training	Formal research training at the graduate level, usually PhD	Bachelor's level training or postbachelor's (or graduate) level training; on-the-job training	Some formal academic programs; certificate programs and on-the-job training
Human subjects review	Always required	Not usually required but dependent on local agency policies	Not usually required but dependent on local agency policies

Note. EBP = evidence-based practice; PDSA = Plan, Do, Study, Act; PICO = P = population/problem, I = intervention, C = comparison/control, O = outcome.

scientific foundations of healthcare, and disseminate new knowledge broadly. The EBP method is a systematic approach to examining a clinical practice issue in a particular setting, comparing it with available evidence on effective strategies, and making a decision about piloting and evaluating a change in practice. A structured approach is applied to adopting, implementing, and evaluating the evidence for a local context with its unique culture, provider expertise, and individuals' values and preferences. The QI method has its roots in industry and was adopted to healthcare many decades ago. The primary goal in QI is to improve processes and outcomes in a local setting. System change, efficiencies, and elimination of waste are stressed in this approach. Each of these methods and its application to the ambulatory setting are discussed in more detail.

Research

The research process is a structured approach to knowledge generation and discovery that follows scientific principles and processes. Table 6.2 outlines the basic steps in the research process. With clinical research and enrollment of human subjects, there are often unexpected realities to the study (eg, participant dropouts, incomplete datasets, nonadherence to the treatment, and/or problems with real-world issues) that cannot always be controlled despite the rigorous implementation of research methods. This work thus requires flexibility and practical or pragmatic considerations in the design and interpretation of study findings.

Research knowledge and skills are learned at the baccalaureate, master's, and doctoral levels of nursing education. Bachelor's degree-prepared nurses learn basic research knowledge and skills. They focus on identifying important clinical questions that can be converted into research questions and may participate on research teams.

Masters-prepared nurses are trained in more research processes and application of research and may lead research studies that are relevant to their specialty practice and to the goal of improving clinical care. They may also serve on research teams, but are not likely to develop a program of research on their own.

Nurses earning the doctoral degree in nursing practice (DNP) are focused on application and evaluation of research in clinical practice settings, including roles as primary investigators in QI or EBP, or as partners with PhD nurse researchers to develop research projects that are embedded in real-world clinical settings. The most intensive research training is acquired through programs at the PhD level and through postdoctoral training and studies designed to advance an area of investigation. Additional competencies are obtained through working with scientific mentors and teams and working through the research process with many different studies. Regardless of the level of preparation, promotion of **nursing research** in a clinical setting requires strong leadership with a vision for nursing as a scientific discipline.

The ambulatory setting has long been included in medical oncology studies and for a number of other medical specialties such as cardiology and endocrinology. However, aside from those specialties, nursing research in the ambulatory setting has been limited. The majority of nursing research has been conducted by faculty from academic settings and most often either in hospitals or in communities outside of the clinic or ambulatory care settings.

Challenges to research in the ambulatory care setting include limited numbers of researchers or clinicians with a research background and lack of time and financial support. However, when research is conducted in the ambulatory setting, ambulatory nurses can collaborate with researchers to identify gaps in research and advocate for resources to support studies that will optimize individuals' health and reduce healthcare expenses.

In spite of the barriers, examples of ambulatory nursing research are growing. In one example, a study in California assessed nurses' activities through the lens of the Nursing Role Effectiveness Model and found that independent nursing activities can have an impact on individuals' outcomes (Rondinelli et al., 2014). These findings also point to more opportunities for chronic disease management and collaboration with other team members. Another example of research led by nurses in the ambulatory setting involved a study on nurse-led

TABLE 6.2 **RESEARCH AND EBP STEPS**

Research Steps	EBP Steps
Step 1—Scientific Gap Identification • Identification of a problem and gap in scientific literature • Research question and hypotheses (if appropriate) are formulated	Step 1—Determine Organizational Readiness • Seek leadership and organizational support for promoting EBP as an approach to providing care

Step 2—Review of Existing Literature
• Extensive review of existing scientific literature to inform research gap and guide study design
• Identification of theoretical framework if indicated
• Research question is refined
	Step 2—Select EBP Model
	• Decide on an EBP model to guide initiatives
	  • Concepts are clear for ambulatory care
	  • Representation of the model allows assimilation of concepts
	  • Steps of EBP are organized and align with the ambulatory care setting and practice model
	  • Model is comprehensive from beginning, through implementation and evaluation of ambulatory care outcomes
	  • Model is easy to use and guides ambulatory care practice changes
	  • Model can be applied to diverse ambulatory populations and practices
	• Educate and disseminate on the chosen model

Step 3—Selection of Research Design • Research proposal is developed • Research design is determined with specific procedures • Human subject protection is assured by review and approval of agency Institutional Review Board	Step 3—Identify Practice Change Needed • Form team for EBP initiative • PICO Question formulated • P = population/problem, I = intervention, C = comparison/control, O = outcome • Search for the best evidence in the literature based on the PICO questions and terms • Critically appraise the evidence • Decide if practice change is warranted and if necessary resources and support are available for the change
Step 4—Study Implementation • Study is launched with recruitment and enrollment • Study procedures and data collection are completed • If intervention is involved, an individual's safety is monitored	Step 4—Implement EBP Change • Develop implementation action plan with timeline and owner for each action • Collect baseline data to evaluate change • Ensure leadership support and visibility • Ensure individual/family preferences and values are honored • Integrate clinician expertise • Monitor integrity of implementation strategies • Solicit stakeholder feedback throughout process
Step 5—Data Analysis and Dissemination • All data collected are analyzed using predetermined statistical plan or qualitative analysis plan • Participant follow-up is completed • Study findings are disseminated locally, at regional and national conferences, and in publications	Step 5—Evaluate EBP Change and Disseminate Lessons • Collect postpractice change data • Evaluate outcome of change • Decide on local roll-out appropriateness • Disseminate outcomes

Note. EBP = evidence-based practice.

self-management support for primary care individuals with anxiety, depression, or somatic symptoms (Zimmerman et al., 2016). Findings indicated significant increases in intervention participants' perceived self-efficacy in managing their symptoms compared with control participants and suggested promise for a nurse-led mental health intervention in primary care.

Evidence-Based Practice

"Evidence-based practice (EBP)" has been a term used in healthcare for more than 20 years. It originated in the medical field and has been adopted in various forms by most healthcare disciplines. Generally speaking, most groups in nursing define EBP as a decision-making approach that includes the healthcare team, individual, and family to apply and adopt the evidence known through scientific discovery within the context of an individual's preferences and values and clinician expertise.

Undergraduate and new nurses often struggle with the distinction between EBP and QI initiatives. EBP is differentiated from research and QI (Table 6.1) primarily through the intent of the initiative. Although there is indeed overlap, the two methods employ different approaches. The aim of EBP is to use a systematic process to support practice changes that are based on published evidence that is integrated with an individual's preferences and values and clinician expertise. The aim of QI is to improve systems and processes unique to an organization. Evidence may be used, but it would generally be internal evidence only.

In general, EBP may be seen as intended for greater dissemination to support or establish specific nursing practices. Although it may be conducted in a specific setting, the intent is to advance or support evidence for a larger audience. In contrast, QI is intended to address a specific problem, challenge, or need identified in the practice site. However, the two approaches may complement each other. For instance, QI tools are sometimes used to sustain EBP changes using local systems and processes, such as with auditing and feedback.

The role of ambulatory registered nurses (RNs) has shifted in the past 10 or more years toward greater scope of practice with more independent nursing functions, and fewer medically delegated tasks with other nonnursing personnel taking those tasks. As a result of these changes, ambulatory RNs today should be familiar with EBP models and trained in EBP processes. This requires leaders who are visionary and proactive and who have expectations for ambulatory care advancement that includes nursing autonomy and independent practice. To be successful in practice changes, ambulatory nurses must be supported with:

1. Training and time to become confident and learn
2. Tools to help guide the processes and champions or mentors who can teach, guide, and keep nurses on pace with an EBP project
3. Access to data to measure outcomes of the process
4. Recognition for the work being advanced
5. Tools for ongoing monitoring to support sustainability of the practice change.

These are no small requests given the legacy culture of ambulatory models and nursing roles and challenges (time, lack of knowledge/confidence, lack of leadership support, organizational culture, etc.) in translating evidence into practice. However, with the need for new healthcare models that advance the outpatient care team scope of practices, these tools and supports will be essential.

EBP is best guided by an EBP model that provides a systematic approach to EBP. Examples of EBP models in nursing include Iowa EBP Model, Johns Hopkins EBP Model, Stetler Model, ACE Star Model, the ARCC Framework, and the PARHIS Framework (Schaffer et al., 2012). The Iowa, Johns Hopkins, ACE Star, and Stetler Models are all process models and provide similar steps to implement an EBP change. Although each model is somewhat unique, all basically cover the steps outlined in Table 6.2. The Promoting Action on Research

BOX 6.1 EBP Model Applied to Ambulatory Care

Huether et al. (2016) implemented a project to reduce fatigue and improve quality of life in cancer patients through physical activity promotion. They followed the Iowa EBP Model to evaluate the research literature on physical activity for cancer patients and used the literature recommendations to design and develop a physical activity intervention and tool kit for patients in a medical oncology survivorship outpatient clinic. Implementation of their intervention resulted in improved outcomes for those in the study and reflected the benefits of nurse-led EBP projects for improving care and patient outcomes among ambulatory patients in busy clinical settings.

Note. EBP = evidence-based practice.

Implementation in Health Services (PARHIS) and Advancing Research and Clinical Practice Through Close Collaboration (ARCC) frameworks are both organizational frameworks that highlight the importance of context, culture barriers, and enablers. The ARCC Framework stresses the importance of organizational readiness, strengths, and weaknesses, whereas the PARHIS Framework focuses on three key factors that influence the success of EBP initiatives: evidence, context, and facilitation. The ambulatory team will need to review the specifics of each model and decide which one is the best fit for their organization. This will be influenced by organizational readiness and presence of strong ambulatory leadership that values EBP. Step two from Table 6.2 provides the considerations involved in selecting an appropriate model.

In understanding the application of EBP to the ambulatory care setting, it can be helpful to understand what has been done in the past. The case described in Box 6.1 provides an example of a project that applied EBP concepts to a specific challenge.

Quality Improvement

Prior to the 20th century, QI in healthcare was implemented by different individuals in different settings with different methods of application. However, one of these individuals, Florence Nightingale, put QI documentation on the map in the 1800s. The 1960s brought about Medicare and Medicaid programs to mitigate the inadequate medical care for the older population and indigent. A number of legislative activities and acts followed, and in 1990 the National Committee for Quality Assurance was established with a key objective of improving healthcare quality (Marjoua & Bozic, 2012). However, one of the most influential trailblazers in QI was physician leader Avedis Donabedian (1968), who created a widely used model measuring the quality of healthcare by observing its structure, processes, and outcomes.

The interest in quality and safety in healthcare was heightened with the publication, by the Institute of Medicine (IOM) in 2000, of *To Err Is Human: Building a Safer Health System* (IOM (US) Committee on Quality of Health Care in America, 2000) followed by the U.S. Patient Safety and Quality Improvement Act in 2005. This act was intended to encourage voluntary reporting of adverse events that ensured confidentiality and the opportunity for improvement.

Batalden and Davidoff (2007) stressed that to meet its full potential, healthcare must embrace change as an intrinsic part of everyone's daily job for the entire system. They defined QI as "the combined and unceasing efforts of everyone—healthcare professionals, individuals and their families, researchers, payers, planners and educators—to make the changes that will lead to better individual outcomes (health), better system performance (care) and better professional development (learning)" (p. 2). This definition is consistent with the quadruple aim (initially forwarded as the Triple Aim by Berwick and colleagues, 2008), which includes population health, individuals' experience of health, cost, and provider experience.

Several models are used in the field of QI, including that of Donabedian (structure, process, and outcomes), the FADE model (Focus, Analyze, Develop, Execute/Evaluate), and Six Sigma (including the steps of define, measure, analyze, improve/design, control/verify). Six

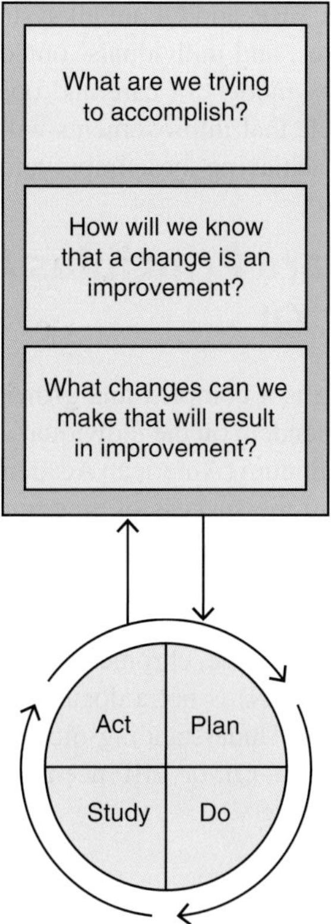

FIGURE 6.1 Plan, Do, Study, Act. (Wiener-Kronish, J. P. [2015]. *Critical care handbook of the Massachusetts general hospital* [6th ed.]. Wolters Kluwer Health.)

Sigma training offers progressive levels of competence and can be a strong resource for nursing leaders. However, for nurses employing QI in the workplace, two commonly applied concepts in QI are Quality and Safety Education for Nurses (QSEN, n.d.) and the Plan, Do, Study, Act (PDSA) method of rapid cycle change.

There are six QSEN competencies, including: (1) patient-centered care, (2) teamwork and collaboration, (3) EBP, (4) QI, (5) safety, and (6) informatics (QSEN, n.d.). The PDSA model is illustrated in Figure 6.1.

In the ambulatory care application of QI, the following is an example of a QI project that used EBP guidelines to support the initiative and illustrates the synergy that can add value to both EBP and QI (Box 6.2).

BOX 6.2 QI Model Applied to Ambulatory Care

A QI project led by Hammelef et al. (2014) aimed to evaluate the feasibility and utility of the NCCN's distress management clinical practice guidelines in ambulatory oncology. The goal of this project was to assess staff implementation of these established guidelines and the impact on individuals' care. Staff were trained to understand, screen (using a distress thermometer), assess, and manage an individual's distress. Following the project initiation, they were surveyed to evaluate effects on workload, perceived benefits, and satisfaction. Overall, the NCCN's distress management guidelines were found to be easy to implement, staff were satisfied with the process, distress was detected, and referral to psychosocial resources was improved, with a higher proportion of individuals being referred to psychosocial services and a shorter time interval between referral and receipt.

Note. NCCN = National Comprehensive Cancer Network; QI = quality improvement.

In summary, research, EBP, and QI are all systematic approaches to improving healthcare knowledge, care processes, and individuals' outcomes. Many ambulatory care settings have been slower to adopt new models of care and operations, but with the push for ambulatory care growth it is inevitable that improvements will be needed, and these skills and tools will provide the methods for achieving these improvements.

Ambulatory Care Principles Applied to Research, EBP, QI

Ambulatory care nursing is a complex and growing care delivery system that encompasses many models that are dependent on the individual's population and the point of an individual's entry across the care continuum (American Academy of Ambulatory Care Nursing [AAACN], 2017). RNs are critical to the success of emerging care delivery models that are needed to provide safe, high-quality care in the outpatient arena. Models of care may vary depending on a wide variety of factors such as severity of illness, facility type and location, practice environment, or population served. The most prevalent models include team-based care, individual-centered medical home, chronic care, and accountable care organizations (ACOs). Strengths-based nursing (SBN) is not a documented model of care but has merit in the discussion of models of care. Understanding models of ambulatory care nursing helps nurses address appropriate research, QI, or EBP needs in various settings toward the common goal of improved healthcare delivery.

Team-Based Care

The principles and concepts of team-based care are more fully addressed in Chapters 10 and 11. In general, it is a concept of care that incorporates the use of team members working at their highest level of practice, with clear roles, while keeping the individual at the center of care decisions. Team-based care may incorporate a number of existing models for implementation and use of tools such as daily huddles, TeamSTEPPS (Team Strategies & Tools to Enhance Performance & Patient Safety), and SBAR (Situation, Background, Assessment, Recommendation). More information about TeamSTEPPS is available on the Agency for Healthcare Research and Quality (n.d.) website, and information on SBAR is available from the Institute for Healthcare Improvement (n.d.) website.

Regardless of the strategies used, a team-based care setting is most enhanced by projects that are grounded in QI or EBP and that address an individual's outcomes, rather than research focused on specific diseases or health challenges.

Patient-Centered Medical Home

The patient-centered medical home (PCMH) (more fully described in Chapter 10) is focused on building partnerships between providers and individuals and families. In this sense, it may be described as both a concept of care and a physical description; many of the concepts behind the PCMH may be applied to other settings, but the key elements of collaboration and communication are specified in the designation of a PCMH. Within the PCMH setting, many of the QI and EBP projects with the same focus as those in the team-based care model would be appropriate. Additionally, the PCMH lends itself well to projects that emphasize communication, workflow, and standardization of care.

Chronic Care Model

The chronic care model (CCM) focuses on diseases that, owing to their chronic nature and sequelae, have a large impact on healthcare costs. These include diagnoses such as diabetes, asthma, and hypertension. One of the strengths of the CCM is nurse-managed protocols. This model lends itself well as the context for nursing research related to specific chronic diseases that can be addressed by nursing interventions.

Accountable Care Organization

Similar to a PCMH, the ACO is a method of organizing healthcare that is specific to a group of healthcare delivery organizations. The ACO designation requires a fiscal collaboration involving primary care clinicians, a hospital, specialists, and other members of the healthcare team who assume joint responsibility for the care of select individuals. This setting is well suited for EBP initiatives that focus on an individual's engagement, reporting quality and financial metrics, and coordinating care, including triage and telehealth.

Strengths-Based Nursing

Strengths-based nursing (SBN) is an approach to care that is grounded in core values that promote empowerment, self-efficacy, and hope and is based on a model of eight values of healthy functioning and healing built on Florence Nightingale's vision (Gottlieb, 2014). In the context of SBN, research initiatives that explore specific interventions to support nursing effectiveness would be valuable to both nursing and an individual's care.

Ambulatory Care Personnel and Roles

A standardized metric to measure workload in ambulatory settings does not exist, unlike the hours per patient day (HPPD) metric commonly used to determine and evaluate appropriate direct nursing care hours for hospitalized individuals. Lack of a metric partially stems from insufficient evidence regarding consistent workflow practices among settings (eg, primary care, specialty care, procedural units, infusion areas) and individual populations, along with differences in skill mix and staffing models that exist between organizations.

Research is not only needed to develop and test metrics to measure workload in various types of ambulatory settings but should also address setting- and individual-specific skill mix. A common misconception is that when delays occur or work is unable to be completed, the solution is to hire additional staff members. Overstaffing brings a whole host of issues, including cost, and the potential to provide inefficient or lower quality care. Benchmarking with reliable sources, such as the Medical Group Management Association (MGMA), is recommended and could assist nursing research efforts related to workload issues.

Workload in ambulatory settings is currently defined by an individual's characteristics, the role of nursing personnel, and the number of individuals (often referred to as units of service or visits) who are being seen. Ambulatory nurses provide care in person, over the telephone, virtually via the Internet, and through other e-technologies (eg, EHR) (AAACN Task Force, 2017). Nurses often have minimal time with each individual and must quickly and efficiently provide and complete individualized, cost-effective nursing care and the associated documentation (Haas et al., 2016; Mastal et al., 2016). Factors that can make this challenging include acuity of the individual, number of scheduled and add-on individuals, hours of business, and a procedure versus clinic environment.

For any project or initiative, whether it be research, QI, or EBP, accurate data collection is essential for success. Frequently, individuals collecting the data are not those who are the primary research investigators or project directors, so it is incumbent on the lead investigators or project directors to support those collecting the data and help them realize the importance of accurate information. Often, an example of ways in which inaccurate data resulted in flawed results may be helpful. The role of those supporting research, QI, or EBP may include varying levels of involvement, depending on the need and institutional support. The specific roles outlined next are more fully described in Chapter 4.

Unlicensed Personnel

In the ambulatory setting, unlicensed personnel are most often Medical Assistants (MAs) who may or may not be regulated, depending on the state of employment. However, in all settings, MAs provide a large proportion of individuals' care. As a result, they can be a valuable resource for the nurse implementing a research, EBP, or QI project.

Registered or Licensed Nurses

As the team leader in the majority of ambulatory care settings, the Registered Nurse (RN)—and often the Licensed Practical Nurse, Licensed Vocational Nurse, or Licensed Nurse (LPN/LVN/LN)—is an essential conduit for information and communication between individuals and families and other members of the healthcare team. The educational preparation for the Bachelor of Science in Nursing (BSN) provides the knowledge and skills that the BSN may need to lead QI and EBP projects, along with QI Leaders described previously, or participate as a research team member.

Advanced Practice Personnel

Advanced practice RNs (Nurse Practitioners, Certified Registered Nurse Anesthetists, Certified Nurse Midwives) and doctorally prepared nurses (PhD—Doctor of Philosophy in Nursing, DNP—Doctor of Nursing Practice) have varying degrees of educational preparation that enable them to advance nursing practice. Research content is a focus in the PhD program, with those graduates involved most heavily in research and external grants. DNP programs generally emphasize practice-related projects as part of an organization's QI program or development and implementation of EBP projects.

Research and EBP Competencies for Nurses and Nurse Leaders

In brief, research and EBP competencies for RNs practicing in ambulatory care settings include the following: identifying clinical problems and opportunities for improvement; reviewing, critiquing, and using the available literature to guide and change practice; implementing practice changes; evaluating process and outcome measures for EBP initiatives to demonstrate impact; and initiating, supporting, and participating in applicable research studies (AAACN, 2017).

Frontline ambulatory RNs are in an ideal position to identify important, clinically relevant topics that can be developed as EBP projects (Balakas et al., 2013; Crabtree et al., 2016; Registered Nurses' Association of Ontario [RNAO], 2013). These frontline RNs are expert clinicians and have the necessary skills to collaborate, problem solve, and identify creative solutions to successfully implement EBP changes and often function as change champions, core group members, opinion leaders, and/or project directors (Balakas et al., 2013; Cullen et al., 2018; Dogherty et al., 2012; Grimshaw et al., 2012; Mark et al., 2014). However, RNs cannot effectively integrate EBP changes into care and be empowered unless sufficient support is provided by nursing leaders (Abdullah et al., 2014; Cullen et al., 2014; Farrington et al., 2015; Walter et al., 2014).

With regard to research studies, frontline RNs in ambulatory settings can function as principal investigators or coprincipal investigators provided that a mentor, someone who is familiar with the research process and organizational requirements related to research, is readily available to assist with all components of the study. In addition to a mentor, these RNs need dedicated time to complete preparatory work, to execute the study, to complete data analysis, and to disseminate results internally and externally. Some of the additional ways that frontline RNs could participate in research studies include participating as research subjects, identifying potential subjects, assisting with the informed consent process, administering the study medication or study intervention, obtaining lab work, collecting data, monitoring individuals, and providing individual/ family education.

Additional research and EBP competencies specific to ambulatory nurse executives, administrators, and managers include facilitating and promoting the use of EBPs in clinical practice and within nursing policies, procedures, and protocols; ensuring researchers follow all regulatory requirements such as obtaining required approvals from the Institutional Review Board and reviewing studies to ensure alignment with organizational goals and priorities relevant to nursing; advocating for resources to allow RNs to participate in EBP and research activities; and recognizing and rewarding RNs for participating in these types of activities (AAACN, 2017).

Nurse managers must develop a clinic culture that supports both innovation and evidence-based care in order to positively impact individuals' outcomes (Aarons et al., 2015; Huis et al., 2013; Ubbink et al., 2013). Nurse managers can facilitate and support EBP by setting clinic expectations; discussing the importance of EBP with clinic nurses and healthcare team members; encouraging and responding to new, innovative ideas; promoting clinicians questioning practice; providing and supporting project work time; promoting the project's importance; tracking progress; facilitating movement of the project through the institutional shared governance approval process; and allocating resources (Paparone, 2015; RNAO, 2013). The nurse manager's commitment to improving quality and safety and to providing performance feedback is critical to project success and can significantly affect project outcomes (McMullan et al., 2013; Paparone, 2015; Stetler et al., 2014).

Clinical nurse specialists (CNSs) and Advanced Practice Providers (APPs) play an important role in project development and are often called on to assist with the most challenging steps in the EBP process, given their educational preparation, clinical expertise, and skills. These individuals often function as opinion leaders, mentors, and facilitators throughout the process (Cullen et al., 2018; Gawlinski & Becker, 2012; McMullan et al., 2013). Research is a component of both the CNS and APP role (Kilpatrick et al., 2014). However, the level of involvement, leading or participating, in research is based on the experience and skill of the individual CNS or APP along with the specific ambulatory setting.

Nurse executives must include EBP and research in the nursing strategic plan and continually advocate for allocation of resources and time for frontline RNs, CNSs, and APPs to complete this important work (Aarons et al., 2014; Clay-Williams et al., 2014; Dogherty et al., 2012; Hauck et al., 2013; Melnyk et al., 2016; Ubbink et al., 2013). In ambulatory and all other healthcare settings, a substantial gap remains in the amount of evidence-based care, from well-developed clinical practice guidelines, that has been implemented and incorporated into day-to-day practice (Shaw et al., 2014). Frontline RNs and nursing leaders of all levels must work together to develop, implement, and sustain effective EBP initiatives that positively impact an individual, clinician, safety, and cost outcomes (Jackson, 2016).

QI Competencies for RNs and Nurse Leaders

Some of the competencies, identified by the AAACN in the QI standard (referred to as the performance improvement [PI] standard by AAACN) are similar to those outlined for research and EBP, whereas others are slightly different. Specific competencies for the ambulatory RN include identifying opportunities for improving clinical outcomes, safety, and the individual's experience; participating in identifying nurse-sensitive indicators (NSIs); leading or participating in QI initiatives; implementing evidence-based improvements; and evaluating QI initiatives and seeking feedback from all key stakeholders (eg, individuals, families, caregivers, visitors, healthcare team members) to ensure an individual's and clinician's safety is maintained (AAACN, 2017).

Additional ambulatory nurse executive, administrator, and manager competencies include:

- soliciting input from key stakeholders to identify improvement opportunities and strategies;
- developing, implementing, and evaluating current and innovative care delivery models;
- setting expectations for all team members regarding QI initiatives;
- providing resources and support for the healthcare team to implement QI initiatives;
- recognizing and rewarding RNs who participate in QI initiatives;
- collecting, analyzing, and benchmarking data related to QI initiatives; and
- evaluating the efficiency and effectiveness of nursing care across the care continuum. (AAACN, 2017)

Within all organizations, it is most often RNs of all levels and positions who are charged with, and responsible for, developing, implementing, and sustaining the quality measures set forth by regulatory agencies such as The Joint Commission (AAACN Task Force, 2012; Patel et al., 2013). Constant vigilance and surveillance must occur by both licensed and unlicensed personnel to proactively identify QI opportunities that impact the six major quality aims outlined by the IOM—safe, effective, individual-centered, timely, efficient, and equitable (IOM, 2001).

Research/QI/EBP Application

The following examples illustrate some of the ways that research, QI, or EBP might be applied within an ambulatory care setting. As the field of ambulatory care nursing expands, there will be many other possibilities for use of these competencies to advance nursing practice.

Triage

Nurse triage and the associated assessments completed over the telephone continue to be an integral component of individualized care in ambulatory settings (Dawson et al., 2011). For nurses to efficiently and effectively perform triage, organizations must ensure the use of readily available, evidence-based nurse triage protocols for adult and pediatric primary care settings, both during office hours and after-hours protocols that can be directly built into the Electronic Health Record (EHR). Additional benefits to using established nurse triage protocols include the protocols being regularly updated, based on new and emerging evidence and research, and inclusion of documentation parameters. Select specialty practice areas (eg, oncology, otolaryngology, and head-neck) have developed and published triage guidelines to assist nurses in performing this role (Dawson et al., 2011; Hickey & Newton, 2012).

Virtual Care

Electronic/virtual visits, individual portals, and other device applications have assisted ambulatory RNs in answering individuals' questions, assessing and documenting individuals' health status, and determining whether individuals are following treatment recommendations, without an actual face-to-face meeting.

Regular encounters with individuals allow the RN to assist them and their families to manage medical and mental health needs and allow the RN to provide assistance for these individuals who may also be facing complex social and family needs, including navigation of the healthcare system (AAACN Task Force, 2017). Comprehensive, timely, evidence-based assessments and follow-up care, completed by RNs, is a guide for providers when prioritizing care, and the backbone of this care is EBP that informs the protocols, assessments, and care provided.

Given that virtual visits and virtual care are relatively new means of clinical interaction between an individual and the healthcare team, research is still needed to determine how individuals perceive this new form of care, to obtain feedback about efficiency and effectiveness from the healthcare team, and to evaluate the impact not only on an individual's outcomes but also on overall healthcare system use.

Care Coordination

Because effective care coordination has been shown to improve individuals' outcomes and to decrease healthcare costs, this is an important area for continued research, QI, and EBP. The goals of care coordination offer potential for multiple types and levels of projects. These goals include the following: addressing systemic problems and identifying solutions to improve care coordination; optimizing communication among all providers; maximizing and providing care coordination efficiently and effectively for each individual every time; optimizing resource utilization and contributing to improving care delivery; reducing length of stay, discharge barriers, and readmission rates by providing continuity that enhances collaboration and partnerships; and minimizing role redundancy and overlap.

Communication, collaboration, and partnerships between the inpatient care coordination team and ambulatory nursing are essential to quality, safety, organizational throughput, discharge planning, readmission prevention, individuals' satisfaction, and employee satisfaction. Identifying an individual's needs in the ambulatory setting prior to admission provides essential information to begin preparations to ensure a safe hospitalization episode (eg, need for fall precautions, baseline cognitive needs for an individual's education, assistive devices, access issues to get home) and ensure posthospitalization needs (eg, ability to take medications, assistive devices, placement need for therapies, need for assistance in the home) are met. As individuals move through the continuum of care, it is essential to utilize and develop technology to maximize nurses' capacity to help develop and communicate safe, seamless, ongoing plans of care. Individual-centered care coordination not only affects and improves nurse-driven individual outcomes but also decreases resource utilization and costs.

Transition Management

Transition management (covered in further detail in Chapter 7) has become increasingly valuable in the context of reduction of readmissions and provision of individual-specific continuity of care. Opportunities for research, EBP, or QI projects related to transition management have often focused on its effectiveness on reducing readmissions, but areas for future work include providing support during the transition to home or assisted living and identification of adverse signs and symptoms with defined follow-up appointments that are within the role and scope of the RN.

Episodic Illness

EBP, as reflected in the use of preestablished order sets and nurse-managed protocols, has been a valuable resource in episodic illness clinics and in ensuring individuals are meeting health maintenance goals. Improved health outcomes have been demonstrated through the use of these types of order sets and protocols (Shaw et al., 2014).

Health Coaching

A prominent RN role in today's healthcare environment is health promotion and health maintenance as a way of promoting healthy people and preventing chronic disease. In terms of practice improvement, health maintenance activities allow primary care clinicians to systematically track evidence-based preventative care recommendations, both procedures and interventions, for select individual populations (eg, hepatitis B vaccine, prostate cancer screening, zoster vaccine, colonoscopy, hemoglobin A_{1c} for an individual with diabetes). Additionally, building the recommendations into the EHR is a quick way to determine whether an individual has received, or when that person should receive, the recommended schedule of preventative care. These activities primarily have resulted from previous EBP initiatives that led to the development of standardized recommendations and protocols. Ongoing development of additional EBP initiatives supports a strong role for the RN in health promotion and maintenance.

Medication Reconciliation

The importance of medication reconciliation is often underestimated as a task appropriate for the RN (versus unlicensed personnel). Because medication adherence is dependent on a number of factors, including education, cognition, and external support, assessing the many reasons for nonadherence is most appropriate for RNs trained in this skill. Research supporting the need for RN-specific competencies in this area can provide evidence for the importance and value of the RN in preventing avoidable medication complications.

Use of Data to Facilitate Research, EBP, and QI

Research, EBP, and QI have a common theme—they all require data to improve individual care. Today's fast-paced healthcare environment increases the need for healthcare provider tools necessary for clinical decision-making providing safe, effective, and quality care. These tools aid in supporting the quadruple aim of improving care quality, individuals' satisfaction, healthcare cost containment, and healthcare provider work life (Bodenheimer & Sinsky, 2014). The following section provides an overview and examples of ways that data may be collected and used in order to facilitate the achievement of the quadruple aim.

Decision-making is supported by data that can be defined as uninterpretable elements such as age or weight. These data are collected (aggregated) to create information (data that are processed giving it meaning). These meaningful data translate into knowledge (about the individual), leading to wisdom—the use of knowledge in making appropriate individual care decisions. This is known as the DIKW process (data/information/knowledge/wisdom) (Nelson & Staggers, 2018).

The DIKW hierarchical model was developed and modified by numerous individuals on the basis of the needs of their discipline, but the model suggests a level of specificity where data provide information that leads to knowledge and, ultimately, wisdom. Nelson and Staggers use the DIKW model in health informatics, articulating a nursing perception where collection

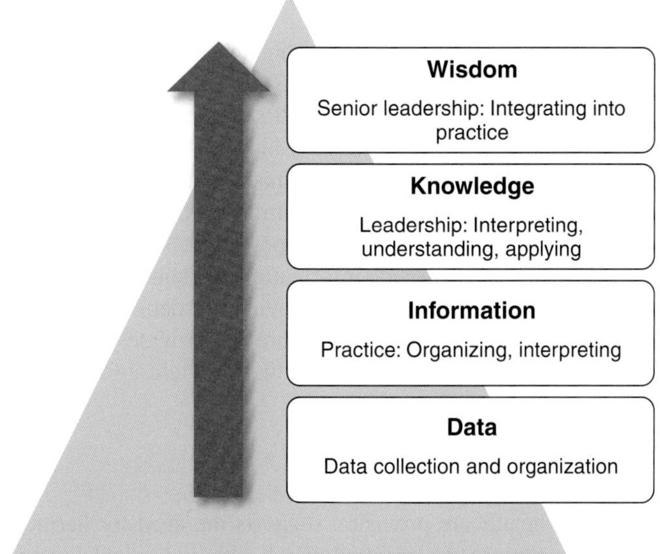

FIGURE 6.2 DIKW (data/information/knowledge/wisdom) model.

of *data* leads to *information* (data organization and interpretation) that informs *knowledge* (understanding and integrating), culminating in *wisdom* (applying and integrative service with compassion) (Nelson & Staggers, 2018). This hierarchical model supports all levels of nursing practice from the associate degree nurse to the PhD and DNP. It provides a complex framework guiding practice (see Figure 6.2).

Nurse-Sensitive Indicators (NSIs)

Ambulatory RNs must continue to partner with regulatory agencies and professional ambulatory nursing organizations to identify specific NSIs, indicators that capture care or outcomes most affected by nursing care, which can be routinely measured and tracked across ambulatory settings to assess the quality of nursing care provided (ANA Care Coordination Quality Measures Professional Issues Panel, 2013; Brown & Aronow, 2016; Haas & Swan, 2014; Martinez et al., 2015; Mastal et al., 2016).

NSIs reflect the **structure, process, and outcomes** of nursing care (ANA Care Coordination Quality Measures Professional Issues Panel, 2013; Brown & Aronow, 2016; Mastal et al., 2016). **Structure** indicators include the supply, skill level, and education and certification of nursing personnel, whereas **process** indicators measure assessment, intervention, and RN job satisfaction (ANA Care Coordination Quality Measures Professional Issues Panel, 2013). Finally, **outcomes** are considered to be nursing sensitive if improvement is seen with either a greater quantity or quality of nursing care (ANA Care Coordination Quality Measures Professional Issues Panel, 2013). Such outcomes are evaluated through valid and reliable data systems that allow for routine and ongoing program and individual care evaluations, as well as for research, QI, and EBP projects.

A significant value of NSIs is that they can provide measurable evidence of the impact nursing can have on an individual's outcomes in the ambulatory care setting. The ongoing identification and classification of NSIs will continue to support the enhanced role of RNs in this field.

Big Data

Big data, a term that has become today's mantra for the rapid generation and use of data, can be described as a collection of data that are too large for typical software to be able to analyze or apply. Electronic medical records (EMRs) provide a large amount of data, but in today's world of wearable and wireless sensors, big data may be gathered from a large variety of sources. A few examples may include cardiac monitors, exercise trackers, and blood pressure or blood glucose measurement. Each day millions of data points are collected on individuals at rapid speeds and types. Various data types are collected from many sources, merged, and, in most cases, analyzed to provide information and knowledge that supports individuals' care. Equally important, many sources that provide big data also allow individuals to participate fully in their own care management. Figure 6.3 provides an overview of the importance of aggregating data for the purpose of providing the right information to the right person at the right time.

Informatics

The variance in healthcare provision suggests the need for harmonization of efforts toward achieving the quadruple aim of population health, individuals' experience of health, cost, and provider experience. One possible solution may be found in the application of informatics. Bakken (2001) suggests the following five key elements needed to interface health informatics with EBP:

1. terminology and structure standardization,
2. digital sources of evidence,
3. interoperability or the ability of systems to share/exchange data,
4. informatics processes that support clinical decision-making, and
5. informatics competencies (Bakken, 2001).

Informatics is not the sole answer to meeting the quadruple aim, but responses to address the elements listed previously are in progress. One important area is data standardization through the use of registered terms (eg, SNOMED [Systematized Nomenclature of Medicine Clinical Terms], common data elements). Terminology standardization allows rapid data aggregation and comparability necessary for determining individual or community trends.

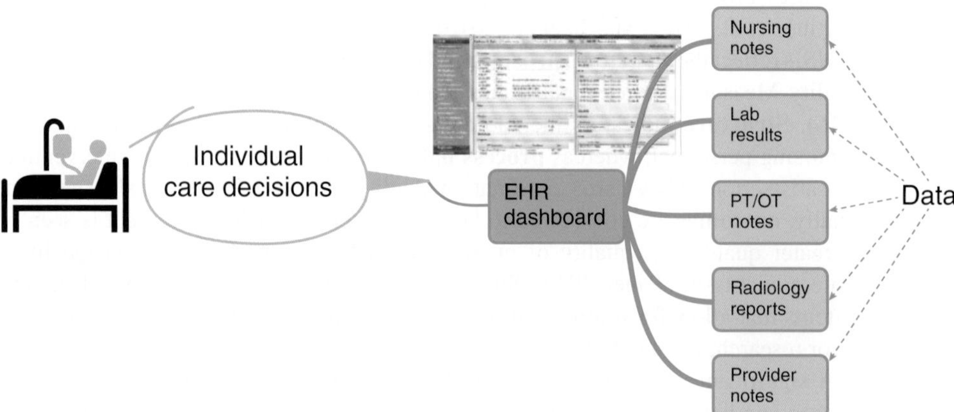

FIGURE 6.3 Use of data to support care decisions for individuals. EHR = electronic health record; OT = Occupational Therapy; PT = Physical Therapy.

Common data elements (CDEs), defined as "variables that are operationalized and measured in identical ways across studies" (Redeker et al., 2015), allow for aggregation and comparability. These elements provide a systematic naming construct defining the context of an individual's care. CDEs are reliable and valid metrics developed by national experts for a transparent and inclusive means of documentation and evaluation of care. A comprehensive list of CDEs can be found at the United States National Library of Medicine (https://cde.nlm.nih.gov).

Electronic health systems provide digital support through rapid access to individuals' information and decision-making support, although the ability of systems to share data between systems is an ongoing challenge. Arguably the most important element, practice standards and competencies, continues to be developed and refined as nurses embrace analytic abilities and incorporate data and information into their practice to support clinical decision-making and EBP.

Electronic Health Record

The American Recovery and Reinvestment Act of 2009 (Pub.L.111-5) mandated that all public and private healthcare providers and other eligible professionals adopt EHRs and demonstrate meaningful use. The EHR is one of the more significant innovations in healthcare but has yet to provide a level of interoperability that would allow unfettered sharing of individual information. A push continues to encourage EHR vendors to reduce system propriety, allowing individual information sharing across institutions for fast, safe, and appropriate individual care.

RNs play a significant role in the development, implementation, and use of EHRs by becoming team members and leaders, thereby ensuring that appropriate data are captured providing adequate information for an individual's care. Healthcare as a whole continues to struggle with the important area of data entry standardization across systems and practices. Maximizing the use of EHR data depends on the data's ability to be machine readable across systems (standardized format that a computer can process) in order to provide interpretable information for delivering rapid care.

Clinical Decision Support Systems

Clinical decision support systems (CDSS) work in concert with EHRs to provide the most current evidence to the healthcare team for immediate and effective care for individuals. They assist in aggregating data, reducing medical errors, and facilitating point-of-care workflow. CDSS incorporate alerts, reminders, clinical guidelines, focused reports on individuals, care-templates, and references. However, they require adequate support from information technology and healthcare providers to ensure accurate documentation. EHRs and CDSS are not the silver bullet for healthcare because they are the direction for improvement of the burgeoning growth of diagnostic and treatment options facing society today.

Federal Regulations

The safety and security of personal health information (PHI) is paramount and governed by federal regulations. The Health Insurance Portability and Accountability Act of 1996 (HIPAA), a congressional mandate, included Privacy and Security rules that established standards for protecting PHI and assuring the security of PHI held electronically. The Health Information Technology for Economic and Clinical Health (HITECH) Act, promulgated under the American Recovery and Reinvestment Act (ARRA) of 2009, led to the expansion of healthcare information technology by expanding the use of EHR. HITECH also expanded the enforcement of HIPAA by imposing penalties for "willful neglect" of HIPAA regulations. Table 6.3 provides a brief overview of the regulation, its responsibility, and the way it affects nursing.

TABLE 6.3 SUMMARY OF FEDERAL REGULATIONS ON INFORMATION TECHNOLOGY

Regulation	Requirement	Application to Nursing
ARRA	Mandated adoption of the EHR and its meaningful use	Provided an electronic version of the medical record with the ability to rapidly share an individual's information, improve healthcare workflow, and increase safety and care quality for the individual
HIPAA	Protection of PHI	Mandate to keep an individual's health information confidential, only to be shared with those documented by the individual
HITECH	Protection and security of the EHR	Mandated EHR security from system breaches, hacks, an unauthorized use of health information

Note. ARRA = American Recovery and Reinvestment Act; EHR = Electronic Health Record; HIPAA = Health Insurance Portability and Accountability Act; HITECH = Health Information Technology for Economic and Clinical Health; PHI = Personal Health Information.

Summary

This chapter has focused on research, EBP, and QI as these problem-solving approaches related to ambulatory nursing care. Each of these approaches has different intentions for their outcomes, yet each can advance ambulatory nursing care. Discovery, application of evidence in practice, and process improvements are all activities in which ambulatory care nurses can engage at some level. Examples of published projects/studies using the different approaches in ambulatory care were provided, and ambulatory staff competencies related research, EBP, and QI were discussed, identifying areas for further development. The chapter concluded with a review of the importance of systems for collecting and aggregating data for evaluating outcomes of any approach.

There is a need for these competencies across the care continuum, including ambulatory care, the fastest growing setting for providing care. Each level of practice in ambulatory care interacts and overlaps with the next, providing an integrated framework epitomizing nursing practice. All levels should include an understanding of research, EBP, QI, and health informatics to ensure quality care for individuals at an appropriate cost and maximizing the provider's ability to practice.

As evidenced by Florence Nightingale, nurses have been engaged from the beginning as leaders in the QI process and key stakeholders in enacting change. The nursing skills of team development and strong leadership are key functions for bringing people together to solve system problems, whether it be through the use of research, QI, or EBP. In the past, much of this work has been driven by hospital teams; however, there are current examples in ambulatory settings of nurses taking leadership roles in these teams. Although movement into the ambulatory setting has not come without challenges, nursing and nonnursing leaders have put forward strong business cases along with quality and safety goals to compel ambulatory model changes.

Case Study

Mary G. is a BSN-prepared RN in the transplant clinic of a large university hospital. She has observed that individuals who come to the clinic for their first appointment after hospital discharge do not have an adequate understanding of postdischarge care. In this clinic, the responsibility of education rests only on the RN, who is often rushed or unable to answer all the individuals' questions.

The purpose of Mary's project was to develop an education curriculum for individuals so that any member of the healthcare team could deliver any portion of the content. In this collaborative manner, a number of interprofessional colleagues would be able to provide timely and appropriate education.

There were well-established evidence-based guidelines for appropriate education, and Mary decided to use the Health Promotion Model as a foundation for her curriculum.

Please discuss the following questions:

1. Would this project be considered research, EBP, or QI? Why?
2. Which colleagues might Mary include as part of the interprofessional team?
3. What contributions would different members of the team be able to provide?
4. How might Mary evaluate the effectiveness of this project?
5. What would be the next steps?

Key Points for Review

- Research, EBP, and QI are essential competencies for RNs to have in order to improve individuals' care and advance the profession of nursing.
- Research is most commonly conducted by nurses at the PhD level; other doctorally prepared nurses collaborate on research or lead in EBP or QI projects.
- Teamwork is an important element of research/EBP/QI, and all members of the healthcare team have areas in which they can contribute.
- Data are essential to successful improvement in healthcare outcomes and may be obtained from EHR as well as the many sources that make up the category of big data.

REFERENCES

Aarons, G. A., Ehrhart, M. G., & Farahnak, L. R. (2014). The Implementation Leadership Scale (ILS): Development of a brief measure of unit level implementation leadership. *Implementation Science, 9*(1), 45. https://doi.org/10.1186/1748-5908-9-45

Aarons, G. A., Ehrhart, M. G., Farahnak, L. R., & Hurlburt, M. S. (2015). Leadership and organizational change for implementation (LOCI): A randomized mixed method pilot study of a leadership and organization development intervention for evidence-based practice implementation. *Implementation Science, 10*(1), 11. https://doi.org/10.1186/s13012-014-0192-y

Abdullah, G., Rossy, D., Ploeg, J., Davies, B., Higuchi, K., Sikora, L., & Stacey, D. (2014). Measuring the effectiveness of mentoring as a knowledge translation intervention for implementing empirical evidence: A systematic review. *Worldviews on Evidence-Based Nursing, 11*(5), 284–300. https://doi.org/10.1111/wvn.12060

Agency for Healthcare Research and Quality. (2017, June). *Ambulatory care safety. Patient Safety Network.* https://psnet.ahrq.gov/primers/primer/16/ambulatory-care-safety

Agency for Healthcare Research and Quality. (n.d.). *About TeamSTEPPS.* https://www.ahrq.gov/teamstepps/about-teamstepps/index.html

American Academy of Ambulatory Care Nursing. (2017). In C. Murray (Ed.). *Scope and standards of practice for professional ambulatory care nursing* (9th ed.). Author.

American Academy of Ambulatory Care Nursing Task Force. (2012). American Academy of Ambulatory Care Nursing position statement: The role of the registered nurse in ambulatory care. *Nursing Economic$, 30*(4), 233–239.

American Academy of Ambulatory Care Nursing Task Force. (2017). American Academy of Ambulatory Care Nursing position statement: The role of the registered nurse in ambulatory care. *Nursing Economic$, 35*(1), 39–47.

ANA Care Coordination Quality Measures Professional Issues Panel. (2013). *Framework for measuring nurses' contributions to care coordination*. American Nurses Association.

Bakken, S. (2001). An informatics infrastructure is essential for evidence-based practice. *JAMA*, 8(3), 199–201. https://doi.org/10.1136/jamia.2001.0080199

Balakas, K., Sparks, L., Steurer, L., & Bryant, T. (2013). An outcome of evidence-based practice education: Sustained clinical decision-making among bedside nurses. *Journal of Pediatric Nursing, 28*(5), 479–485. https://doi.org/10.1016/j.pedn.2012.08.007

Batalden, P. B., & Davidoff, F. (2007). What is "quality improvement" and how can it transform healthcare? *Quality & Safety in Health Care,* 16(1). https://doi.org/10.1136/qshc.2006.022046

Berwick, D. M., Nolan, T. W., & Whittington J. (2008). The Triple Aim: Care, health, and cost. *Health Affairs, 27*(3), 759–769. https://doi.org/10.1377/hlthaff.27.3.759

Bodenheimer, T., & Sinsky, C. (2014). From triple to quadruple aim: Care of the patient requires care of the provider. *Annals of Family Medicine, 12*(6), 573–576. https://doi.org/10.1370/afm.1713

Brown, D. S., & Aronow, H. U. (2016). Ambulatory care nurse-sensitive indicator series: Reaching for the tipping point in measuring nurse-sensitive quality in the ambulatory surgical and procedure environments. *Nursing Economic$, 34*(3), 147–151.

Clay-Williams, R., Nosrati, H., Cunningham, F. C., Hillman, K., & Braithwaite, J. (2014). Do large-scale hospital-and system-wide interventions improve patient outcomes: A systematic review. *BMC Health Services Research, 14*, 369. https://doi.org/10.1186/1472-6963-14-369

Crabtree, E., Brennan, E., Davis, A., & Coyle, A. (2016). Improving patient care through nursing engagement in evidence-based practice. *Worldviews on Evidence-Based Nursing, 13*(2), 172–175. https://doi.org/10.1111/wvn.12126

Cullen, L., Dawson, C. J., Hanrahan, K., & Dole, N. (2014). Evidence-based practice: Strategies for nursing leaders. In D. L. Huber (Ed.), *Leadership and nursing care management* (5th ed., pp. 274–290). Elsevier.

Cullen, L., Hanrahan, K., Farrington, M., Deberg, J., Tucker, S., & Kleiber, C. (2018). *Evidence-based practice in action: Comprehensive strategies, tools and tips from the University of Iowa Hospitals and Clinics*. Sigma Theta Tau International.

Dawson, C. J., Hickey, M. M., & Newton, S. (Eds.). (2011). *Telephone triage for otorhinolaryngology and head-neck nurses*. Oncology Nursing Society.

Dogherty, E. J., Harrison, M. B., Baker, C., & Graham, I. D. (2012). Following a natural experiment of guideline adaptation and early implementation: A mixed-methods study of facilitation. *Implementation Science*, *7*, 9. https://doi.org/10.1186/1748-5908-7-9

Donabedian, A. (1968). The evaluation of medical care programs. *Bulletin of the N Y Academy of Medicine, 44*, 117–124.

Farrington, M., Hanson, A., Laffoon, T., & Cullen, L. (2015). Low-dose ketamine infusions for postoperative pain in opioid-tolerant orthopaedic spine patients. *Journal of PeriAnesthesia Nursing, 30*(4), 338–345. https://doi.org/10.1016/j.jopan.2015.03.005

Gawlinski, A., & Becker, E. (2012). Infusing research into practice: A staff nurse evidence-based practice fellowship program. *Journal for Nurses in Staff Development, 28*(2), 69–73. https://doi.org/10.1097/NND.0b013e31824b418c

Gawlinski, A., & Rutledge, D. (2008). Selecting a model for evidence-based practice changes. *AACN Advanced Critical Care, 19(3), 291–*300. https://doi.org/10.4037/15597768-2008-3007

Gottlieb, L. N. (2014). Strengths-based nursing. *American Journal of Nursing, 114*(8), 24–32. https://doi.org/10.1097/01.NAJ.0000453039.70629.e2

Grimshaw, J. M., Eccles, M. P., Lavis, J. N., Hill, S. J., & Squires, J. E. (2012). Knowledge translation of research findings. *Implementation Science, 7*, 50. https://doi.org/10.1186/1748-5908-7-50

Haas, S. A., & Swan, B. A. (2014). Developing the value proposition for the role of the registered nurse in care coordination and transition management in ambulatory care settings. *Nursing Economic$, 32*(2), 70–79.

Haas, S. A., Vlasses, F., & Havey, J. (2016). Developing staffing models to support population health management and quality outcomes in ambulatory care settings. *Nursing Economic$, 34*(3), 126–133.

Hammelef, K. J., Friese, C. R., Breslin, T. M., Riba, M., & Schneider, S. M. (2014). Implementing distress management guidelines in ambulatory oncology: a quality improvement project. *Clinical journal of oncology nursing*, 18 Suppl, 31–36. https://doi.org/10.1188/14.CJON.S1.31-36

Hauck, S., Winsett, R. P., & Kuric, J. (2013). Leadership facilitation strategies to establish evidence-based practice in an acute care hospital. *Journal of Advanced Nursing, 69*(3), 664–674. https://doi.org/10.1111/j.1365-2648.2012.06053.x

HealthIT.gov. (2015, February 6). *Meaningful use definitions and objectives. EHR Incentives and Certifications.* https://www.healthit.gov/providers-professionals/meaningful-use-definition-objectives

Hickey, M., & Newton, S. (Eds.). (2012). *Telephone triage for oncology nurses* (2nd ed.). Oncology Nursing Society.

Huether, K., Abbott, L., Cullen, L., Cullen, L., & Gaarde, A. (2016). Energy Through Motion©: An Evidence-Based Exercise Program to Reduce Cancer-Related Fatigue and Improve Quality of Life. *Clinical journal of oncology nursing*, 20(3), E60–E70. https://doi.org/10.1188/16.CJON.E60-E70

Huis, A., Holleman, G., van Achterberg, T., Grol, R., Schoonhoven, L., & Hulscher, M. (2013). Explaining the effects of two different strategies for promoting hand hygiene in hospital nurses: A process evaluation alongside a cluster randomised controlled trial. *Implementation Science, 8*, 41. https://doi.org/10.1186/1748-5908-8-41

Institute for Healthcare Improvement. (n.d.). *SBAR communication technique.* http://www.ihi.org/Topics/SBARCommunicationTechnique/Pages/default.aspx

Institute of Medicine. (2001). *Crossing the quality chasm: A new health system for the 21st century.* The National Academies Press.

Institute of Medicine (US) Committee on Quality of Health Care in America; Kohn, L. T., Corrigan, J. M., & Donaldson, M. S., (Eds.). (2000). *To err is human:*

Building a safer health system. National Academies Press (US). https://www.ncbi.nlm.nih.gov/books/NBK225182/

Jackson, N. (2016). Incorporating evidence-based practice learning into a nurse residency program: Are new graduates ready to apply evidence at the bedside? *Journal of Nursing Administration, 46*(5), 278–283. https://doi.org/10.1097/NNA.0000000000000343

Kilpatrick, K., Kaasalainen, S., Donald, F., Reid, K., Carter, N., Bryant-Lukosius, D., Martin-Misener, R., Harbman, P., Anne Marshall, D., Charbonneau-Smith, R., & DiCenso, A. (2014). The effectiveness and cost-effectiveness of clinical nurse specialists in outpatient roles: A systematic review. *Journal of Evaluation in Clinical Practice, 20,* 1106–1123. https://doi.org/10.1111/jep.12219

Marjoua, Y., & Bozic, K. J. (2012). Brief history of quality improvement in US healthcare. *Current Reviews in Musculoskeletal Medicine, 5,* 265–273. https://doi.org/10.1007/s12178-012-9137-8

Mark, D. D., Latimer, R. W., White, J. P., Bransford, D., Johnson, K. G., & Song, V. L. (2014). Hawaii's statewide evidence-based practice program. *Nursing Clinics of North America, 49*(3), 275–290. https://doi.org/10.1016/j.cnur.2014.05.002

Martinez, K., Battaglia, R., Start, R., Mastal, M. F., & Matlock, A. M. (2015). Nursing-sensitive indicators in ambulatory care. *Nursing Economic$, 33*(1), 59–66.

Mastal, M., Matlock, A. M., & Start, R. (2016). Ambulatory care nurse-sensitive indicators series: Capturing the role of nursing in ambulatory care—The case for meaningful nurse sensitive measurement. *Nursing Economic$, 34*(2), 92–97, 76.

McMullan, C., Propper, G., Schuhmacher, C., Sokoloff, L., Harris, D., Murphy, P., & Greene, W. H. (2013). A multidisciplinary approach to reduce central line-associated bloodstream infections. *Joint Commission Journal on Quality and Patient Safety, 39*(2), 61–69. https://doi.org/10.1016/S1553-7250(13)39009-6

Melnyk, B. M., Gallagher-Ford, L., Thomas, B. K., Troseth, M., Wyngarden, K., & Szalacha, L. (2016). A study of chief nurse executives indicates low prioritization of evidence-based practice and shortcomings in hospital performance metrics across the United States. *Worldviews on Evidence-Based Nursing, 13*(1), 6–14. https://doi.org/10.1111/wvn.12133

Nelson, R., & Staggers, N. (2018). *Health informatics: An interprofessional approach.* Elsevier.

Paparone, P. (2015). Supporting influenza vaccination intent among nurses: Effects of leadership and attitudes toward adoption of evidence-based practice. *Journal of Nursing Administration, 45*(3), 133–138. https://doi.org/10.1097/NNA.0000000000000172

Patel, M. S., Arron, M. J., Sinsky, T. A., Green, E. H., Baker, D. W., Bowen, J. L., & Day, S. (2013). Estimating the staffing infrastructure for a patient-centered medical home. *The American Journal of Managed Care, 19*(6), 509–516.

Quality and Safety Education for Nurses. (n.d.). http://qsen.org/

Redeker, N., Anderson, R., Bakken, S., Corwin, E., Docherty, S., Dorsey, S., Heitkemper, M., Jo McCloskey, D., Moore, S., Pullen, C., Rapkin, B., Schiffman, R., Waldrop-Valverde, D., & Grady, P. (2015). Advancing symptom science through use of common data elements. *Journal of Nursing Scholarship, 47,* 379–388. https://doi.org/10.1111/jnu.12155

Registered Nurses' Association of Ontario. (2013). Developing and sustaining nursing leadership (2nd ed.). Author.

Rondinelli, J. L., Omery, A. K., Crawford, C. L., & Johnson, J. A. (2014). Self-reported activities and outcomes of ambulatory care registered nurses: An exploration. *The Permanete Journal, 18*(1), E108–E115. https://doi.org/10.7812/TPP/13-135

Schaffer, M. A., Sandau, K. E., & Diedrick, L. (2012). Evidence-based practice models for organizational change: Overview and practical applications *Journal of Advanced Nursing, 69*(5), 1197–1209. https://doi.org/10.1111/j.1365-2648.2012.06122.x

Shaw, R. J., McDuffie, J. R., Hendrix, C. C., Edie, A., Lindsey-Davis, L., Nagi, A., Kosinski, A. S., & Williams, J. W. (2014). Effects of nurse-managed protocols in the outpatient management of adults with chronic conditions: A systematic review and meta-analysis. *Annals of Internal Medicine, 161*(2), 113–121. https://doi.org/10.7326/M13-2567

Stetler, C. B., Ritchie, J. A., Rycroft-Malone, J., & Charns, M. P. (2014). Leadership for evidence-based practice: Strategic and functional behaviors for institutionalizing EBP. *Worldviews on Evidence-Based Nursing, 11*(4), 219–226. https://doi.org/10.1111/wvn.12044

Ubbink, D. T., Guyatt, G. H., & Vermeulen, H. (2013). Framework of policy recommendations for implementation of evidence-based practice: A systematic scoping review. *BMJ Open, 3*(1). https://doi.org/10.1136/bmjopen-2012-001881

Walter, M. R., Aucoin, J., Brown, R., Thompson, J. A., & Sullivan, D. T. (2014). A multimodal approach to EBP. *Nursing Management, 45*(1), 14–17. https://doi.org/10.1097/01.NUMA.0000440638.48766.a7

Zimmerman, T., Puschmann, E., van den Bussche, E., Wiese, B., Ernst, A., Porzelt, S., Scherer, M. (2016). Collaborative nurse-led self-management support for primary care patients with anxiety, depressive or somatic symptoms: Cluster-randomised controlled trial (findings of the SMADS study). *International Journal of Nursing Studies, 63,* 101–111. https://doi.org/10.1016/j.ijnurstu.2016.08.007

UNIT 3

Fundamentals for Ambulatory Care Nursing

7

Engaging Individuals and Families in Health

Anne T. Jessie

PERSPECTIVES

"Shared decision-making is critically important for healthcare delivery. Many decisions require an understanding of how individuals value potential benefits and harms of care. The only way to get at this is through shared decision-making. An added benefit is that involving individuals in their care is the best way to engage them in care and make sure they follow through on care decisions."

Alex H. Krist, MD, MPH, professor of family medicine and population health at Virginia Commonwealth University and an active clinician and teacher at the Fairfax Family Practice Residency. Codirector of the Virginia Ambulatory Care Outcomes Research Network and director of community-engaged research at the Center for Clinical and Translational Research.

LEARNING OBJECTIVES

Upon completion of this chapter, the reader will be able to:

1. Describe the role of individual and family engagement in ambulatory care nursing practice.
2. Understand the defining elements of activation, empowerment, engagement, and shared decision-making, especially within the context of individuals and families, environment, and nursing role.
3. Discuss how guiding principles for engaging individuals and families foster effective engagement of consumers across healthcare settings.
4. Apply tools, principles, and methods for fostering behavioral change.
5. Explain the importance of incorporating individual values, goals, and preferences in developing knowledge, skills, and attitudes that support self-care management.
6. Discuss the role of advisory councils in fostering individual and family engagement.

KEY TERMS

Activation
health literacy
Patient engagement
Person-centered care
Self-care management
Shared decision-making

Introduction

The advancement of health science and technology has accelerated over the past half-century, along with the needs of an increasingly diverse and aging population. Care has become extremely complex and costly from both a health and healthcare delivery perspective and is fraught with fragmentation, medical errors, overutilization, and often poor quality (American Nurses Association Executive, 2012; Humowiecki et al., 2018; Sofaer & Schumann, 2013). Concurrently, the incidence and prevalence of chronic health conditions have increased, with conditions such as diabetes, heart disease, cancer, hypertension, stroke, arthritis, obesity, renal disease, and respiratory diseases leading the way as the most common causes of illness, long-term disability, reduced quality of life, and death (Centers for Disease Control and Prevention [CDC], 2018; Raghupathi & Raghupathi, 2018). Chronic health conditions or diseases are defined as conditions that last a minimum of a year, require ongoing medical management, and are the leading drivers of the $3.3 trillion spent annually on healthcare in the Unites States (CDC, 2018). Nearly half (45%) of all Americans—133 million people—suffer from at least one chronic disease (Raghupathi & Raghupathi, 2018).

Individuals experiencing chronic health conditions are living longer, thus ensuring the need for sustained interactions with healthcare delivery systems that often increase in frequency, duration, and intensity over time. Individuals with significant chronic conditions and those with multiple comorbid conditions are managed by primary care providers in combination with other medical and surgical specialists, often crossing state lines and healthcare systems. This sets up a care environment with multiple silos in which different providers make medical decisions without complete information about an individual's condition, medical history, medications ordered, care managed, or services rendered in numerous care settings by multiple clinicians (Krist et al., 2017).

Quality Context for Engaging Individuals and Families

These increasingly complex and diverse care environments, involving multiple specialists, present a varied menu of diagnostic and treatment options requiring individuals, families, and/or caregivers to assimilate data and information needed in order to make care and treatment decisions. Once treatment and care decisions are made, individuals must possess a level of knowledge and understanding of their role in care management in order to comply with prescribed treatments, medications, and rehabilitation. In 2001, the Institute of Medicine (IOM) produced a groundbreaking report, *Crossing the Quality Chasm: A New Health System for the 21st Century*, that identified patient-centeredness as foundational to quality healthcare. Included in the report were 10 new rules to redesign and improve care along with the recommendation that private and public purchasers, healthcare organizations, clinicians, and individuals work together in the redesign of healthcare delivery (IOM, 2001). The IOM report endorsed "six patient-centeredness dimensions that stipulated that care must be: respectful to patients' values, preferences, and expressed needs; coordinated and integrated; provide information, communication, and education; ensure physical comfort; provide emotional support; and involve family and friends" (Tzelepis et al., 2015, p. 831). In 2015, the Institute for Healthcare Improvement (IHI) released *10 New Rules to Accelerate Healthcare Redesign* providing an update to the IOM recommendations from 2001. In Table 7.1, the IOM and IHI rules are compared to illustrate the evolutionary focus for redesign in an era of healthcare and payment reform. Influenced by the current focus on payment reform and emphasis on value over volume, the IHI's guiding principles emphasized the need for meaningful partnerships with individuals, families, and care providers to effectively engage all stakeholders in thinking

TABLE 7.1 COMPARISON OF IHI AND IOM

IHI 10 New Rules to Accelerate Healthcare Redesign	IOM Formulating New Rules to Redesign and Improve Care
1. Change the balance of power. Coproduce health and well-being in partnership with patients, families, and communities.	1. Care based on continuous healing relationships. Patients should receive care whenever they need it and, in many forms, not just face-to-face visits. This rule implies that the healthcare system should be responsive at all times (24 hours a day, every day) and that access to care should be provided over the Internet, by telephone, and by other means in addition to face-to-face visits.
2. Standardize what makes sense. Standardize what is possible to reduce unnecessary variation and increase the time available for individualized care.	2. Customization based on patient needs and values. The system of care should be designed to meet the most common types of needs but have the capability to respond to individual patient choices and preferences.
3. Customize to the individual. Contextualize care to an individual's needs, values, and preferences, guided by an understanding of what matters to the person in addition to "what's the matter?"	3. The patient as the source of control. Patients should be given the necessary information and the opportunity to exercise the degree of control they choose over healthcare decisions that affect them. The health system should be able to accommodate differences in patient preferences and encourage shared decision-making.
4. Promote well-being. Focus on outcomes that matter the most to people, appreciating that their health and happiness may not require healthcare.	4. Shared knowledge and the free flow of information. Patients should have unfettered access to their own medical information and to clinical knowledge. Clinicians and patients should communicate effectively and share information.
5. Create joy in work. Cultivate and mobilize the pride and joy of the healthcare workforce.	5. Evidence-based decision-making. Patients should receive care based on the best available scientific knowledge. Care should not vary illogically from clinician to clinician or from place to place.
6. Make it easy. Continually reduce waste and all non–value-added requirements and activities for patients, families, and clinicians.	6. Safety as a system property. Patients should be safe from injury caused by the care system. Reducing risk and ensuring safety require greater attention to systems that help prevent and mitigate errors.
7. Move knowledge, not people. Exploit all helpful capacities of modern digital care and continually substitute better alternatives for visits and institutional stays. Meet people where they are, literally.	7. The need for transparency. The healthcare system should make information available to patients and their families that allows them to make informed decisions when selecting a health plan, hospital, or clinical practice or choosing among alternative treatments. This should include information describing the system's performance on safety, evidence-based practice, and patient satisfaction.
8. Collaborate and cooperate. Recognize that the healthcare system is embedded in a network that extends beyond traditional walls. Eliminate silos and tear down self-protective institutional or professional boundaries that impede flow and responsiveness.	8. Anticipation of needs. The health system should anticipate patient needs, rather than simply reacting to events.

(*continued*)

TABLE 7.1 COMPARISON OF IHI AND IOM (CONTINUED)

IHI 10 New Rules to Accelerate Healthcare Redesign	IOM Formulating New Rules to Redesign and Improve Care
9. Assume abundance. Use all the assets that can help to optimize the social, economic, and physical environment, especially those brought by patients, families, and communities.	9. Continuous decrease in waste. The health system should not waste resources or patient time.
10. Return the money. Give the money from healthcare savings to other public and private purposes (Loehrer et al., 2015, pp. 66–68).	10. Cooperation among clinicians. "Clinicians and institutions should actively collaborate and communicate to ensure an appropriate exchange of information and coordination of care" (IOM, 2001, p. 67).

Note. IHI = Institute for Healthcare Improvement; IOM = Institute of Medicine.

differently about healthcare delivery in order to improve the overall health of individuals and communities.

Nationally, individual and family engagement has become a major focus of healthcare reform and policy development with a growing body of literature that suggests that strengthening individual engagement in **self-care management** and **shared decision-making** contributes to improved health outcomes and care experiences, as well as to cost containment (American Academy of Ambulatory Care Nursing [AAACN], 2017a; Greene et al., 2015; Krist et al., 2017). This call to action advocates for the inclusion of individuals, families, and/or caregivers in the design of care based on values, goals, and preferences that are collaborative, responsive to individual needs, integrated, and accessible. Such shifts in care delivery processes require a focus on individual strengths, valuing individuals and families as members of the team and "doing care 'with me' and not 'to me'" (Swartwout et al., 2016, p. S11). Krist and colleagues further stated that "**patient engagement** demarcates an increasing shift from more paternalistic models of care in which clinicians tell patients what they should do (and often ineffectively), to one in which clinicians' partner with patients" (Krist et al., 2017, p. 106). As the largest and most respected group of healthcare professionals in the United States, nurses play a critical role in ensuring that individuals are fully engaged and active in managing their personal health and care (Brenan, 2018).

Why Engaging Individuals and Families Is Nursing's Priority

For 17 consecutive years, the profession of nursing has been recognized as the most honest and ethical profession among a diverse group of top professions within the United States (Brenan, 2018). The nursing profession has a long history of caring for individuals in a holistic manner, taking into consideration interventions that address identified needs of the individual as a whole person: body, mind, and spirit. This includes integrating traditional healthcare with person-centered approaches that are focused on health and healing, integrating and incorporating interventions from a variety of healthcare disciplines, and providing care that is based on the individual's specific care needs.

Nurses at all levels and in all care settings are uniquely poised and ethically bound to support individuals and families in successful engagement and self-care management activities and to advocate for inclusion in shared decision-making based on informed consent (AAACN, 2017a, 2017b; Krist et al., 2017; Sofaer & Schumann, 2013). Historically, nursing has focused on **person-centered care** as a care delivery model, empowering individuals and leading the healthcare team through education and culturally sensitive care programs and interventions (Pelletier & Stichler, 2013). In 2007, Cronenwett and colleagues solidified person-centered care as a core competency for nurses through inclusion in *Quality and Safety Education for Nurses* (QSEN). These competencies apply not only to undergraduate students but also to nurses engaged in graduate education, as well as ongoing competency development for all nurses actively engaged in nursing practice. The definition of QSEN's patient-centered care competency is to: "Recognize the patient or designee as the source of control and full partner in providing compassionate and coordinated care based on respect for patient's preferences, values, and needs" (Cronenwett et al., 2007, p. 123).

Nowhere is this competency more critical than in the ambulatory care setting, where registered nurses (RNs) work independently and collaboratively, partnering with individuals, families, providers, and other healthcare professionals in the design and provision of care. The context of the ambulatory care environment is ever expanding, complex, rapidly changing, and often difficult to navigate across varied and diverse care settings. In addition to the need for competency development in person-centered care and engaging individuals and families in self-care management and shared decision-making, RNs practicing in ambulatory care settings need to have awareness and a level of understanding of the scope and standards of nursing practice in ambulatory care. The American Academy of Ambulatory Care Nursing (AAACN), the specialty nursing organization for RNs practicing in ambulatory care settings, has defined the scope and standards of practice that provide a foundation for nurses engaging with individuals and families in the provision of care (AAACN, 2017c).

"Across the continuum of care, ambulatory care RNs work independently and collaboratively, partnering with patients, caregivers, providers, and other healthcare professionals in the design and provision of care in an ever-expanding array of settings" (AAACN, 2017a, p. 1). Ambulatory care RNs, functioning within expanded roles, are well positioned to collaborate in redefined interprofessional relationships and to design and deliver care that is inclusive of individual and family values, goals, and preferences (AAACN, 2017a). These roles include responsibility for (1) engaging individuals in self-care management, (2) coordinating care with individuals and families among increasingly diverse and complex populations, and (3) navigating transitions of care and healthcare encounters that range from simple to highly complex.

Scope and Standards of Practice

The AAACN's evidence-based standards support effective leadership and clinical management of ambulatory care RNs practicing in increasingly complex environments and executing roles and responsibilities within a constantly evolving healthcare environment. "Ambulatory care RNs, acting as partners, advocates, and advisors, assist and support patients/families in the optimal management of their healthcare, respecting their culture and values, individual needs, health goals, and treatment preferences" (AAACN, 2017c, p. 6). Each standard for ambulatory professional nursing practice defines the scope and standards of practice for ambulatory care RNs regardless of organizational practice settings. Ambulatory care RNs partner with individuals, families, and caregivers; other healthcare professionals; a variety of community-based agencies; and lead interprofessional teams. Associated competencies for the ambulatory care RN, as well as additional competencies for nurse executives, administrators, and managers can be found in the *Scope and Standards of Practice for Professional Ambulatory Care Nursing* (2017c) publication. A subset of standards and competencies particularly applicable to engaging individuals and families is highlighted in Table 7.2.

TABLE 7.2 AMBULATORY CARE NURSING STANDARDS AND COMPETENCIES FOR INDIVIDUAL AND FAMILY ENGAGEMENT

Standard	Competencies
1. Assessment	• "Establish a therapeutic rapport with patient and caregivers as well as determine patient's perception of his or her immediate needs and concerns. • Identify barriers to providing optimal care (e.g., language, culture, and behavioral health issues). • Prioritize data collection activities based on the patient's, groups, or population's immediate health need or the nurse's clinical expertise of anticipated patient needs. • Prioritize the data and information collected based on the patient's or population's condition and preferences, situation, and/or anticipated needs." (AAACN, 2017c, p. 21)
2. Diagnosis	• Identify, state, and "validate the diagnoses and/or issues with the patient, caregivers, and other members of the interprofessional healthcare team when appropriate. • Prioritize the diagnoses based on the patient's condition, expectations and preferences, situation, cultural and age-specific considerations, and/or anticipated needs." (AAACN, 2017c, p. 22)
3. Outcomes Identification	• "Involve the patient, family, and healthcare team in formulating measurable expected outcomes. • Define expected outcomes in terms of the patient values, preferences, spiritual, emotional, cultural and ethical considerations, age-related issues and situational environment. • Specify a time estimate for attainment of measurable expected outcomes. • Modify measurable expected outcomes based on changes in the status of the patient or reevaluation of the plan of care." (AAACN, 2017c, p. 23)
4. Planning	• "Develop an individualized ambulatory care nursing plan for patients seeking care for health promotion, health maintenance, or health-related problems. • Include the patient, family or caregivers as appropriate and the healthcare team in making shared decisions about prioritizing plans and strategies. • Consider the economic impact of the plan on patient and family resources." (AAACN, 2017c, p. 24)
5. Implementation	• "Prioritize interventions based on the patient's health status, preferences, resources, motivation, and anticipated needs. • Provide age-appropriate, population-specific care in a compassionate, holistic, culturally and ethically sensitive manner, with a focus on the patient's communication preferences. • Advocate for the health needs of individuals and diverse populations across the lifespan and the continuum of care." (AAACN, 2017c, p. 25)
5a. Coordinating Care	• "Facilitate patients' and/or populations' progress toward positive person-centered clinical outcomes. • Utilize an interprofessional approach to engage patient, caregivers, and providers in implementing the plan of care across care settings. • Educate and activate patient and caregivers for optimal disease management by promoting healthy lifestyle changes in the prevention of illness across population(s)." (AAACN, 2017c, p. 26)
5b. Health Teaching and Health Promotion	• "Assess a group or patient's learning needs, abilities, readiness, preferences, and barriers to learning. • Utilize health teaching and health-promotion strategies which support the patient's learning needs, values, preferred language, socioeconomic status, cultural, and spiritual preferences. • Continuously evaluate learner comprehension and effectiveness of teaching strategies and nursing interventions based on feedback from patient, caregivers, and healthcare team." (AAACN, 2017c, p. 27)

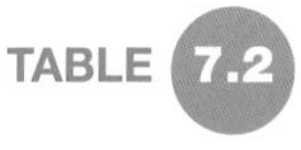

AMBULATORY CARE NURSING STANDARDS AND COMPETENCIES FOR INDIVIDUAL AND FAMILY ENGAGEMENT (CONTINUED)

Standard	Competencies
5c. Telehealth Services	• "Utilize current and evolving electronic information and telecommunication technologies to minimize time and distance barriers for the delivery of nursing care. • Coordinate interprofessional services across the care continuum." (AAACN, 2017c, p. 29)
6. Evaluation	• "Include patient, caregivers, and all others involved in the care of the patient in the evaluation process. • Consider patient and family values, preferences, socio-economic, political, religious, cultural, and environmental factors in evaluating the expected outcomes of the plan of care." (AAACN, 2017c, p. 30)

Note. American Academy of Ambulatory Care Nursing. (2017). In C. Murray (Ed.), *Scope and standards of practice for professional ambulatory care nursing* (9th ed.). Author. Used with permission of American Academy of Ambulatory Care Nursing (AAACN), aaacn.org

Defining Individual and Family Engagement

For decades, nursing has focused on individual and family-centered care as a model of care delivery, leading interprofessional healthcare teams and providing education and culturally sensitive care (Pelletier & Stichler, 2013). Increasingly, individual and family engagement has been linked to better quality healthcare, more efficient and effective provision of care, improved population health, improved provider and individual satisfaction with care delivery experiences, and decreased healthcare costs (Greene et al., 2015; Krist et al., 2017; Sofaer & Schumann, 2013). Definitions of individual and family engagement and the conceptualization of how it contributes to healthcare vary. A sample of definitions and concepts highlighting both the variation and commonality of concepts may be found in Appendix 7.1 (see pp. 144–145).

Engagement can range from consultation to partnership and can

> occur across the healthcare system, from the direct care setting to incorporating patient engagement into organizational design, governance, and policy making, with the term *patient engagement* used for simplicity but synonymous with those who engage and are engaged: patients, families, caregivers, and other consumers and citizens. (Carman et al., 2013, p. 224)

Perspectives around individual and family engagement require that all nurses—and, in particular, ambulatory care nurses working across diverse settings of care—understand that values, cultural context, preferences, goals, potential contributions, social determinants of health, and unique health profiles are central to person-centered care with individuals as active decision-makers in the design of their own care (Sofaer & Schumann, 2013). To assist in understanding the complexity of individual and family engagement, the contexts within which it occurs, and the identification and impact of influential factors, a conceptual framework has been developed and applied to practice.

Framework for Individual and Family Engagement

In 2013, Carman and colleagues proposed a conceptual framework, with an updated approach by Carman and Workman (2017), to include the involvement of individual and consumer engagement in the design, planning, interpretation, and dissemination of research findings as they relate to engagement. A myriad of definitions for individual and family engagement currently exist and are shared elsewhere in this chapter. However, for the purpose of describing the conceptual framework, individual and family engagement is defined as "patients, families, their representatives, and health professionals working in active partnership at various levels across the health system—direct care, organizational design and governance, and policy making—to improve health and healthcare" (Carman & Workman, 2017, p. 25). Development of collaborative partnerships between individuals, families, consumers, and healthcare professionals is the focal point and ultimate objective of engagement (Carman & Workman, 2017). These partnerships should ultimately lead to improved outcomes through efficient and effective care management strategies and interventions, appropriate and timely use of limited societal and individual resources, as well as an improvement in the overall population health.

The foundational framework's principles reveal that engagement takes place along a continuum, from direct care settings to larger organizational systems, influencing healthcare policy development. The framework posits that individuals and healthcare professionals share responsibility, in full partnership, to achieve safe, high-quality, efficient, and person-centered care (Carman & Workman, 2017). The intent of the framework is to present the various forms that individual engagement can demonstrate in the evolution from consultation to partnership through shared leadership and decision-making. Figure 7.1 represents a continuum of engagement activities, different levels at which engagement occurs, and factors that affect an individual's willingness and ability to engage (Carman et al., 2013; Carman & Workman, 2017).

The framework highlights three primary implications for developing interventions that promote individual and family engagement:

1. The continuum of engagement helps characterize the extent to which patients are involved in decision-making.
2. This framework underscores the possibility that a greater impact could be achieved by implementing interventions across multiple levels of engagement.
3. Interventions can be designed to address the factors that influence patient engagement. (Carman et al., 2013, p. 227)

Robust measures are also needed to monitor and link engagement interventions and participation to improved individual clinical outcomes, which include assessing an individual's interest and capacity for engagement. Ambulatory nurses are uniquely positioned to influence individual and family engagement through care management activities that occur across the continuum of care.

Levels of Engagement

Individual engagement occurs across a continuum, characterized by the flow of information between the individual and their provider, the individual's level of participation in care decisions, as well as how involved the individual or organization is in policy making or decisions made by healthcare systems (Carman et al., 2013). At the lower end of the continuum, individuals have constrained decision-making authority and may also have limited input into the plan of care. Information typically flows to the individual from providers, healthcare organizations, and systems and may or may not include individual input flowing to the patients and back to the system. Shared power and responsibility, with individuals as active participants in care decisions, occurs at the higher end of the continuum, with bidirectional communication and shared decision-making occurring throughout. At the partnership end of the continuum, individuals have direct access to their medical records, with the record reflecting the perspectives of both the individual and clinical providers in shared decisions made collaboratively with all relevant information included (Carman et al., 2013). Although it may sound ideal to always engage individuals and clinician perspectives collaboratively in shared decision-making, it may not always be appropriate based on the unique circumstances of an individual. However, striving for engagement and inclusion of individuals and families in shared decision-making ensures that individual values, goals, and preferences are honored in care delivery design.

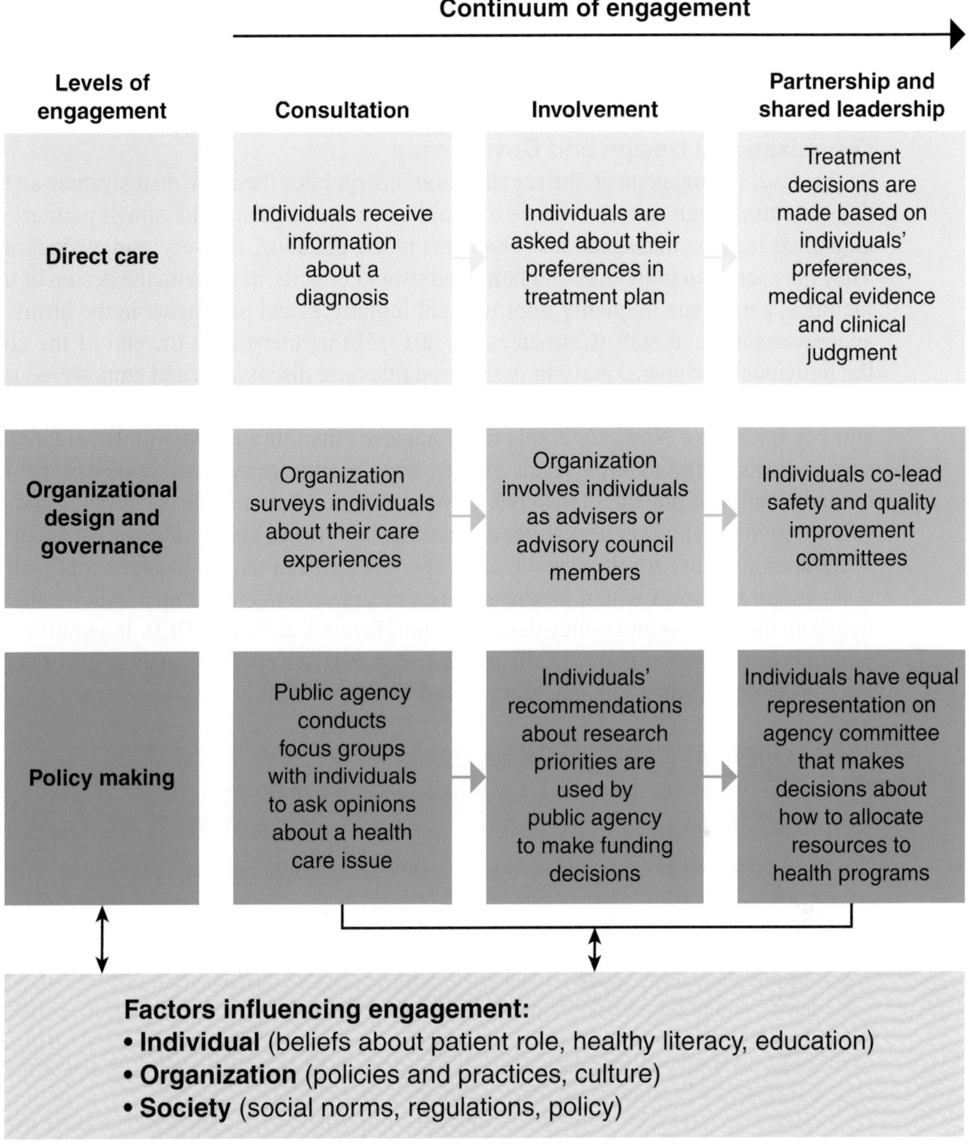

FIGURE 7.1 Continuum of engagement. From Carman, K. L., & Workman, T. A. (2017). Engaging patients and consumers in research evidence: Applying the conceptual model of patient and family engagement. *Patient Education and Counseling*, *100*, 25–29.

Direct Care

At the direct care level, engagement does not have to involve clinicians but could include an individual engaging in groups and health-related community-based resources, seeking information about health-related conditions and treatments, and participating in self-management support groups (Carman et al., 2013). More advanced involvement moves the individual from simply being the recipient of information to actively participating as a member of the health-care team. This enhanced involvement includes setting goals, making decisions, and proactively managing health using timely, complete, and understandable information. Decisions will incorporate the individual's values, beliefs, and preferences while evaluating risk tolerance in order to make fully informed treatment decisions (Carman et al., 2013). An example might be that an individual could go online to explore treatment options, the risks and benefits of various treatments, and associated clinical and quality-of-life considerations. Armed with the new knowledge, the individual might further discuss important considerations with their family and provider and ultimately decide on a treatment approach that considers the individual and family life circumstances, values, preferences, goals, and risk tolerance for adverse outcomes (Carman et al., 2013).

Organizational Design and Governance

At this level of engagement, the organization incorporates the individual's values and perspectives into the design and governance of healthcare organizations. Individuals partner with organizational leaders, managers, and clinicians in the planning, delivery, and evaluation of care. They may serve on individual and family advisory councils, assist with the design of healthcare facilities, participate in quality improvement initiatives, and participate in the hiring, training, and development of staff (Carman et al., 2013). In partnership at the end of the continuum, the individual is engaged early in design and planning discussions and empowered to develop agendas, set priorities, and have shared decision-making authority to guide the organization and key initiatives. Nowhere is this more apparent than through the implementation of advisory councils across multiple levels of care: large healthcare systems, acute care facilities, and outpatient clinical practices (Haycock & Wahl, 2013). Many healthcare systems and providers still question the appropriateness of empowering individuals and families as equal partners who share accountability for their health and experience within the healthcare system. However, it is no longer the norm within progressive healthcare systems to exclude individuals and families from discussions and policy development (Haycock & Wahl, 2013). Integrating individual preferences is foundational to healthcare delivery. Box 7.1 provides an example of components for consideration when implementing an individual and family advisory council.

BOX 7.1 Components for Launching an Individual and Family Advisory Council

- Develop an evidence-based introduction/background/rationale for establishing an advisory council
- Conduct an organizational analysis to include opportunities for inclusion of individuals and families in existing structures: committees, task forces, internal boards
- Perform a feasibility study for launching a formal advisory council
- Identify and prioritize opportunities for integration based on likelihood of successful adaptation and acceptance
- Create an implementation guide
  - Sample policy and procedure for the advisory council
  - Outline leadership strategies for hospital, provider, and community leaders as representative members of the council
  - Develop a council orientation guide
- Outline measure of success
  - Goals
  - Structure, process, outcome measures
  - Define interval and frequency for reporting
- Develop a communication strategy, talking points templates, newsletter templates, reporting templates and plan, with messaging that targets key stakeholders
- Develop a recruitment strategy and plan that includes identifying key attributes and characteristics of council members and create recruiting materials
- Create an orientation manual that includes roles, responsibilities, and expectations
- Design a council charter to define goals and objectives, with a timeline for achieving deliverables

Note. Adapted from Haycock, C., & Wahl, C. (2013). Achieving patient and family engagement through the implementation and evolution of advisory councils across a large healthcare system. *Nursing Administration Quarterly, 37*(3), 242–246. https:/doi.org/10.1097/NAQ.0b013e318295f54c

Policy Making

Individuals collaborate with leaders and policy makers through the development, implementation, and evaluation of local, state, and national healthcare policy and programs (Carman et al., 2013). At the advanced end of the continuum, individuals partner to set priorities, develop policy, and make program decisions. Federal advisory committees often include consumer representatives to contribute to recommendations on policies that promote adaptation of programs or technologies, especially when they pertain to individual and family engagement.

Factors That Influence Engagement

Understanding what factors influence individual and consumer engagement can lead to identifying strategies that are effective in enabling meaningful partnerships between individuals and healthcare providers to improve individual health outcomes and the healthcare system as a whole (Carman & Workman, 2017).

The Individual

Factors unique to individuals that can influence their ability to engage as partners in healthcare delivery and self-management include motivation; willingness and ability to engage across settings of care and levels of organizations; knowledge, skills, attitudes, culture, and personal beliefs; and **health literacy**, mental, and functional status. Individuals from vulnerable populations, such as older adults or those with limited English proficiency, of lower socioeconomic status, or who are declining cognitively can be exceptionally challenging to engage.

The Organization

Organizational characteristics and polices can directly influence an individual's ability to engage as advisors, participants in quality initiatives, and in individual and family-centered councils. For example, organizations survey recipients of care about their care experience and involve individuals in advisory councils that develop action plans to address survey responses. In addition, recipients of care are coleading quality and safety improvement committees.

Society

Organizations and individuals operate within a broad social and political context that is influenced by social norms, payers, regulators, and national, state, and local policies (Carman et al., 2013). In addition, community and social norms directly influence an individual's confidence in the ability to contribute to their care, how they interact with the organizations and individuals that care for them, and whether they can contribute to or influence insurance coverage benefit design and policy development and application.

Person- and Family-Centered Care

Pelletier and Stichler (2013) define person- and family-centered care

> as care that is (1) considerate and respectful of patients' beliefs, values, and personal meanings associated with their state of wellness or illness; (2) inclusive of patients' personal and social support systems; (3) delivered in the context of a caring, therapeutic partnership between patient and provider; (4) integrated and coordinated across a continuum of services, providers, and settings; (5) empowering with the education, information, and evidence necessary to enable and engage patients in their own healthcare; and (6) activating by facilitating patients' use of internal and external resources to manage their own care. (p. 52)

Empowerment

Empowerment authorizes individuals to receive access to education, information, and support and to develop skills that enable them to participate in full partnership with healthcare and service providers in decision-making and actions impacting their healthcare. Individual empowerment and engagement are foundational in leading to **activation** and participation in decision-making and self-care management (Krist, 2017).

Engagement

Engagement has become a major focus and an increasingly important component of healthcare reform strategies, contributing to growing evidence that improved health outcomes, improved satisfaction with the care experience, clinician satisfaction, and lower costs are associated with increased engagement (Greene et al., 2015; Hibbard & Greene, 2013; Krist et al., 2017). Emphasis on increased individual engagement is a departure from historically paternalistic models of care in which providers tell individuals what should be done. Increased engagement involves partnering with individuals to make healthcare decisions, providing education on managing health conditions, and developing systems to support, activate, and sustain individual participation in ongoing care. The need for engagement is fundamental, as most adults do not spend time in healthcare facilities, are often on their own to make appropriate healthcare decisions, and ultimately have responsibility for chronic disease management and health behavior change (Krist et al., 2017). Furthermore, individual engagement has "a) an ethical basis, supporting patient autonomy, b) interpersonal basis, promoting confidence and trust in the individual-provider relationship, and c) educational basis, improving knowledge, setting reasonable expectations, and reducing decisional conflict" (Krist et al., 2017).

Improved health outcomes have been noted when individuals are effectively engaged in self-management, including "reduction of decisional conflict; improved treatment adherence to asthma pharmacology; improved likelihood of receiving guideline-concordant depression care and improved symptoms; improved confidence in dealing with breathing problems and clinical care for patients with COPD" (Grande et al., 2014, p. 282). Despite evidence that supports success, most methods have failed implementation in routine, real-world clinical settings. Workload pressures, including provider perception of lack of time during clinical encounters, as well as limited application of engagement methods and the complexity of healthcare organizational systems, have contributed as barriers to implementation of engagement strategies. Table 7.3 outlines the benefits and barriers to engagement.

To support the feasibility of implementing individual engagement methodologies, Grande and colleagues described how using a classification system of engagement, tools or strategies can be applied as part of the clinical workflow and support individuals as involved partners in their care and decision-making activities (Grande et al., 2014). This classification model of individual engagement methods and assessment of feasibility categorizes methods based on the provision of information, individual activation, and individual–provider collaboration. High and low feasibility of implementation in clinical settings is considered, along with the extent of extra work required by the individual, provider, or clinical system. Successful implementation of methods is highly dependent on the ability to integrate their use with existing workflows that require proportional work to be completed by the individual.

Categories that illustrate increasing levels of activation and collaboration include:

- Passive information provision—unidirectional sharing of information such as educational booklets, one-page leaflets, web-based content, videos, and the electronic medical record to passively transmit information to the individual;
- Information and activation—individuals are prompted, coached, encouraged, and supported to perform specific engagement behaviors during the clinical encounter, including

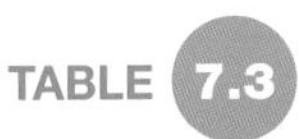

BENEFITS AND BARRIERS TO INDIVIDUAL ENGAGEMENT

Barriers	Benefits
Individual Barriers • Personal and professional commitments • Lack of time and resources to allow for individual participation • Health status and self-confidence • Time to manage diagnosis/clinical condition • Lack of financial resources • Inability to appreciate potential for personal benefit • Participation fatigue • Difficulty in coordinating personal/work schedule to allow for participation	Individual Benefits • Improved communications • Improved understanding of health services • Commitment to contribute • Empowerment and valued for skills and expertise • Ability to network with others with similar challenges and diseases
Providers Barriers • Negative attitude toward individual involvement • Lack knowledge of possibility of individual involvement • Dismissive of value of individuals' contributions, not forthcoming with resources/information • Unable/unwilling to explain complex terminology • Threatened by potential reduction of influence and change in traditional models of medical care delivery • Impact on individual/provider relationships • Reluctant to relinquishing power	Provider Benefits • Builds trust and improves communication between individuals and clinical staff • Incorporates information around patient experience, informing planning and service improvement • Supports provision of accessible and responsive services based on local resources and individual needs • Enhances individual confidence in the healthcare system
Leader/Institutional Barriers • Negative attitudes around individual involvement • Lack of knowledge/understanding of how to involve individuals and lack of training/guidance for professionals partnering with individuals • Leadership may be questioned	Leader/Institutional Benefits • More appropriate, higher quality, and relevant services • Services provided are responsive to individual needs • Policy, research, practice, and individuals' information includes input from consumers and their ideas and concerns

Note. Adapted from Burns, K. K., Bellows, M., Eigenseher, C., & Gallivan, J. (2014). "Practical" resources to support patients and family engagement in healthcare decisions: A scoping review. *BioMed Central Health Services Research, 14*(175), 1–15.

methods focused on enhancing communication skills, tools for formulating questions in advance, and developing confidence to participate in the clinical encounter;

- Information, activation, and collaboration—fosters the individual–provider relationship, building upon previous categories and methods, with the addition of collaboration using decision support tools (Decision Boxes, Option Grids, Issue Cards) to facilitate communication and foster shared decision-making (Elwyn et al., 2012; Giguere et al., 2012; Grande et al., 2014).

Table 7.4 further describes the feasibility of methods of individual engagement framed within the classification categories and includes delivery mediums or methods, resource descriptions, level of work required, and overall feasibility for use.

The term *engagement* is sometimes used synonymously with activation and person- and family-centered care. Although these concepts are related, they are not identical. Individual engagement is a broader concept that encompasses activation and an individual's resulting

TABLE 7.4 FEASIBILITY OF METHODS OF INDIVIDUAL ENGAGEMENT

Classification	Delivery Medium and/or Method	Description	Patient Work Required?	Additional Human Resources Required?	Fit Within Existing System?	Overall Feasibility?
Passive information provision	Text-based information	A document with either general or specific health-related information (any media)	Variable	No	Good	High
	Audiovisual information	Audiovisual information describing, teaching, or demonstrating	Variable	No	Good	High
	Combination text based and audiovisual information	Multifaceted information to read, view, and practice	High	Variable	Poor	Low
Information + activation	Text-based prompts to action	List of questions prepare patients, give feedback to provider	Low	Yes	Good	High
	Human interaction	Consultation with professional previsit	Moderate	Yes	Fair	Low
	Human interaction and text-based prompts to action	Consultation with professional previsit, prepare questions for visit, feedback to provider	High	Yes	Poor	Low
	Text-based information and human interaction	A document with either general or specific health-related information (any media) completed with assistance by a professional previsit	High	Yes	Fair	Low
Information + activation + collaboration	Point-of-care engagement tools	Tools/methods focused on supporting, creating, and maintaining collaboration within the clinical encounter; may be designed for multiple points of engagement and allow for patient and provider input	Moderate	No	Good	High

Note. Grande, S. W., Faber, M. J., Durand, M., Thompson, R., & Elwyn, G. (2014). A classification model of patient engagement methods and assessment of their feasibility in real-world settings. *Patient Education and Counseling, 95*, 281–287.

behavior. Focusing on engagement and activation instead of compliance—emphasis on following health advice versus individual self-management—recognizes that individuals make decisions daily to manage their own health, affecting their health outcomes and impacting costs (Hibbard & Greene, 2013).

Activation

Individual activation is defined as "understanding one's role in care processes and having the knowledge, skills, and individual's knowledge, and confidence to manage one's health and healthcare" (Hibbard & Greene, 2013, p. 207). In 2005, the short form of the Patient Activation Measure (PAM) was refined and validated as a reliable instrument to measure an individual's knowledge, self-management skills, and confidence in health and healthcare management decision-making (Hibbard et al., 2005). Well-researched and validated, PAM has demonstrated applicability across different cultures, languages, demographic groups, and populations of individuals with differing health status and is the most commonly used metric for quantifying individual engagement, activation, and self-care management abilities (Greene et al., 2015; Hibbard & Green, 2013). PAM is considered a "latent construct," meaning the variable cannot be measured directly but is assessed through a series of questions that link to an individual's perception of self as a manager of their own health and healthcare (Hibbard & Greene, 2013). The PAM tool is scored using a range from 0 to 100, with results falling into one of four levels of engagement where level one is the least activated and level four the most activated. Each engagement level is predictive of varied individual health behaviors and can be used to target healthcare interventions (Greene et al., 2015; Hibbard & Greene, 2013; Hibbard et al., 2009). Table 7.5 provides a detailed description of each level of activation.

The construct of activation is not condition specific and is broader than the concepts of self-efficacy, readiness to change, and locus of control that focus on changing one specific behavior. Activation is associated instead with a wider range of outcomes (Greene et al., 2015). Individuals who are more activated, as assessed by PAM, more effectively use healthcare services and resources, as well as engage in more positive health behaviors as compared to those who have not been assigned an activation level (Hibbard & Greene, 2013). Examples include the following:

- Individuals with higher levels of activation are more likely to have established relationships with healthcare providers and regularly and appropriately access care; are twice as likely to prepare questions prior to an encounter with a provider, understanding treatment guidelines for their condition; participate in preventive care; engage in healthy behaviors

TABLE 7.5 PATIENT ACTIVATION MEASURE LEVELS OF ACTIVATION

Level 1	Individuals tend to be passive, lack knowledge and confidence in managing their own health. They may not understand their role in the care process and prefer the doctor take charge of managing their health.
Level 2	Individuals have some knowledge but large gaps remain. They can set simple goals toward achieving health but require significant coaching.
Level 3	Individuals have knowledge of health needs and are self-managing. They are goal oriented and participate with the healthcare team with minimal coaching.
Level 4	Individuals have acquired knowledge and are motivated to self-manage. They demonstrate many of the behaviors needed to support their health acting as their own advocate. May need coaching and support in times of stress or change.

Note. Adapted from Hibbard, J. H., & Gilbert, H. (2014). *Supporting people to manage their health: An introduction to patient activation*. The Kings Fund. http://www.kingsfund.org.uk/sites/files/kf/field/field_publication_file/supporting-people-manage-health-patient-activation-may14.pdf such as maintaining a healthy diet and regular exercise; do not experience delays in care; and report more positive care experiences (Greene et al., 2015; Hibbard & Green, 2013).

- Less activated individuals have low confidence in their ability to manage their health and often feel overwhelmed with the task(s).
- Individuals who are less activated are three times more likely to have unmet healthcare needs and twice as likely to delay seeking medical care, are less likely to ask questions during medical encounters, do not independently seek out health information or guidelines specific to their medical condition, are more likely to engage in health-damaging behaviors such as smoking and illicit drug use, and are twice as likely to be readmitted to the hospital within 30 days of discharge (Greene et al., 2015; Hibbard & Green, 2013).
- Individuals with chronic health conditions who are at a higher level of activation are more likely than those at lower activation levels to participate in the development of and adherence to treatment plans; obtain regular chronic care, such as lab monitoring and disease-specific testing and screening; and perform regular self-monitoring (Greene et al., 2015; Hibbard & Green, 2013).

Research findings demonstrate that an individual's activation level or self-management capability, when controlling for baseline chronic disease status, is predictive of future disease progression and burden, as well as predictive of costly care utilization that could be avoided (Hibbard et al., 2017). A growing volume of interventional studies are providing evidence that individual activation is changeable and can be modified over time, progressing to increased activation levels using specific interventions (Greene et al., 2015; Hibbard & Greene, 2013; Shane-McWhorter et al., 2015; Shively et al., 2013). In addition, a recently conducted longitudinal study demonstrated that directional changes in PAM scores were associated with improved clinical outcomes and costs (Greene et al., 2015). Table 7.6 lists examples of focused areas of interventions that have been shown to increase individual activation.

Finally, efficiencies can be gained through identifying individual behaviors or patterns of healthcare services utilization with appropriate, targeted interventions applied to individuals

TABLE 7.6 FOCUSED AREAS OF INTERVENTIONS LINKED TO INCREASED ACTIVATION LEVELS

Focused Area	Exemplars
Skill Development, Problem Solving, Peer Support	• Diabetes self-management program, using trained lay leaders in community settings, to facilitate workshops to educate and support chronically ill individuals in disease management, problem solving, improving provider communication and engaging in exercise (Lorig & Alvarez, 2011). • Skill developments in a safety-net clinic, such as question formulation, were shown to improve individual's skills, participation in care, and activation levels (Deen et al., 2011).
Changing the Social Environment	Interventions that seek to change the social environment such that individual's experience changes in beliefs, skills, and social norms and participate in healthy behaviors. • Health classes; work-based environmental changes; posters and informational campaigns; personal coaching for high-risk employees (Hibbard & Greene, 2013).
Tailoring Support to Individual's Activation Level	Encouraging less activated individuals to take actions where they are likely to succeed, using small incremental, manageable steps, while supporting more activated individuals to make substantial behavioral changes (Hibbard & Greene, 2013).

who are the most impactable—who offer the greatest opportunity for management and healthcare cost reduction (Hibbard et al., 2017). New opportunities exist to identify individuals at risk for poor outcomes early to support the ability to initiate early interventions. Innovative healthcare delivery systems are using PAM to individualize care and strengthen an individual's role in improving outcomes through tailored coaching, education, and skill building. These delivery systems are also making more efficient use of healthcare resources by providing more support to individuals with heavier disease burdens and those lacking self-management skills and less support for those with higher levels of activation and more developed skills (Hibbard & Greene, 2013). Understanding an individual's capability for self-management is key to preventing declining health, improving health outcomes, and avoiding unnecessary and preventable healthcare utilization.

Shared Decision-Making

At its core, shared decision-making is an interpersonal, interdependent process in which clinicians and individuals share the best available evidence, relating to, influencing, and supporting each other collaboratively to consider options in making decisions about the individual's healthcare (Elwyn et al., 2012; Legare & Wittman, 2013). Nurses practicing in ambulatory care settings, as well as clinicians and healthcare system leaders, must view consumers of healthcare as competent to make decisions about their own health and healthcare and worthy of the opportunity to become well-informed and supported in making decisions (Sofaer & Schumann, 2013).

Elwyn and colleagues (2012) outlined three key steps involved in shared decision-making: choice talk, option talk, and decision talk. *Choice talk* is the step taken to ensure that individuals understand that reasonable options are available. *Option talk* provides detailed information on treatment options available. *Decision talk* is the step that further explores what matters most to an individual and encompasses support for consideration of individual goals and preferences (Elwyn et al., 2012). Some healthcare decisions can be straightforward with one clear choice, but many vary in complexity with wide-ranging advantages and disadvantages to consider and discuss. In order for an individual to fully engage in discussions that center on treatment options, there is an inherent need for some level of patient health literacy. All decision steps in the process should be approached with attention to an individual's literacy needs and assess the individual's knowledge and understanding throughout the process (Krist et al., 2017). Common examples of healthcare decisions include whether and how to make a behavior change, when and how to start to get preventive screening, management of acute and chronic conditions, how to prioritize competing health needs, and when to change or stop a treatment (Krist et al., 2017). Circumstances that may prohibit individuals from engaging in shared decision-making may include poor health or functional status, low level of education, lack of financial resources, frail health, cognitive impairment, mental health issues, or language barriers. These factors should not prevent individuals or their designee from participating in shared decision-making (Sofaer & Schumann, 2013). It is important to recognize that an individual's capacity to engage may also change over time, as stages of illness progress. When individuals are unable to engage, the ambulatory care RN and others on the interprofessional care team use agents or trusted family members, empowered by the individual either formally or informally, to act on their behalf. Considerations, barriers, and benefits of engagement in shared decision-making can be found in Box 7.2.

Shared decision-making requires that ambulatory care RNs, providers, and the larger healthcare team possess specific knowledge, skills, and attitudes in order to effectively engage individuals and families. Individuals can play one of three roles in improving the quality of their care. In the *informed choice role*, individuals consider the quality of care as key for choosing providers, health plans, and hospitals. In the *coproducer role*, individuals assist

BOX 7.2 Considerations for Individual and Family Engagement

Effectively engaging individuals in their care is essential to improve health outcomes, improved satisfaction with care experience, reduce costs, and improved provider satisfaction (Krist, 2017).

Considerations

- Systems are required to better support individual engagement.
- How do social determinants of health influence individual engagement?
- Approaches that demonstrate how to better engage individuals in their health and well-being.
- Relationship between health literacy and individual engagement is particularly important for:
  - (1) Decision-making, (2) health behavior change, (3) chronic disease management

Benefits

- Participating patients have

  higher levels of satisfaction with their care; have increased knowledge about conditions, tests, treatment; have more realistic expectations about benefits and harms; are more likely to adhere to screening, diagnostic, or treatment plans; have reduced decisional conflict and anxiety; are less likely to receive unnecessary test and procedures which may be unnecessary (Krist et al., 2017, p. 107).

Strategies

- Ensure that engagement activities are appropriate to an individual's health literacy.
  - Adapting and simplifying language to reduce misunderstanding
  - Provide examples relevant to lifestyle and cultural context
  - Use visual media to represent data
  - Integrate decision aids
  - Presented in a manner that facilitates understanding of material that spans clinical settings where care is delivered—home, community, and clinical settings.

Barriers

- Time
- Expense
- Clinician training
- Perceived legitimacy
- Patient characteristics
  - Comfort with decision aids
- Clinical situations
  - Capacity
  - Ability to integrate into existing workflows

in achieving an improved health state by acting as effective partners with providers. In the *evaluator role*, individuals provide data on the performance of providers and systems, and participate in defining what constitutes quality care (Bernabeo & Holmboe, 2013). Providers must agree that individuals should be part of the decision-making process, and healthcare systems must move toward stronger support of interprofessional collaboration and teamwork that includes individuals and families, grounded in shared decision-making competencies. Table 7.7 describes competencies that are imperative to the success for engaging stakeholders in shared decision-making.

Historically, clinicians engage individuals and families in shared decision-making during in-person visits. Use of decision aids can be an extension of face-to-face clinical encounters and can aid in the support of the "decision journey" over time, allowing individuals to contemplate options, discuss with family, consider additional information, and address personal

TABLE 7.7 EXAMPLES OF INDIVIDUAL, PHYSICIAN, AND SYSTEM COMPETENCIES FOR SHARED DECISION-MAKING

Patient Competencies	Physician Competencies	System Competencies
Define the preferred doctor–patient relationship; find a physician and establish, develop, and adapt a partnership	Develop a partnership with the patient	Provide overarching support for physician's and patient's increased and timely access to patient-centered services
Articulate health problems, feelings, beliefs, and expectations in an objective and systematic manner	Establish or review the patient's preferences for information about his or her health or treatment plan	Restructure reimbursement schemes to provide sufficient time and incentive for physicians to counsel and engage patients
Share relevant information with the physician clearly and at the appropriate time in the medical interview	Establish or review the patient's preferred role in decision-making and any uncertainty about the course of action to take; ascertain and respond to the patient's ideas, concerns, and expectations	Create innovative models for redesigning care delivery in office settings to facilitate communication and optimize efficiency
Access information	Identify choices and evaluate the research evidence in relation to the individual patient	Implement new information systems to link patients with the best resources and decision aids available
Evaluate information	Present evidence, taking into account the patient's competencies, framing effects, etc.	Increase access to understandable information about risks and benefits of therapy and diagnostic procedures
Negotiate decisions with the physician, give feedback, resolve conflict, and agree on a care plan	Help the patient reflect on and assess the impact of alternative decisions with regard to his or her values and lifestyle; negotiate decisions with the patient, resolve conflict, agree on a care plan, and arrange for follow-up	Add professional staff to help patients achieve self-management and health literacy; implement interprofessional collaboration and teamwork; reward and acknowledge high levels of professionalism

Note. Adapted from Bernabeo, E., & Holmboe, E. S. (2013). Patients, providers, and systems need to acquire a specific set of competencies to achieve truly patient-centered care. *Health Affairs, 32*(2), 250–258. https:/doi.org/10.1377/hlthaff.2012.1120. Modified from Towle, A., & Godolphin, W. (1999). Framework for teaching and learning informed decision making. *British Medical Journal, 319*, 766–769.

concerns. Figure 7.2 outlines how specific variables might influence an individual as they seek information. Examples of how the ambulatory care RN might incorporate decision aids and facilitate shared decision-making into practice are listed in Box 7.3.

National Alliance for Quality Care (NAQC) Guiding Principles for Consumer Engagement

NAQC, an organization composed of 22 national nursing associations and consumer advocacy groups, published a white paper entitled *Fostering Successful Patient and Family Engagement: Nursing's Critical Role* with the charge to all nurses to commit to the effective engagement of individuals and families across all healthcare settings. Box 7.4 lists principal assumptions that serve to guide NAQC, care delivery providers, and other consumer stakeholders to ensure that all healthcare provided is person-centered. These guiding principles constitute a healthcare reform imperative, providing a basis for how nursing contributes to fostering effective engagement of consumers across healthcare settings (Sofaer & Schumann, 2013).

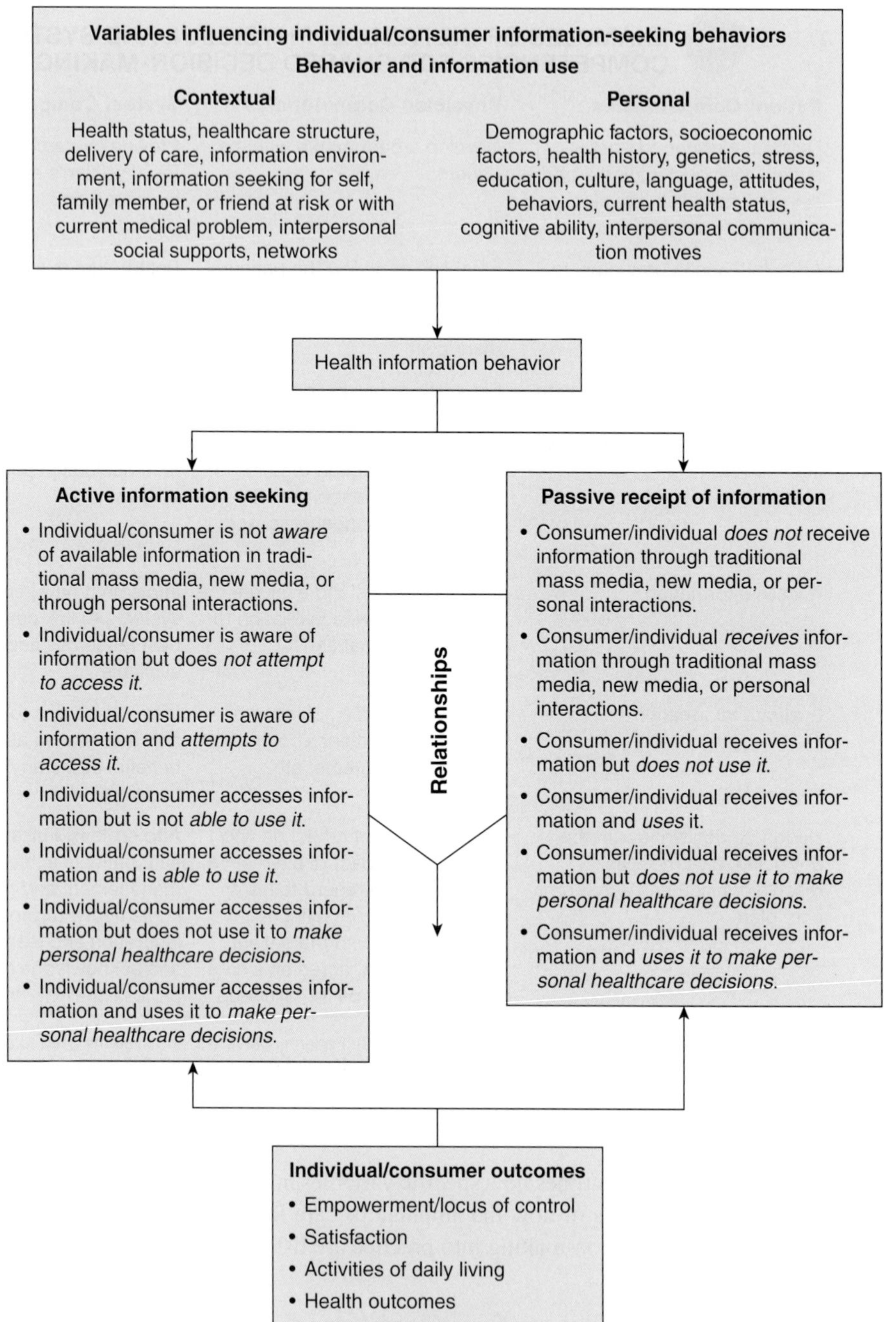

FIGURE 7.2 Model to describe patient's health information–seeking behaviors. (From Longo, D. R., Schubert, S. L., Wright, B. A., LeMaster, J., Williams, C. D., & Clore, J. N. [2010]. Health information seeking, receipt, and use in diabetes self-management. *Ann Fam Med, 8*[4], 334–340. Copyright ©2010 American Academy of Family Physicians. All Rights Reserved.)

BOX 7.3 Examples of How the Ambulatory Care RN Prepares Individuals for Shared Decision-Making

- Individuals with decision support needs can be identified using electronic medical record data and outreached outside of an office visit, using the patient portal, telephonically or face-to-face, RN to initiate consideration of decision options.
- Using the portal, telephone outreach of face-to-face, the RN assesses the individual's personal preferences, knowledge, needs, and readiness to make a decision.
- The RN provides additional sources of educational information using websites, videos, and various modalities to communicate with the individual: portal, the telephone, text, and mobile applications.
- The RN provides personalized educational material tailored to the individual's preferences and decision stage.
- The individual shares preferences and decision needs with clinician via portal or with the RN.
- The clinician prepares for the individual's office encounter by reviewing information and the individual's needs.
- A shared clinical decision is made jointly based on information.
- The RN follows up with both the clinician and individual to ensure that decisions acted upon are consistent with the individual's wishes.

Note. RN = registered nurse.

BOX 7.4 Guiding Principles for Consumer Engagement

Patient engagement is a critical cornerstone of patient safety and quality. The NAQC has grounded its approach to this topic by recognizing the primary importance of *relationships* between engaged patients and families and their clinicians, including but not limited to nurses. The following are principal assumptions that guide NAQC in addressing care that is patient-centered.

1. There must be an active partnership among patients, their families, and the providers of their healthcare.
2. Patients are the best and ultimate source of information about their health status and retain the right to make their own decisions about care.
3. In this relationship, there are shared responsibilities and accountabilities among the patient, the family, and clinicians that make it effective.
4. While embracing partnerships, clinicians must nevertheless respect the boundaries of privacy, competent decision-making, and ethical behavior in all their encounters and transactions with patients and families. These boundaries protect recipients as well as providers of care. This relationship is grounded in confidentiality, where the patient defines the scope of the confidentiality.
5. This relationship is grounded in an appreciation of patient's rights and expands on the rights to include mutuality. Mutuality includes sharing of information, creation of consensus, and shared decision-making.
6. Clinicians must recognize that the extent to which patients and family members are able to engage or choose to engage may vary greatly based on individual circumstances, cultural beliefs, and other factors.
7. Advocacy for patients who are unable to participate fully is a fundamental nursing role. Patient advocacy is the demonstration of how all of the components of the relationship fit together.
8. Acknowledgment and appreciation of culturally, racially, or ethnically diverse backgrounds is an essential part of the engagement process.
9. Healthcare literacy and linguistically appropriate interactions are essential for patient, family, and clinicians to understand the components of patient engagement. Providers must maintain awareness of the language needs and healthcare literacy level of the patient and family and respond accordingly.

Note. NAQC = National Alliance for Quality Care. Sofaer, S., & Schumann, M. J. (2013). *Fostering successful patient and family engagement: Nursing's critical role*. Nursing Alliance for Quality. http://www.naqc.org/WhitePaper-PatientEngagement

In order to successfully foster individual engagement in health and healthcare, the following conditions must be met:

- Nurses must practice a fully patient-centered approach to healthcare delivery;
- Nurses must embrace and support fully the belief that patients and families are or can become competent to engage fully in making informed decisions about their own health and healthcare; and,
- Nurses must be willing to fully support patients as they encounter obstacles in the healthcare system. (Sofaer & Schumann, 2013, p. 14)

Logic Models

Expanding upon the guiding principles and the conditions to be realized to successfully foster engagement, NAQC also created logic models to describe development of engagement strategies, behaviors, and outcomes, as well as to outline how to maximize the contributions of nurses to individual engagement.

Development and Outcomes for Patient Engagement

The first logic model, *Development and Outcomes for Patient Engagement*, is given in Table 7.8 and identifies engagement strategies, behaviors, and outcomes for successful

TABLE 7.8 DEVELOPMENT AND OUTCOMES OF PATIENT ENGAGEMENT

Engagement Strategies	Underlying Orientation to Engagement	Engagement Behaviors	Outcomes
Tailoring treatment plans to patient's level of activation Chronic disease self-management Shared decision-making Motivational interviewing Health coaching Family rounding Bedside change of shift Redesigned discharge protocols Information exchanges Decisions aids Public reporting of comparative performance information	Measured by the PAM Patient at the center of the decision-making process for his/her healthcare	Frameworks for observing behaviors Center for Advancing Health Framework—40+ behaviors in 10 areas, such as: • Find safe, decent care • Communicate with health professionals • Organize healthcare • Pay for healthcare • Make good treatment decisions • Participate in treatment • Promote health • Get preventive healthcare • Plan for the end of life • Seek health knowledge • Reduction of health risk behaviors • Self-management of preventive health strategies • Self-management of episodic illness	• Absence of harm as a result of care received • Improvements in health for patients/consumers of care • Improved biometrics • Improved functional status • Improved quality of life • Improved population health • Improved health risk behavior profile • Improved and safe work environments for healthcare professionals

Note. PAM = Patient Activation Measure. Sofaer, S., & Schumann, M. J. (2013). *Fostering successful patient and family engagement: Nursing's critical role.* Nursing Alliance for Quality. http://www.naqc.org/WhitePaper-PatientEngagement

engagement. The context for the model notes that healthcare providers and the healthcare team recognize that individuals are central to all decision-making; stipulates that individuals become increasingly well-informed about health and healthcare choices and consequences to making decisions; measures the individual's level of engagement by PAM; and asserts that based on the PAM activation level, strategies and interventions are individualized to support success.

Maximizing the Contributions of Nurses to Patient Engagement

The second logic model, *Maximizing the Contributions of Nurses to Patient Engagement*, given in Table 7.9, outlines six strategies, as well as tactics needed by nurses to influence and achieve the three conditions previously described. The model also addresses the need for changes in awareness and behaviors among nurses in order to achieve the proximate, intermediate, and longer-term outcomes outlined. These strategies, leveraged both nationally and locally, will support understanding of nursing's roles and responsibilities in fostering individual and family engagement (Sofaer & Schumann, 2013).

The following activities can be leveraged through work environments regardless of care settings to positively impact behaviors that foster engagement and lead to improved outcomes for individuals:

- Broad alignment of the organization's mission, vision, and values with patient-centered care;
- Inclusion to reflecting individual engagement practices in job descriptions, hiring, promotion, and clinical ladder criteria for all health professionals;
- Advocate for inclusion of language specifically requiring evidence of effective individual engagement as part of the Centers for Medicare and Medicaid Services "conditions of participation";
- Recognition of interventions that foster successful individual engagement, such as motivational interviewing (MI), health coaching, and shared decision-making, and incorporate interventions across primary care practices and consider financial incentives the support adaptation (Sofaer & Schumann, 2013).

Health Literacy

A critical step in engaging individuals and families in their care and shared decision-making is health literacy. The IOM report, *Implications of Health Literacy for Public Health: Workshop Summary*, defined health literacy as "the degree to which individuals have the capacity to obtain, process, and understand basic health information and services needed to make appropriate health decisions" (IOM, 2014, p. 1). According to the U.S. Department of Health and Human Services (2019), health literacy is dependent on both individual and system factors such as communication skills, knowledge of health topics, culture, and healthcare and public health system demands. Health literacy affects an individual and family's ability to share personal health information, navigate the healthcare system and locate and access needed services, engage in self-care and chronic disease management, as well as measure blood sugar, understand nutrition labels, measure medications, and negotiate healthcare coverage options (U.S. Department of Health and Human Services, 2019). Healthcare information can overwhelm individuals with advanced literacy skills as well as those who function at lower literacy levels and is further impacted by an individual's native language, cultural beliefs, values, attitudes, and traditions.

The Health Literate Care Model is a tool that incorporates health literacy principles into the Care Model, formally Wagner's Chronic Care Model, infusing literacy language into the foundational framework for cross-continuum care delivery (Koh et al., 2013). Figure 7.3 provides a visual, incorporating literacy principles within the framework.

TABLE 7.9 MAXIMIZING THE CONTRIBUTIONS OF NURSES TO PATIENT ENGAGEMENT

Domains of Strategy	Changes in Awareness of Nurses	Changes in Behaviors Among Nurses	Outcomes
Ensuring that all nursing education emphasizes patient engagement Amplifying the professional standing of nurses as champions of patient engagement Strengthening support for nurses as advocates in the care environment of patients Aligning incentives to encourage patient engagement Elevating regulatory expectations and standards that support patient engagement principles in practice Intensifying efforts to conduct and disseminate research on patient engagement	All nurses respect patient/consumer place at the center of healthcare decision-making and in accordance with principles of patient-centered care All nurses embrace the belief that patients and families are or can become competent to engage fully in making informed healthcare decisions All nurses recognize their own important role in supporting patients who are encountering obstacles in the healthcare system Nurses at front lines: • Recognize that patient goals, values, preference, cultural context, and particular circumstances must be incorporated into the care plan • Recognize that when the patient perspective is not being honored, they will need to be active as an advocate, preferably with rather than for the patient/family Nurses in managerial roles: • Recognize the impact of organizational structure and culture on the likelihood that engagement will be easy and well supported • Recognize the role of rewards and incentives in shaping an organization moving in the direction of fuller engagement Nurses in executive/policy roles: • Recognize the relationship of patient engagement to achieving Goals of National Quality Strategy • Recognize that they may need to lead transformation to achieve full engagement	**At the front lines:** • Listening • Speaking in the language of the patient/family (plain English, Spanish, etc.) • Using Motivational Interviewing and other methods of eliciting patient goals/values • Seeing the world from the "shoes" of the patient • Using key engagement strategies such as bedside and family rounds, bedside change of shift, shared decision-making • Incorporating patients into advisory committees and QI teams • Ensuring patient friendliness of information and technology; facilitating their use by patients • Ensuring authenticity of informed consent • Advocating effectively whenever necessary for the patient and family **In managerial, executive, and policy roles:** • Becoming a "champion" for patient engagement and shared decision-making • Building small "p" political support for engagement, including use of "business cases" • Analyzing barriers and facilitators of engagement from the nursing and patient perspectives • Advocating for needed reforms and research	**Proximate** • Increases in scores of nurses on the Clinical Support for Patient Activation Measure • Higher nurse work satisfaction, better assessments of work environment, nurse retention • Higher scores on Patient Activation Measure • Higher prevalence of CFAH "engagement behaviors" among patients/family • More self-management of chronic conditions • Greater use of evidence in treatment decision-making **Intermediate** • Improved patient experience of care scores • Increased professional standing of nursing • Supportive care environments where nurses advocate for patients **Longer term** • Improved quality and safety • Decreased/eliminated disparities in care and health across age, gender, race, ethnicity, etc. • Reduced overuse of unneeded tests and treatments • Increased use of evidence-based services • Lower costs • Improved population health

Note. QI = Quality Improvement; CFAH = Center for Advancing Health. Sofaer, S., & Schumann, M. J. (2013). *Fostering successful patient and family engagement*: Nursing's critical role. Nursing Alliance for Quality. http://www.naqc.org/WhitePaper-PatientEngagement

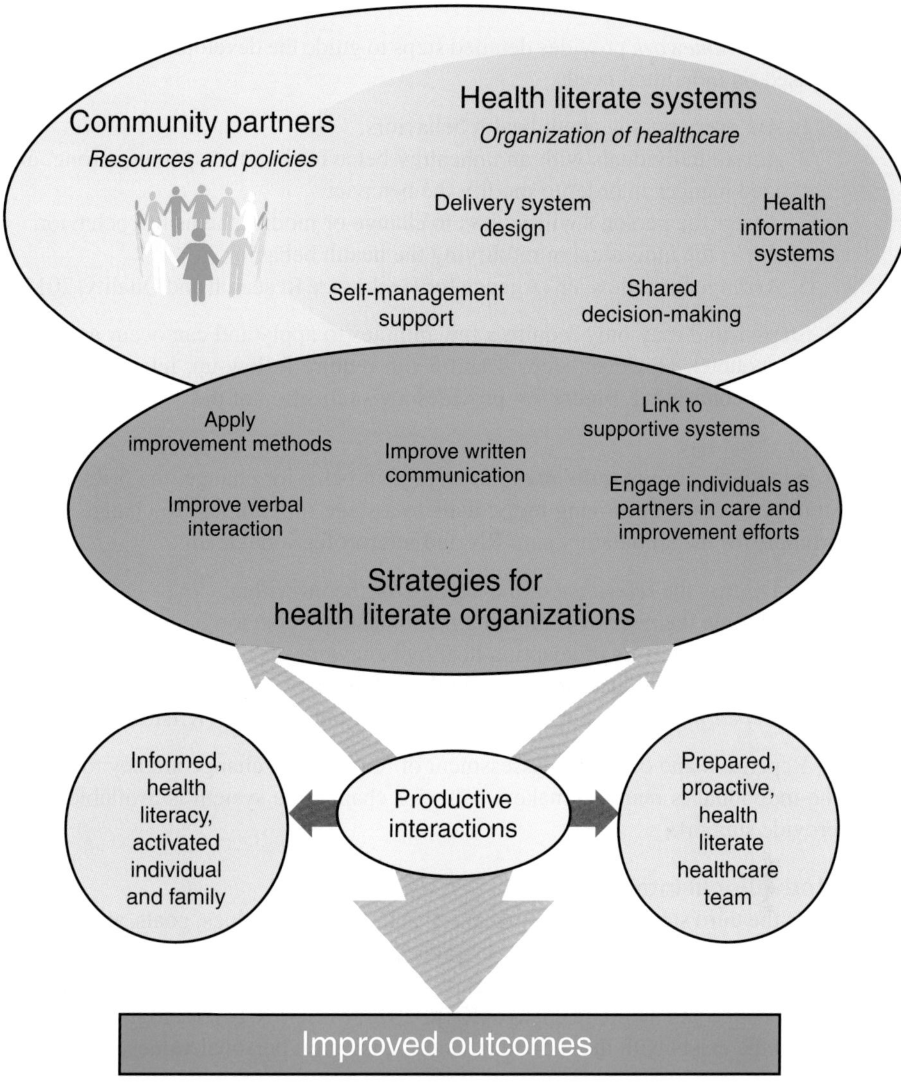

FIGURE 7.3 Health Literacy Care Model. (From Koh, H. K., Brach, C. M., Harris, L. M., & Parchman, M. L. [2013]. A proposed "health literacy care model" would constitute a systems approach to improving patients' engagement in care. *Health Affairs* [*Millwood*], *32*[2], 357–367. https:/doi .org/10.1377/hlthaff.2012.1205)

The Health Literacy Care Model seeks to encourage clinicians to approach all individuals as being at risk for not understanding their healthcare condition(s), treatment options, and role in managing their chronic disease(s), as well as confirming and ensuring individuals' understanding with a focus on enhancing health literacy through assisting individuals in making appropriate health decisions and improving processes that contribute to the quality of care (Krist et al., 2017).

Strategies, Tools, and Methods for Behavior Change

In support of the framework previously shared, core strategies, tools, and methods facilitate successful engagement. Strategies include the 5 As, the 5 Rs, and MI, all of which require the healthcare team to elicit an individual's readiness to change in order to incorporate reasons to change as part of the plan to influence behavior change.

5 As Framework

The *5 As Framework* provides detailed steps to guide the development of interventions that are focused on individual needs.

1. *Ask* every person about health behaviors.
2. *Advise* individuals with an unhealthy behavior in a transparent, strong, and individualized manner in order to modify the behavior.
3. *Assess* the person's willingness to change or modify the health behavior.
4. *Assist* the individual in modifying the health behavior.
5. *Arrange* for follow-up (Agency for Healthcare Research and Quality, 2012; Krist, 2017).

Steps 1 to 3 may only require a few minutes to apply and can occur as part of one healthcare encounter. However, steps 4 and 5 can require follow-up, intensive support, as well as extended counseling. Figure 7.4 provides a visualization of the 5 As Framework.

5 Rs Strategy

If individuals are not quite ready to engage in behavior change, the 5 Rs can be an effective strategy to assist in moving individuals to a stage of readiness to change. The 5 Rs serve as prompts for the ambulatory care RN and interprofessional team to:

1. Discuss the *relevance* of the change for the individual.
2. Outline the *risks* of continuing the unhealthy behavior.
3. List the *rewards* of adapting healthy behavior.
4. Identify *roadblocks* to changing the behavior.
5. *Repeating* the personalized 5 Rs message at each visit (Krist, 2017).

Repetition and continued assessment of readiness to change are key to ensuring that when the individual is ready to make a behavior change the system is available and positioned to provide support.

Motivational Interviewing

MI is the third strategy that incorporates an individual's values, goals, and preferences in order to influence and initiate behavior change. This person-centered, collaborative approach seeks to harness intrinsic motivation to explore ambivalence and strengthen motivation to resolve ambivalence and facilitate change (Krist, 2017; Miller, 2016). Recognizing that the true power of change exists with the individual and focusing on personal values, goals, and preferences,

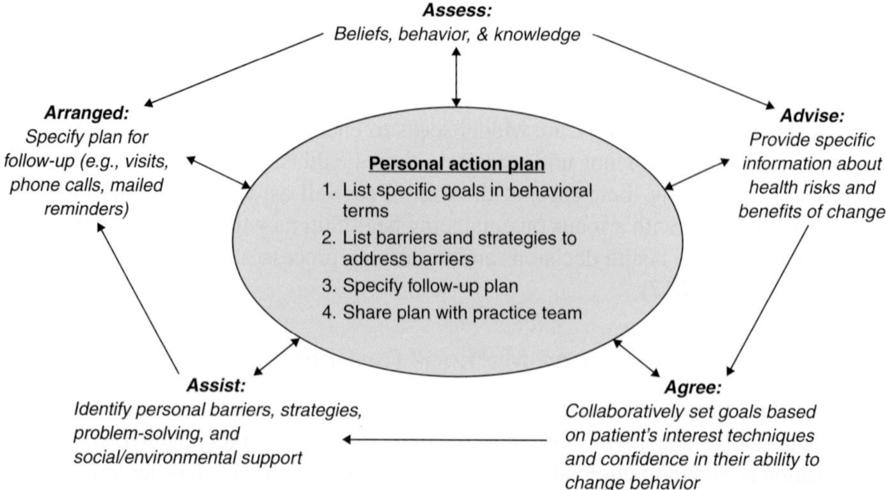
Assess:
Beliefs, behavior, & knowledge
Arranged:
Specify plan for follow-up (e.g., visits, phone calls, mailed reminders)
Advise:
Provide specific information about health risks and benefits of change
Personal action plan
1. List specific goals in behavioral terms
2. List barriers and strategies to address barriers
3. Specify follow-up plan
4. Share plan with practice team
Assist:
Identify personal barriers, strategies, problem-solving, and social/environmental support
Agree:
Collaboratively set goals based on patient's interest techniques and confidence in their ability to change behavior

FIGURE 7.4 5 As behavior change model. (Adapted for Self-Management Support Improvement. Glasgow, R. E. [2002]. *Self-management aspects of the improving chronic illness care breakthrough series: Implementation with diabetes and heart failure teams*. Springer Science + Business Media.)

the MI approach is one of respect and builds upon rapport that is developed as part of the individual and care team relationship. MI is intended to be a short intervention to be delivered in two to four sessions (Miller, 2016). Core to MI is the identification, examination, and resolution of ambivalence about behavior change.

Readiness for change has three essential elements: (1) MI is a conversation about change; (2) MI is a collaborative, person-centered partnership that honors individual autonomy; and (3) MI evokes an individual's intrinsic motivation and commitment to change (Miller, 2016). A foundational component is an individual's ability to develop intrinsic motivation, which is predicated on their knowledge of how behavior change directly impacts personal goals. To achieve success, an individual must be able to relate the change to their sense of self, their view of self within the context of family and community, their roles and personal values, and their belief that self-management and behavior change are possible (self-efficacy) (Miller, 2016). The ambulatory care RN and larger healthcare team use five general principles to guide MI:

1. Express empathy through reflective listening, communicating respect, and understanding of an individual's experience, which includes exploring an individual's personal reasons for making a change.
2. Explore discrepancies between individual's current behaviors and identified goals, highlighting the individual's awareness of the consequences of problematic behaviors and motivating change.
3. Avoid argument over current behaviors as it is counterproductive to change.
4. Roll with resistance instead of confronting behaviors by acknowledging an individual's perception or disagreements, work to deescalate, and have the individual define the problem and develop their own solutions.
5. Self-efficacy is predicated on the probability of change, allowing the individual, with support of the ambulatory care RN and healthcare team, to have confidence and optimism that achieving change is possible (Miller, 2016).

MI techniques include OARS:

1. *Open-ended questions* are not easily answered by yes or no and that aid in exploration of reasons for change.
2. *Affirmations* are genuine and acknowledge individual difficulties.
3. *Reflections* repeat, mirror back, and rephrase content, encouraging individuals to synthesize and process content.
4. *Summaries* are used to demonstrate clinician interest and understanding of the conversations, focus on important elements of the discussions, serve to highlight the individual's ambivalence, and assist the individual to move forward (Miller, 2016). Table 7.10 outlines questions for consideration in guiding MI conversations. Box 7.5 describes eight strategies for evoking "change talk."

SMART Goals

SMART is an acronym for a process that provides a structure for clearly defining objectives and goals and includes guiding questions that explore barriers and facilitators that can support or prevent achievement of objectives and goals (Bjerke & Renger, 2017; Doran, 1981). Originally designed for application in the business sector, the principles and processes have been expanded for use in realms such as healthcare design and delivery and as a component of educational delivery models. The SMART goal acronym is defined as follows:

S—Identify a goal that is *specific*.
M—Determine methods to quantify and *measure* progress toward the goal(s).
A—Ensure that the goals can be *achieved* by identifying both barriers and facilitators for success.
R—Goals are *relevant* to the individual.
T—Goals are *time-bound* and can be realized within the planned time frame.

TABLE 7.10 MOTIVATIONAL INTERVIEWING QUESTIONS

1. What changes would you most like to discuss?
2. What have you noticed about …?
3. How important is it for you to change?
4. How confident do you feel about changing …?
5. How do you see the benefits of …?
6. How do you see the drawback of …?
7. What will make the most sense to you …?
8. How might things be different for you …?
9. In what way …?
10. Where does this leave you now?

Note. Adapted from Rollnick, S., Butler, C. C., Kinnersley, P., Gregory, J., & Mash, B. (2010). Motivational interviewing. *BMJ* Publishing Group Ltd.

BOX 7.5 Eight Strategies for Evoking Change Talk

Ask Evocative Questions

- Open-ended questions.
- Why would you want to make this change?

Elaboration

- When a change talk theme emerges, ask for details.
- When and how do you think this change will happen?

Examples

- When was the last time you attempted to make a change?

Looking Back

- Describe how things were better in the past.

Looking Forward

- What would happen if things stay the same?
- If you were 100% successful in making the change, how would your life be different?

Query Extremes

- Ask about best- and worst-case scenarios.
- What is the best/worst thing that would happen if you did/didn't make the change?

Use Change Rules

- Use open-ended questions for individuals to rank themselves on a scale from 1 to 10 from least important or most important it is to change…

Explore Goals and Values

- What do you really want in life?
- What activities that you used to participate in would you like to be able to do again?

Come Along Side

- Side with the negative side of ambivalence—"maybe smoking is so important to you that you won't give it up no matter what the cost/outcome."

Note. Adapted from Miller, R. (2016). *Motivational interviewing and stages of change theory*. Sage Publications. https://www.sagepub.com/sites/default/files/upm-binaries/65225_Jones_Smith_Chapter_10.pdf

TABLE 7.11 SMART GOALS

Specific	What exactly do you want to accomplish (who, what, when, why, how)?
Measurable	How will you know when you have reached this goal (measure/quantify) progress?
Achievable	Is achieving this goal realistic with the level of effort and commitment required? Do you have the skills/resources to achieve this goal? If not, how will you get them?
Relevant	Why is this goal significant to your life?
Time-Bound	When will this goal be achieved? Is the timeline realistic?

Note. Adapted from Bjerke, M. B., & Renger, R. (2017). Being smart about writing SMART objectives. *Evaluation and Program Planning, 61*, 125–127. https://www.ncbi.nlm.nih.gov/pubmed/28056403

Table 7.11 lists suggested questions for the ambulatory care nurse to use in order to elicit information from individuals during the goal development process. Finally, when engaging individuals and providers in collaborative decision-making and care delivery design, it is often helpful to delineate responsibilities and establish a formal commitment to ensure success. This can be achieved through use of an informal contract or agreement process, or by using a pledge for both individuals and providers. Table 7.12 provides an example of a participation pledge that could be utilized as part of nursing practice.

TABLE 7.12 PLEDGE TO PARTNER

As Your Healthcare Partner We Pledge To	As a Patient I Pledge To
• Include you as a member of the team	• Be a responsible and active member of my healthcare team
• Treat you with respect, honesty, and compassion	• Treat you with respect, honesty, and consideration
• Always tell you the truth	• Always tell you the truth
• Include your family or advocate when you would like us to	• Respect the commitment you have made to healthcare and healing
• Hold ourselves to the highest quality and safety standards	• Give you the information that you need to treat me
• Be responsive and timely with our care and information to you	• Learn all that I can about my condition
• Help you to set goals for your healthcare and treatment plans	• Participate in decisions about my care
• Listen to you and answer your questions	• Understand my care plan to the best of my ability
• Provide information to you in a way you can understand	• Tell you what medications I am taking
• Respect your right to your own medical information	• Ask questions when I do not understand and until I do understand
• Respect your privacy and the privacy of your medical information	• Communicate any problems I have with the plan for my care
• Communicate openly about benefits and risks associated with any treatments	• Tell you if something about my health changes
• Provide you with information to help you make informed decisions about your care and treatment options	• Tell you if I have trouble reading
• Work with you, and other partners who treat you, in the coordination of your care	• Let you know if I have family, friends, or an advocate to help me with my healthcare

Note. Copyright © 2008 by National Patient Safety Foundation. Printed with permission of the Institute for Healthcare Improvement (IHI), ©2019.

As noted by Krist and colleagues (2017), engaging individuals and families in self-care management—occurring across the life span, settings of care, and spectrum of disease—is critical to disease prevention and chronic disease control. From a conceptual model perspective, individual engagement is predicated on relationships between individuals, health professionals, and healthcare systems. It should include full partnership and shared leadership in designing models of care delivery, influencing how individuals and families are integrated within healthcare encounters and processes, and creating healthcare policies at local, state, and national levels (Carman & Workman, 2017). Incorporating individuals and families as part of care delivery redesign holds vast potential for widespread healthcare system transformation founded on individual needs and preference for care. As outlined in Table 7.13, continued actions related to practice, education, research, and policy development are essential in order to advance individual and family engagement. Broad implementation of individual- and family-engaged care holds promise to incorporate both evidence-based and experience-based elements that address areas previously overlooked, such as dimensions of workplace culture, new approaches to communication, the quality of human interactions, as well as physical environment design (Frampton et al., 2017). All impact quality, healthcare culture, value, and experience for both individuals and providers, and cannot be accomplished without effective partnerships among healthcare executives, policy makers, and individual and family leaders.

TABLE 7.13 ACTION STEPS FOR THE ADVANCING INDIVIDUAL AND FAMILY ENGAGEMENT

Practice	• Reach consensus on standard conceptual definitions for patient-centered care/individual and family engagement/activation; • Integrate engagement measures in electronic healthcare systems; • Identify and develop professional nursing models for patient-centered care/individual and family engagement/activation; • Develop competencies for nurses and members of the interprofessional team for patient-centered care/individual and family engagement/activation; • Outline specific roles for nurses to ensure that patient-centered/individual and family engagement/activation are incorporated across all settings and models of care; • Establish patient-centered care/individual and family engagement/activation as a core element of nursing practice in all care settings; and • Link nursing-specific interventions for patient-centered/individual and family engagement and activation.
Research	• Develop instruments to measure patient-centered care/individual and family engagement/activation; • Develop assessment measures linking patient-centered care/individual and family engagement/activation to health outcomes; • Continue development and refinement of evidence-based tools and methodologies to support patient-centered care/individual and family engagement/activation; and • Fund nursing and interprofessional research to support patient-centered care/individual and family engagement/activation.
Education	• Focus interprofessional education on best practices, competencies, tool and methodology use, and skill building to support patient-centered care/individual and family engagement/activation; • Develop setting-specific strategies for educating interprofessional staff to support patient-centered care/individual and family engagement/activation; and • Recommend adoption of QSEN competencies in academic and service organizations.
Policy	• Engage consumers in policy development; • Develop financial incentives for nurses with successful patient-centered care/individual and family engagement/activation; and • Advocate for funding of nursing research and performance measure development to support patient-centered care/individual and family engagement/activation.

Note. QSEN = Quality and Safety Education for Nurses. Adapted from Pelletier, L. R., & Stichler, J. F. (2013). Action brief: Patient engagement and activation: A health reform imperative and improvement opportunity for nursing. *Nursing Outlook*, 61(1), 51–54.

Case Study

Ella is a 60-year-old woman experiencing obesity, who is not established with a primary care physician. During a recent health event, Ella participated in diabetes lab screening. The result was a hemoglobin A1C of 12. Ella's sole focus had been on raising her five children.

You are the RN assigned to follow up on Ella's A1C and arrange to meet Ella for an assessment and care planning. As a nurse, you recognize the importance of understanding Ella's activation level. Ella is assessed at PAM Level 2: some knowledge of diabetes but large gaps in understanding treatment. At Level 2, you will need to set simple goals toward achieving health and provide significant coaching and support. Open-ended MI questions and use of "change talk" techniques help to determine what is most important to Ella and you use the SMART goal framework to begin. Two goals are identified: testing and logging her blood sugar daily and using a food log to track food intake. Ella commits to both, and you schedule time the following week to review. In addition, you schedule a new patient appointment with a provider who is convenient to where Ella lives and at a time that suits her family responsibilities.

1. How will you continue to support Ella to have the confidence and knowledge to self-manage her diabetes?
2. What additional community-based resources or activities or interventions could be incorporated to support Ella in the management of her diabetes?

Key Points for Review

- Individual engagement refers to the knowledge skills, ability, and willingness to manage one's own healthcare.
- Active collaboration between individuals and providers is essential to design, implement, and manage engagement practices in order to achieve health outcomes, manage associated healthcare costs, and influence policy development that supports a culture of individual and family engagement.
- Due to the breadth and diversity of care settings that extend well beyond traditional acute care environments, as well as the constant evolution of care delivery methodologies, ambulatory care nurses must foster individual and family engagement as an element of daily practice.
- Ambulatory care nurses must develop an understanding of core elements, principles, strategies, tools, and methodologies and develop competencies in order to foster behavior change and engage individuals in self-management.

REFERENCES

Agency for Healthcare Research and Quality. (2012). *Five major steps, to intervention (The "5A's")*. https//:www.ahrq.gov/professionals/clinicians-providers/guidelines-recommendations/tobacco/5steps.html

American Academy of Ambulatory Care Nursing. (2017a). *American Academy of Ambulatory Care Nursing position paper: The role of the registered nurse in ambulatory care. Nursing Economic$*. https://www.aaacn.org/sites/default/files/documents/PositionStatementRN.pdf

American Academy of Ambulatory Care Nursing. (2017b). Position statement on the role of the registered nurse in ambulatory care nursing. *Nursing Economic$, 35*(1), 39–47.

American Academy of Ambulatory Care Nursing. (2017c). In C. Murray (Ed.), *Scope and standards of practice for professional ambulatory care nursing* (9th ed.). Author.

American Nurses Association Executive. (2012). *The value of nursing care coordination*. https://www.nursingworld.org/~4afc0d/globalassets/practiceandpolicy/health-policy/care-coordination-white-paper-3.pdf

Bernabeo, E., & Holmboe, E. S. (2013). Patients, providers, and systems need to acquire a specific set of competencies to achieve truly patient-centered care. *Health Affairs, 32*(2), 250–258. https://doi.org/10.1377/hlthaff.2012.1120

Bjerke, M. B., & Renger, R. (2017). Being smart about writing SMART objectives. *Evaluation and Program Planning, 61*, 125–127. https://www.ncbi.nlm.nih.gov/pubmed/28056403

Brenan, M. (2018). *Nurses again outpace other professions for honesty, ethics. GALLUP*. https://news.gallup.com/poll/245597/nurses-again-outpace-professions-honesty-ethics.aspx

Carman, K. L., Dardess, P., Maurer, M., Sofaer, S., Adams, K., Bechtel, C., & Sweeney, J. (2013). Patient and family engagement: A framework for understanding the elements and developing interventions and policies. *Health Affairs, 32*(2), 223–231. https://doi.org/10.1377/hlthaff.2012.1133

Carman, K. L., & Workman, T. A. (2017). Engaging patients and consumers in research evidence: Applying the conceptual model of patient and family engagement. *Patient Education and Counseling, 100*, 25–29. https://doi.org/10.1016/j.pec.2016.07.009

Centers for Disease Control and Prevention. (2018). *About chronic disease*. National Center for Chronic Disease Prevention and Health Promotion. https://www.cdc.gov/chronicdisease/about/index.htm

Cronenwett, L., Sherwood, G., Barnsterner, J., Disch, J., Johonson, J., Mitchell, P., Sullivan, T., & Warren, J. (2007). Quality and safety education for nurses. *Nursing Outlook, 55*(3), 122–131. https://doi.org/10.1016/j.outlook.2007.02.006

Deen, D., Lu, W. H., Rothstein, D., Santana, L., & Gold, M. R. (2011). Asking questions: The effect of a brief intervention in community health centers on patient activation. *Patient Education, 84*(2), 257–260. https://doi.org/10.1016/j.pec.2010.07.026

Doran, G. T. (1981). There's a S. *M. A. R.* T. way to write management's goals and objectives. *Management Review, 70*(11), 35–36.

Elwyn, G., Frosch, D., Thompson, R., Joseph-Williams, N., Lloyd, A., Kinnersley, P., Cording, E., Tomson, D., Dodd, C., Rollnick, S., Edwards, A., & Barry, M. (2012). Shared decision making: A model for clinical practice. *Journal of General Internal Medicine, 27*(10), 1361–1367. https://doi.org/10.1007/s11606-012-2077-6

Elwyn, G., Lloyd, A., & Joseph-Williams, N. (2013). Option grids: Shared decision making made easier. *Patient Education and Counseling, 90*, 207–212. https://doi.org/10.1016/j.pec.2012.06.036

Frampton, S. B., Guastello, S., Hoy, L., Naylor, M., Sheridan, S., & Johnston-Fleece, M. (2017). Harnessing evidence and experience to change culture: A guiding framework for patient and family engaged care. *National Academy of Medicine*, 1–38. https://doi.org/10.31478/201701f

Giguere, A., Legare, F., Grad, R., Pluye, P., Haynes, R. B., Cauchon, M., Rousseau, F., Argote, J. A., & Labreque, M. (2012). Decision boxes for clinicians to support evidence-based practice and shared decision making: The user experience. *Implementation Science, 7*(72). https://doi.org/10.1186/1748-5908-7-72

Grande, S. W., Faber, M. J., Durand, M., Thompson, R., & Elwyn, G. (2014). A classification model of patient engagement methods and assessment of their feasibility in real-world settings. *Patient Education and Counseling, 95*, 281–287. https://doi.org/10.1016/j.pec.2014.01.016

Greene, J., Hibbard, J. H., Sacks, R., Overton, V., & Parrotta, C. (2015). When patient activation levels changes, health outcomes and costs change, too. *Health Affairs, 34*(3), 431–437. https://doi.org/10.1377/hlthaff.2014.0452

Haycock, C., & Wahl, C. (2013). Achieving patient and family engagement through the implementation and evolution of advisory councils across a large healthcare system. *Nursing Administration Quarterly, 37*(3), 242–246. https://doi.org/10.1097/NAQ.0b013e318295f54c

Hibbard, J. H., & Greene, J. (2013). What the evidence shows about patient activation: Better health outcomes and care experiences: Fewer data on costs. *Health Affairs, 32*(2), 207–214. https://doi.org/10.1377/hlthaff.2012.1061

Hibbard, J. H., Greene, J., & Overton, V. (2013). Patients with lower activation associated with higher costs. *Health Affairs, 32*(2), 216–222. https://doi.org/10.1377/hlthaff.2012.1064

Hibbard, J. H., Greene, J., Sacks, R. M., Overton, V., & Parrotta, C. (2017). Improving population health management strategies: Identifying patients who are more likely to be users of avoidable costly care and those more likely to develop a new chronic disease. *Health Services Research, 52*(4), 1297–1309. https://doi.org/10.1111/1475-6773.12545

Hibbard, J. H., Greene, J., & Tusler, M. (2009). Improving the outcomes of disease-management by tailoring care to the patient's level of activation. *American Journal of Managed Care, 15*, 353–360.

Hibbard, J. M., Mahoney, E. R., Stockard, J., & Tusler, M. (2005). Development and testing of a short form of the Patient Activation Measure. *Heath Services Research, 40*(6), 1918–1930. https://doi.org/10.1111/j.1475-6773.2005.00438.x

Humowiecki, M., Kuruna, T., Sax, R., Hawthorne, M., & Cullen, K. (2018). *Blueprint for complex care: Advancing the field of care for individuals with complex health and social needs*. https://www.nationalcomplex.care/our-work/blueprint-for-complex-care/

Institute of Medicine. (2001). *Crossing the quality chasm: A new health system for the 21st century*. National Academies Press. https://pubmed.ncbi.nlm.nih.gov/25057539/

Institute of Medicine. (2014). *Implications of health literacy for public health: Workshop summary*. National Academies Press. https://doi.org/10.17226/18756

Koh, H. K., Brach, C. M., Harris, L. M., & Parchman, M. L. (2013). A proposed "health literacy care model" would constitute a systems approach to improving patients' engagement in care. *Health Affairs (Millwood), 32*(2), 357–367. https://doi.org/10.1377/hlthaff.2012.1205

Krist, A. H., Tong, S. T., Aycock, R. A., & Longo, D. R. (2017). Engaging patients in decision-making and behavioral change to promote prevention. *Information Services & Use, 37*, 105–122. https://doi.org/10.3233/ISU-170826

Krist, A. H., Tong, S. T., Aycock, R. A., & Longo, D. R. (2017). Engaging patients in decision-making and behavior change to promote prevention. *Studies in Health Technology and Informatics*, 240, 284–302. https://doi.org/10.3233/978-1-61499-790-0-284

Legare, F., & Wittman, H. (2013). Shared decision making: Examining key elements and barriers to adoption into routine practice. *Health Affairs, 32*(2), 276–284. https://doi.org/10.1377/hlthaff.2012.1078

Loehrer, S., Feely, D., & Berwick, D. (2015). 10 new rules to accelerate healthcare redesign. *Healthcare Executive, 30*(6), 66–69. http://www.ihi.org/resources/Pages/Publications/10NewRulesAccelerateHealthcareRedesign.aspx

Lorig, K. R., & Alvarez, S. (2011). RE: Community-based diabetes education for Latinos. *Diabetes Education, 37*(1), 128. https://doi.org/10.1177/0145721710393089

Miller, R. (2016). *Motivational interviewing and stages of change theory*. Sage Publications. https://www.sagepub.com/sites/default/files/upm-binaries/65225_Jones_Smith_Chapter_10.pdf

Pelletier, L.R., & Stichler, J. F. (2013). Action brief: Patient engagement and activation: A health reform imperative and improvement opportunity for nursing. *Nursing Outlook, 61(1)*, 51–54. https://doi.org/10.1016/j.outlook.2012.11.003

Raghupathi, W., & Raghupathi, V. (2018). An empirical study of chronic diseases in the United States: A visual analytics approach to public health. *International Journal of Environmental Research and Public Health, 15*(431). https://doi.org/10.3390/ijerph15030431

Shane-McWhorter, L., McAdam-Marx, C., Petersen, M., Woolsey, S., Coursey, J. M., Whittaker, T. C., Hyer, C., LaMarche, D., Carroll, P., & Chuy, L. (2015). Pharmacist-provided diabetes management and education via a telemonitoring program. *Journal of the American Pharmacy Association, 55*(5), 516–526. https://doi.org/10.1331/JAPhA.2015.14285

Shively, M. J., Gardetto, N. J., Kodiath, M. F., Kelly, A., Smith, T. L., Stepnowsky, C., Maynard, C., & Larson, C. B. (2013). Effect of patient activation on self-management in patients with heart failure. *Journal of Cardiovascular Nursing, 28*, 20–34. https://doi.org/10.1097/JCN.0b013e318239f9f9

Sofaer, S., & Schumann, M. J. (2013). *Fostering successful patient and family engagement: Nursing's critical role*. Nursing Alliance for Quality. https://www.nursingworld.org/~4aa949/globalassets/naqc/naqc_patientengagement whitepaper.pdf

Swartwout, E., Drenkard, K., McGuinn, K., Grant, S., & El-Zein, A. (2016). Patient and family engagement summit. Needed changes in clinical practice. *Journal of Nursing Administration, 46*(35), S11–S18. https://doi.org/10.1097/NNA.0000000000000317

Tzelepis, F., Sanson-Fisher, R. W., Zucca, A. C., & Fradgley, E. A. (2015). Measuring the quality of patient-centered care: Why patient-reported measures are critical to reliable assessment. *Patient Preference and Adherence, 9*, 831–835. https://doi.org/10.2147/PPA.S81975

U.S. Department of Health and Human Services. (2019). *Quick guide to health literacy*. Office of Disease Prevention and Health Promotion. https://health.gov/communication/literacy/quickguide/factsbasic.htm

APPENDIX 7.1 DEFINITIONS OF INDIVIDUAL AND FAMILY ENGAGEMENT

Definition and Context	Source
1. "A 'patient-centered' view of patient engagement requires that it will only happen if health professionals, organizations and policies (1) create clear opportunities for engagement; (2) make clear that they welcome engagement; and (3) provide the support that people need in order to engage."	Sofaer and Schumann (2013, p. 9)
2. "A partnership among practitioners, patients, and their families (when appropriate) to ensure that decisions respect patients' wants, needs, and preferences and that patients have the education and support they need to make decisions and participate in their own care."	IOM (2001, p. 7)
3. "Patient and family-centered care is defined as care that is: (1) considerate and respectful of patients' beliefs, values, and personal meanings associated with their state of wellness or illness; (2) inclusive of patients' personal and social support systems; (3) delivered in the context of a caring, therapeutic partnership between patients' and provider; (4) integrated and coordinated across a continuum of services, providers, and settings; (5) empowering with education, information, and evidence necessary to enable and engage patients in their own health care; and (6) activating by facilitating Patients' use of internal and external resources to manage their own care."	Pelletier and Stichler (2013, p. 52)
4. Focus on relationship between patients and healthcare providers as they work together to "promote and support active patient and public involvement in health and healthcare to strengthen their influence on healthcare decisions at both the individual and collective levels."	Carman et al. (2013, p. 223) and Coulter (2011, p. 10)
5. Model of public engagement organized around settings in which engagement occurs: during care experience, within microsystem of clinic or hospital room, within the larger healthcare organization, within the larger community.	Carman et al. (2013)
6. "Patients, families, their representatives, and health professionals working in active partnership at various levels across the health care system—direct care, organizational design and governance, and policy making—to improve health and health care."	Carman et al. (2013)
7. "Patient engagement is the involvement in their own care by individuals (and other they designate to engage on their behalf), with the goals that they make competent, well-informed decisions about their health and health care and take action to support those decisions."	Sofaer and Schumann (2013, p. 9)

APPENDIX  DEFINITIONS OF INDIVIDUAL AND FAMILY ENGAGEMENT (CONTINUED)

Definition and Context	Source
8. Engagement is "a set of behaviors by patients, family members, and health professionals and a set of organizational policies and procedures that foster both the inclusion of patients and family members as active members of the health care team and collaborative partnerships with providers and provider organizations...the desired goals of patient and family engagement include improving the quality and safety of health care."	Maurer et al. (2012, p. 9)
9. "Patient engagement has multiple definitions but has broadly been defined as the process of actively involving and supporting patients in health care and treatment decision making activities. Patient engagement can target professionals, patients, the organizational environment and the intervention itself."	Grande et al. (2014, p. 281)

8

Care Coordination

Mary Hines Vinson, Beth Ann Swan, and Caroline Varner Coburn

PERSPECTIVES

"Care coordination is needed today more than ever, especially for persons with chronic conditions and the families and significant others who assist with their care. Care coordination by nurses in all health care settings focuses on education, coaching and counseling to enhance understanding and execution of the plan of care. Nurses providing care coordination identify each person's values, goals and preferences for care, as well as, best evidence-base[d] practices for populations and advocate for them as needed within the interprofessional health care team and with those responsible for costs of care."

Sheila A. Haas, PhD, RN, FAAN, Dean and Professor Emeritus, Loyola University Chicago, Niehoff School of Nursing

LEARNING OBJECTIVES

Upon completion of this chapter, the reader will be able to:

1. Understand the context of care coordination within the current healthcare delivery system, the profession of nursing, and the practice of ambulatory care nursing.
2. Understand the differences among the following roles: case manager, care manager, transitional care nurse, nurse navigator, care coordinator, care coordination and transition management (CCTM) registered nurse (RN).
3. List specific knowledge, skills, and attitudes required for the practice of care coordination in ambulatory care nursing.
4. Identify sources of professional practice standards for RNs in care coordination roles.
5. Define and describe types of care coordination models.

KEY TERMS

Care continuum
Care coordination
Care management
Case management
Health information technology
Transition management
Transitional care

Care Coordination in U.S. Healthcare

Care coordination has in recent years emerged as one of the most rapidly expanding areas of nursing practice. Seen as a foundational element of healthcare reform, much attention has been directed toward defining and measuring specific processes and quality outcomes related to care coordination (Bower, 2016; Swan et al., 2019b). Government agencies, health systems, insurers, and quality programs across the United States are focused on improving care and reducing costs, particularly for high-risk and vulnerable populations that consume healthcare resources. There is an urgency within the healthcare community to make progress in this rapidly evolving area of nursing care.

Healthcare services in the United States are among the most expensive in the world, yet the quality of care has been negatively impacted by increasing complexity, decentralization, fragmentation of services, and failure to engage individuals and families in their care. Individuals often see multiple providers and receive a variety of services with rapid turnover, leading to confusion and difficulty managing complex plans of care. These factors ultimately affect health outcomes. Care coordination has been recognized as a key strategy for addressing these issues, and registered nurses (RNs) are well positioned to lead this initiative.

Historical Perspective

Although the awareness of nursing's significant contributions to care coordination in healthcare may be recent, RNs have, in fact, been providing care coordination for decades with little recognition of the processes inherent in the provision and organization of these services. In recent history, this began with the advent of diagnosis-related groups (DRGs) in the 1980s and managed care in the 1990s. At that time, health plans began to require primary care "gatekeepers" to oversee access to expensive specialist care. **Care management** evolved as a way for hospitals to control cost and reduce length of stay. RNs were deployed as case managers, both by hospitals and in community settings, where they followed high-risk individuals in an effort to reduce costs and prevent readmission. Health plans created utilization management roles to audit hospital care and coordinate postdischarge services (Zazworsky & Bower, 2016).

These payer-driven changes in care delivery increased the visibility of and payment for specific treatments and interventions. One downstream effect of these changes was that care coordination activities that may be wide-ranging and difficult to ascribe to a single diagnosis became increasingly critical, yet often unrecognized and undervalued. This attention to cost and quality in healthcare provided the foundation for today's focus on RN care coordination. Readers are referred to Chapter 2 for a full discussion of national strategies and payment models driving the need for care coordination.

Nursing Perspective

In 2012, the American Academy of Nursing (AAN) put forth policy recommendations to the Centers for Medicare and Medicaid Services (CMS), urging them to move quickly to adopt clear and consistent definitions for care coordination and **transitional care** and to implement reimbursement models for these services at the community level. Further, the AAN recommended that such models be sustainable and replicable. The policy statement urged the government to allocate funding for the development of performance measures and information technology to ensure consistent outcome measurement. Finally, they recommended that the government invest in workforce development directly related to care coordination and transition services (Cipriano, 2012). In 2013, AAN published the American Nurses Association's (ANA's) white paper, *The Value of Nursing Care Coordination*, highlighting the numerous accomplishments of the profession of nursing in promoting, practicing, and leading care coordination in diverse settings and on behalf of a wide variety of individual populations.

The authors illustrated the importance of care coordination in healthcare reform with its potential to support the goals of better quality, more efficient use of resources, and reduced cost (Camicia et al., 2013).

In 2014, ANA convened the Care Coordination Task Force (CCTF) to review evidence and seminal documents related to care coordination in nursing. This group put forth recommendations for federal policy priorities to address goals of healthcare reform and advance nursing's contributions to effective care coordination. An interprofessional, collaborative approach was recommended that would prioritize individual, family, and population-specific approaches to care. The task force outlined policy priorities to reduce barriers related to scope of practice. Specific recommendations included a call for an acceleration of the design and implementation of evidence-based care coordination measures, as well as consistent reimbursement for care coordination services across all qualified health professionals (Lamb et al., 2015).

The American Academy of Ambulatory Care Nursing (AAACN) was quick to recognize the need for competencies to guide ambulatory care RNs in the evolving area of practice of care coordination. Between 2011 and 2014, thought leaders within the organization organized members and stakeholders nationwide in a call to action to define the roles and competencies needed for care coordination and transitional care across the **care continuum** (Haas et al., 2013).

Care Continuum, Care Coordination, and Proliferation of Terms

Within the framework of a longitudinal approach to chronic health issues, it is important for care coordinators to look beyond current or immediate needs of individuals and to incorporate past and anticipated future challenges. The continuum of care is a concept that describes a system that guides and tracks individuals over time through a comprehensive array of health services spanning all levels and intensity of care (Healthcare Information and Management Systems Society, 2018). The notion of a care continuum that includes care across time and place, between and during care delivery encounters and care providers, has existed for many decades. However, dramatic changes in healthcare service delivery, augmented by innovative technology advances, have resulted in a continuum of care today that is much more complex than in the past. Care is offered in a variety of settings and must address not only physical health but also psychosocial, environmental, and economic issues.

Today's care continuum includes assessment of healthcare services, social determinants of health, and community resources, all factors that impact the health and well-being of individuals and families. Care coordination is essential in navigating these and other influences on the continuum of care. A variety of terms and roles related to care coordination have proliferated over the last 15 years; their definitions and differentiation are described in what follows. It is essential for RNs in ambulatory care and all practice settings to understand the full scope of care coordination and comprehend the differences between care management/manager, **case management**/manager, nurse navigator, transitional care, and **transition management**.

Care Coordination

The most recent definition from the National Quality Forum's (NQF) Care Coordination Endorsement Maintenance Project 2016 to 2017 is "a multidimensional concept that includes effective communication among healthcare providers, patients, families, caregivers (regarding chronic conditions); safe care transitions; a longitudinal view of care that considers the past, while monitoring present delivery of care and anticipating future needs; and the facilitation of linkages between communities and the healthcare system to address medical, social, educational and other support needs that align with patient goals" (National Quality Forum, 2017).

Care Management

Care management is "a process designed to assist patients and their support systems in managing their medical/social/mental health conditions more efficiently and effectively" (Agency for Healthcare Research and Quality, 2014). Care management at the individual practice level refers to team-based approaches to care whose purpose is to assist individuals and their caregivers in managing health-related conditions across providers and services (Tomoaia-Cotisel et al., 2018).

Care managers identify target groups within the practice along with the defined responsibilities of team members and activities performed. Care management is most successful when services are provided by high-functioning interprofessional teams characterized by shared values, clearly defined roles, and effective communication skills (Tomoaia-Cotisel et al., 2018). Care management differs from care coordination in that care management is a more episodic approach.

Case Management

The Case Management Society of America defines case management as "a collaborative process of assessment, planning, facilitation and advocacy for options and services to meet an individual's health needs through communication and available resources to promote quality cost-effective outcomes" (2017). The primary focus in case management is to help the individual navigate from one level of care to another. For instance, the case manager may coordinate complicated home care needs for recovery after surgery until individuals resume their previous level of independence. Another focal area of case management is utilization review. Case management differs from care coordination in that case management is episodic, spanning only the time frame defined by a health service encounter, until an individual is transitioned from one level or site of service to another (Ahmed, 2016).

Nurse Navigation

One example of nurse navigation is an oncology nurse navigator (ONN), who is "a professional registered nurse with oncology-specific clinical knowledge who offers individualized assistance to patients, families, and caregivers to help overcome healthcare system barriers. Using the nursing process, an ONN provides education and resources to facilitate informed decision-making and timely access to quality health and psychosocial care throughout all phases of the cancer continuum" (Oncology Nursing Society, 2017, p. 6). The limited ONN role is focused on education and engagement, access, and standardized communication between providers and settings regarding individual needs and issues. Nurse navigation is different than care coordination in that nurse navigation is a singular intervention not encompassing all the dimensions and activities of care coordination (Haas et al., 2019).

Transitional Care

Transitional care is defined as "a broad range of time-limited services designed to ensure health care continuity, avoid preventable poor outcomes among at-risk populations, and promote the safe and timely transfer of individuals from one level of care to another or from one type of setting to another" (Naylor et al., 2011, p. 747). Transitional care is a short-term process as an individual moves from one level of care to another. An example of transitional care may be ensuring full communication and support for an individual who needs temporary care in a skilled nursing facility (SNF) and who will be returning home at a previous level of health. Transitional care differs from care coordination in that transitional care is time limited, involving a single transfer.

Transition Management

Transition management is defined "in the context of RN practice in multiple settings as the ongoing support of individuals and their families over time as they navigate care and relationships among more than one provider and/or more than one healthcare setting and/or more than one health care service. The need for transition management is not determined by age, time, place, or healthcare condition, but rather by individuals' and/or families' needs for support for ongoing, longitudinal individualized plans of care and follow-up plans of care within the context of healthcare delivery" (Swan et al., 2019a, p. 3). This concept of transition management is specific to the care coordination and transition management (CCTM) model developed by AAACN and described more fully next. Inherent in this model is the management of care on an ongoing basis across the continuum of care.

The Care Coordination and Transition Management Model

The CCTM model provides a blueprint for the RN practice of CCTM. Theoretical foundations of the CCTM model include the chronic care model (Wagner, 1998) and the quality and safety education for nurses (QSEN) framework that serve to further refine knowledge, skills, and attitudes related to each dimension (Cronenwett et al., 2007). The CCTM model includes nine dimensions with competencies for each dimension. This model is summarized in Box 8.1.

The work of AAACN in developing the CCTM model reflects the goals of the *Future of Nursing* report (Institute of Medicine, 2011) by advocating for RNs to serve in roles that allow them to practice to the full extent of their preparation and licensure and by challenging professional nurses to lead change in healthcare. In addition, the identification of unique roles as providers of care coordination services speaks to the Institute of Medicine's (IOM's) call for RNs to seek higher levels of education and to be full participating partners in healthcare redesign.

BOX 8.1 Nine Dimensions/Competencies of Care Coordination and Transition Management (CCTM)

Advocacy
Education and engagement of individuals and families
Coaching and counseling of individuals and families
Person-centered care planning
Support for self-management
Nursing process
Teamwork and collaboration
Cross-setting communications and care transitions
Population health management

Note. American Academy of Ambulatory Care Nursing. (2017). In C. Murray (Ed.), *Scope and standards of practice for professional ambulatory care nursing* (9th ed). Author. Used with permission of American Academy of Ambulatory Care Nursing (AAACN), aaacn.org

Scope and Standards of Practice for Care Coordination and Transition Management

The ANA delineates expectations for all RNs in its *Scope and Standards of Practice*, and standard 5A is defined as coordination of care (ANA, 2015). As in any professional specialty, RNs in CCTM must be guided by universally accepted standards of practice. The knowledge, skills, and attitudes associated with CCTM must be defined and embraced by the profession and employed in measuring performance, as well as in determining payment for care coordination services (Lamb & Newhouse, 2018). In 2016, AAACN published standards that provide detailed authoritative statements describing the responsibilities that RNs specializing in CCTM are accountable for, including nurse executives, administrators, and managers. The domain of *Clinical Practice* includes six standards that address the nursing process, describing its application specifically in the practice of CCTM. The domain of *Professional Performance* includes 10 professional practice standards that describe professional behaviors associated with the practice of CCTM (AAACN, 2016). A summary of these standards is found in Box 8.2.

BOX 8.2 Scope of Practice for Registered Nurses in Care Coordination and Transition Management (CCTM) from the American Academy of Ambulatory Care Nursing

Clinical Practice Standards	Professional Performance Standards
Assessment: systematically collects data related to the involved patient or population as they move across the care continuum.	**Ethics:** applies the nursing code of ethics to all areas of practice.
Nursing Diagnosis: analyzes data to identify diagnosis or issues to facilitate the appropriate level of care.	**Education:** maintains ongoing knowledge and competence of current evidence-based practice.
Outcomes Identification: identifies expected outcomes for the patient, group, or population.	**Research and Evidence-Based Practice:** integrates relevant research to maintain and optimize best practices, promote improvement, and advance the profession.
Planning: develops patient- and/or population-centered plan of care that identifies and advocates for strategies and alternatives to achieve the expected outcomes.	**Performance Improvement:** enhances quality and effectiveness of practice, systems, and population health outcomes.
Implementation: implements the developed plan of care (including subsets of care coordination, health teaching or promotion, and consultation).	**Communication:** communicates effectively through a variety of formats to build relationships and deliver care.
Evaluation: evaluates the status and progress of the patient or population and communicates the status and progress to relevant professionals across the care continuum.	**Leadership:** acquires and utilizes leadership behaviors in all settings and across the care continuum.
	Collaboration: interacts with patient, family, caregivers, and other professionals to improve health outcomes.
	Professional Practice Evaluation: evaluates the nurse's own practice in relation to patient outcomes and relevant policies, standards, procedures, regulations, and statutes.

(continued)

BOX 8.2 Scope of Practice for Registered Nurses in Care Coordination and Transition Management (CCTM) from the American Academy of Ambulatory Care Nursing (*continued*)

Clinical Practice Standards	Professional Performance Standards
	Resource Utilization: utilizes appropriate resources that are safe, effective, and fiscally responsible.
	Environment: engages in initiatives to maintain an environment that is safe, confidential, and comfortable for patients, visitors, and staff.

Note. Adapted with permission of American Academy of Ambulatory Care Nursing. (2016). *Scope and standards of practice for registered nurses in care coordination and transition management* (1st ed.). Author. Used with permission of American Academy of Ambulatory Care Nursing (AAACN), aaacn.org

Roles of Registered Nurses in Care Coordination

The roles of RNs in care coordination continue to evolve. In 2012, AAN recommended guiding principles for implementation, evaluation, and payment for care coordination and transitional care (Cipriano, 2012). The principles suggested that successful models offer care tailored to individual and family needs and preferences provided by interprofessional teams. The teams are highly collaborative, allowing for leadership to shift between disciplines based on the individual situation. Shared decision-making is a core foundation, and the expertise of RNs is visible.

In 2015, representatives from the American Organization for Nursing Leadership (AONL) (formerly the American Organization of Nurse Executives) and AAACN came together to discuss the role of nurse leaders in CCTM across the healthcare continuum. This dialogue resulted in a joint statement, *The Role of the Nurse Leader in Care Coordination and Transition Management Across the Health Care Continuum* (AAACN, 2015). The statement included the following six major areas:

- Know how care is coordinated in your setting.
- Know who is providing care coordination in your organization.
- Establish relationships with multiple stakeholders to improve CCTM systems.
- Understand the value of technology and its impact on workflow and roles.
- Engage individuals and families.
- Engage all team members in care coordination.

Although the foregoing principles were addressed to nurse leaders, the concepts are applicable to any RN working in care coordination. The following section describes the application of care coordination in the clinical setting.

Nursing Process and Care Coordination

Care coordination begins with the nursing process, as reflected in the six standards of clinical practice for CCTM listed in Box 8.2. The nursing process represents the essential core that unites all nursing practice and serves as the common thread across the profession and the care continuum, providing a framework to guide practice in diverse practice settings and across populations and developmental stages (ANA, 2017). With its roots in the scientific process, these steps guide the nurse through an evidence-based process in providing care.

Person-centered and population-based assessment and care planning are the foundation of care coordination. RNs performing care coordination activities utilize a longitudinal care planning process that involves a deliberate and in-depth approach to assessment, planning for individual needs across time and place to achieve or maintain health and wellness. A variety of assessment tools are employed to gather information and contribute to a comprehensive picture of individual and family needs, priorities, preferences, and desired outcomes. The RN analyzes information gathered during the assessment to determine care priorities. Using an interprofessional approach, the RN identifies goals that are realistic, measurable, time sensitive, and reportable (AAACN, 2016). Interventions in care coordination are based on current evidence and best practices. The RN explores opportunities for self-management support, involving the individual and family in choosing specific goals for improving health status and well-being. Collaborative and interprofessional contributions to care are an essential part of the longitudinal plan. Care coordination is based on shared decision-making with individuals and families, as well as involving them in evaluating the effectiveness of care and services. Goals are established through collaboration between the individual/family, RN, and other members of the healthcare team. An important aspect of internal communication includes documenting goals and expectations in the electronic health record to encourage individual/family and interprofessional participation in achieving and evaluating outcomes.

RN Care Coordination in Ambulatory and Primary Care

Public policy changes such as the Affordable Care Act (ACA) have resulted in millions of additional people seeking primary care, many with complex chronic healthcare needs. To respond to this increasing need, RNs are working in expanded and enhanced roles in ambulatory and primary care, coordinating care and managing chronic diseases, particularly for high-risk individuals and populations. High-quality primary care models, such as the Patient-Centered Medical Home (PCMH), have emerged with new opportunities for nurse leaders and RNs to advance care models supported by interprofessional care teams and preventive approaches to care (Bodenheimer & Mason, 2017). Most primary care practices today are incorporating principles of disease prevention and care coordination, with a concurrent increase in RNs providing care at their full scope of practice. This approach to primary care is discussed in more detail in Chapter 10.

RNs performing care coordination in primary care settings describe a variety of activities, including: (1) identifying individuals in need of care coordination, (2) performing outreach to individuals by telephone and/or electronically, (3) providing face-to-face nurse visits, (4) providing support for self-management and social support, (5) managing cross-setting communication, (6) coaching and counseling individuals and families, (7) triaging contacts by individuals, and (8) participating in group visits (Friedman et al., 2016). Most care coordination roles include medication management and going beyond simply determining whether an individual's medication list is current. In the context of care coordination, RNs review medications for appropriate use, situations that may have changed the need for a particular medication, unrecognized side effects, and other implications for care. Protocols and guidelines may be employed for medication adjustment and refills.

The most consistent use of RNs coordinating care is related to long-term management of chronic conditions. In one review of RN roles in primary care, the most prevalent chronic diseases reported were diabetes, hypertension, and asthma (Norful et al., 2017). The authors found that for all chronic diseases, RNs reported care coordination roles using standard clinical practice guidelines, under which they were able to perform risk assessment and care coordination by reviewing laboratory and diagnostic tests and identifying individuals with abnormal findings requiring follow-up. Under appropriate scope of practice, RNs performed these care coordination tasks for the purpose of coordinating next steps in the individual's care, rather than making treatment adjustments.

RNs providing care coordination to underserved populations in primary care face significant challenges. One study that exemplified the common challenges in this setting described efforts to improve outcomes for diabetic patients at a Federally Qualified Health Center (FQHC), where care coordinators at the FQHC contacted participants and offered appointments within 2 to 5 days of referral. They found that persistent efforts on the part of care coordinators contributed to improved outcomes for those patients who continued with care at the FQHC (Mehta et al., 2016). A more complete discussion of care for underserved populations is found in Chapter 12.

Roles of Registered Nurses During Care Transitions

A care transition occurs when an individual moves from one setting of care to another. This includes movement to and from a hospital, between ambulatory care practices or specialty care practices, short- or long-term care, home health, or rehabilitation facilities. Early research related to care transitions focused largely on the discharge processes from the acute care environment, but current evidence reveals a high level of vulnerability for errors in care transitions of all types at all points on the care continuum. This realization has led to calls for increased awareness and more research to define strategies for improved processes and enhanced communication at every transition of care (Rattray et al., 2017; Sheikh et al., 2018).

Transition: Leaving or Returning to Acute Care

Discharge from the acute care hospital environment to the ambulatory environment continues to be the most common transition, primarily because of the significant opportunity for improving quality of care and reducing costs (Adams et al., 2019). Acute care transitions focus on care that is transferred to the individual's primary or specialty care provider, an alternate care facility, supported home care, or home. This focus has, in part, been driven by penalties applied to hospitals for inappropriate readmission rates. However, a trend toward decrease in the length of hospital stay also means that individuals may be discharged without a full understanding of or having support for their required follow-up care.

A variety of innovations to address the challenges of care transition from the hospital continue to be explored. For example, an RN may serve as a transition manager in order to identify individuals at high risk for readmission and to provide specific interventions during both hospitalization and postdischarge follow-up. Clearly defined roles and improved linkages between RNs in these diverse care delivery environments would contribute greatly to creating more seamless care. The following are examples of transitions from acute or ambulatory care to different settings and their associated challenges.

Acute Care to Home

Arguably the most common care transition is from the hospital to an individual's home, with follow-up provided by the individual's care provider. For individuals with an uncomplicated hospital stay and few to no comorbidities, transition is likely to be seamless. For individuals who do not fall into that category, the skills of care transition outlined previously become more important. Effective communication between the acute care facility and the primary care provider is essential. The RN who provides discharge planning in the hospital is well positioned to ensure that the individual's primary care provider is notified of the individual's hospital admission and subsequent discharge.

Acute Care to Skilled Nursing Facilities

Transitions between acute care and long-term care environments are associated with significant risk, particularly for frail older adults with comorbidities and limited social support. It is estimated that two million older adults receive postacute care in SNFs annually in the United States (Toles et al., 2016). SNF residents are highly vulnerable, often because of age, cognitive impairment, and the presence of one or more chronic diseases. Adequate communication from the hospital is essential to avoid poorly executed care transitions and poor outcomes from medication errors and delays in treatments.

A retrospective medical record audit of 155 charts transferred from acute care hospitals to one SNF reported deficiencies that included missing transferring physician contact information and incomplete medication lists. Missing medication information included instructions for steroid tapering, as well as details related to administration of antiarrhythmic and anticoagulant medications, adding significant risk for adverse drug events (Jusela et al., 2017). In addition to SNFs that are intended for long-term stay, annually in the United States, 1.8 million older adults transfer from acute care hospitals to short-term postacute rehabilitative services following surgery. Expectations among payers to reduce inpatient hospital length of stay have led to a growing need for short-term SNF settings to provide care during the recovery period. This population is highly vulnerable, with one in seven readmitted after major surgery and one in five experiencing an adverse event within 30 days (Davidson et al., 2017).

In this setting, transitional care that is specific to postdischarge needs becomes especially important, especially related to postoperative infection. One study found that among Medicare patients undergoing vascular surgery who were transferred to an SNF, the most common reason for hospital readmission was postoperative infection (Fernandes-Taylor et al., 2018). These and other complications may be a factor of inappropriate transition referral to facilities that are not equipped to handle the patient's needs. Consequently, the authors suggested that there is a need for processes to match short-term SNF capabilities to individuals' postoperative care needs.

Ambulatory Care, Primary Care, or Skilled Nursing Facility to Acute Care

The responsibility of ambulatory care, primary care, or SNF teams to coordinate care during transitions to the acute care environment is often overlooked. Acute care RNs have responsibility for creating a plan of care at admission but often have incomplete information regarding the individual's prior health status, socioeconomic status, family support systems, cultural preferences, and coping mechanisms (Adams et al., 2019). RNs in ambulatory care, primary care, or SNF settings can improve care transitions by initiating a collaborative process of information exchange on behalf of the individual. Providing a complete list of medications, including over-the-counter medications and supplements, is important, especially if the hospital and ambulatory/primary care practice do not share a common electronic health record system. A designated member of the ambulatory/primary care team should be responsible for all care transitions, with RNs who have expertise in care coordination often being best suited for this role.

Transition: Between Nonacute Settings and Providers

The transitional care literature does not include transitions between nonacute care settings. However, this type of care transition is addressed by the CCTM model, described previously, with transition management working in tandem with care coordination. CCTM defines the ongoing support of individuals, families, and populations as they navigate multiple systems of care delivery over time. Unique to the CCTM model is the notion that CCTM are dynamic "integrated functions that may occur simultaneously or separately and are not time limited" (Swan et al., 2019a, p. 3). RNs performing CCTM activities follow individuals and families across time and place, reflecting various levels of care, for example, transitions between different ambulatory providers, changing developmental needs, and episodic needs requiring hospitalization. Especially in individuals most needing CCTM, it is common to find frequent movement between different nonacute facilities with varying skilled care levels. These individuals with complex care needs benefit from a system that ensures the communication and coordination principles inherent in quality care transitions.

Skilled Nursing Facilities to Home

The challenges of transition from hospital to SNF have been noted; however, challenges also are reported in the transition of frail older adults from the SNF to home. One systematic review reported poor outcomes within 90 days, including emergency department visits, hospital readmission, and increased risk of mortality. The authors reported promising but limited evidence of transitional care interventions associated with lower rates of rehospitalization and improved physical function (Toles et al., 2016). In a review of existing transitional care models, recommendations included that the discharge summary from the SNF to home should include identification and availability of a caregiver, a report of baseline cognitive status and cognitive status at discharge, and identification of the primary care provider to link with home care services for ongoing care (Sheikh et al., 2018). Another descriptive study added that SNF cultures that promote staff engagement with individuals and families appear to improve the ability of staff to deliver evidence-based transitional care services (Toles et al., 2016). Successful transition from the SNF to home includes the already identified themes of support for the individuals when they return home, involvement of family, and communication with primary care providers and may also include population-specific recommendations of cognitive evaluation and availability of a caregiver.

Ambulatory/Primary Care to Palliative Care or End-of-Life Services

Health systems frequently offer palliative care and end-of-life services in order to improve quality of care and continuity for individuals and families. Palliative care is described as "a medical subspecialty focused on providing relief from the symptoms, pain, and stress of serious illness. The goal is to improve quality of life for both the patient and the family. It is appropriate at any age and any stage of illness and can be provided along with curative treatment" (Spaulding et al., 2016, p. 189). Although, as noted, palliative care can be provided at any stage of illness, end-of-life or hospice care is provided when the individual's death is imminent.

In the U.S. healthcare system of today, individuals generally do not completely transition to a palliative care team; often their care continues to be overseen by their primary or specialty provider. However, when palliative care is initiated it may become the primary source of care coordination for that individual during the time that it is needed, and this is especially true for individuals who transition to end-of-life care.

Successful transition to palliative care providers includes the essential concepts of communication and support, but with the added focus on the highest possible quality of life, regardless of the expected outcome. Depending on those expected outcomes, transition to this care may require a higher level of emotional support from both the RN coordinating care and provider and the palliative care team. Attention to this emotional support is even more important in the transition to end-of-life care.

Ambulatory/Primary Care to Specialty Care

Referrals from primary care providers to specialists represent a high-volume care transition between and among ambulatory care practices. When there is a care transition between primary care and specialty care, both communication, including robust use of the electronic health record, and collaborative relationships between specialists and primary care providers are important in minimizing gaps in care because of silos created by multiple care providers. Consultative services provided by specialists may be episodic in nature with a focus on a single issue. However, the specialist who has long-term or permanent involvement in the individual's care may make decisions that would overlap with or affect those of the primary care provider. In these situations, it is especially important for the RN to be involved in coordinating care and managing the transition by assuring information flow and the integration of the specialist plan into the longitudinal plan of care. There may be a specific transitional care RN role in these practices.

Care Coordination and Care Transition Tools

The transition from one care setting to another is inherently vulnerable to breakdowns or errors in communication, and evidence has demonstrated that poor communication between service providers at times of transition has contributed to negative patient outcomes. Poorly executed care transitions often result in negative impacts for individuals and their families, as well as downstream effects, including increased costs and risk of rehospitalization (Sheikh et al., 2018). There is evidence that as many as 20% of individuals discharged from acute care hospital settings experience an adverse event within 3 weeks of discharge, 66% of which are medication related (Jusela et al., 2017).

Some contributing factors to poor communication are easily identifiable, such as language barriers, cultural differences, and health literacy. Other factors, however, may be systematic and require the use of standardized tools to ensure that essential aspects of care transitions are not overlooked. It is imperative for healthcare organizations to place a priority on improving processes related to care transitions, particularly between acute care hospitals and the ambulatory care practice environment. Standardization of communication processes and discharge tools has been recognized as a strategy for improving care transitions between hospital and home or next level of care. Some examples are provided in the following section.

Better Outcomes for Older Adults Through Safe Transitions

The Better Outcomes for Older Adults Through Safe Transitions (BOOST) model is a nationally recognized quality improvement program for reducing hospital readmissions and includes use of the 8Ps screening tool and the universal patient discharge checklist and general assessment of preparedness (GAP) (Society of Hospital Medicine, n.d.). The tools assess social determinants of health, predict risk of adverse events postdischarge, and provide risk-specific evidence-based interventions. These tools are available online at https://www.hospitalmedicine.org/globalassets/clinical-topics/clinical-pdf/8ps_riskassess-1.pdf. Outcomes reported across participating organizations include reduced 30-day readmission rates and improved communication between hospital and primary care providers (Hansen et al., 2013; Robertson, 2017).

Project Reengineered Discharge

Project Reengineered Discharge (RED), an innovative discharge approach developed by the research group at Boston University Medical Center, is characterized by a standardized discharge process to ensure individuals are prepared when leaving the hospital. This model includes: (1) tailored education to meet literacy needs and postdischarge care, (2) an emergency plan for the individual and family/caregiver, and (3) an individualized discharge plan and follow-up telephone contact for reinforcement of instructions (Stubenrauch, 2015). The tool kit is available at https://www.bu.edu/fammed/projectred/toolkit.html. Project RED outcomes include improved experience of care, decreased emergency department utilization, decreased readmissions, and decreased costs (Cancino et al., 2017; Stubenrauch, 2015).

STate Action on Avoidable Rehospitalizations

The STate Action on Avoidable Rehospitalizations (STAAR) model was developed by a team at the Institute for Healthcare Improvement (IHI) with the goal of improving transitions from hospital to community settings and reducing avoidable readmissions. The key design elements of this model include individual and family engagement, cross-continuum team collaboration, health information exchange, and shared care plans (Boutwell et al., 2009). Key elements in the ideal transition from acute care hospital to office practice include the assurance of timely access to care following hospitalization, use of standardized communication processes, and adjustment of postdischarge care based on risk. Postdischarge calls focus on medications, self-care, symptom management, and confirmation of follow-up between hospitalist and primary care provider as well as an emphasis on structured elements of posthospital follow-up appointments (Bates et al., 2014). Supporting materials and tools may be found at http://www.ihi.org/Engage/Initiatives/Completed/STAAR/Pages/Materials.aspx.

Integrated Care Transitions Approach

Unlike the three tools described previously, the Integrated Care Transitions Approach (ICTA) is designed to improve transitions across the care continuum between and among ambulatory and primary care, home care, skilled care, and acute care. The seven components of the model are: (1) communicating effectively among provider teams, (2) discussing goals of care and advance directives, (3) assessing function, (4) reconciling medications, (5) implementing a coordinated plan of care, (6) providing timely and complete discharge summaries, and (7) developing person-centered instructions and risk-related education (Sheikh et al., 2018).

The Role of Health Information Technology in Care Coordination

The term "**health information technology (HIT)**" refers to the application of computers and technology in the provision of healthcare. HIT supports care coordination activities by enabling the transfer of information and enhancing communication between providers in different locations, as well as providing clinicians with tools for managing care using distance technology (Austin et al., 2019). The growing use of mobile devices allows on-demand access to health information and enhances communication with individuals through automated reminders.

Advancing the role and use of HIT in improving CCTM within and across settings, disciplines, and with individuals, families, and caregivers must be a priority (Swan et al., 2019b).

HIT is intended to support and complement the practice of CCTM by providing continuous access to information that improves efficiency of care. Information systems have considerable potential to make care coordination more effective, and further development is needed to create systems that reflect the team-based nature of care coordination. Progress is dependent on the creation of standard data formats (domains) related specifically to care coordination, as well as the ability of information systems to transmit this data within and across care settings (interoperability).

More work is needed to create tools that document important care coordination processes and interventions. Domains with the largest gaps include information transfer, monitoring systems, tools to track progress toward self-management goals, and direct links to community resources for individuals, families, and caregivers (Samal et al., 2016). These are significant areas of concern that will continue to hamper progress in accurately documenting, measuring, and reporting care coordination processes, outcomes, and effectiveness.

Care Coordination and Technology-Mediated Information Sharing

Legislation and initiatives related to healthcare reform have ensured that electronic health records are well embedded in the U.S. healthcare system. Electronic health records contain comprehensive, longitudinal information about individuals that supports care across settings and providers. The electronic health record supports documentation, reduces redundancy, and improves accessibility to information across the continuum. Electronic health records also enable individuals to access their health information by way of portals that provide a direct link to secure personal health information (PHI) such as test results and visit notes as well as to scheduling and billing activities. Although portals are an extension of the electronic health record, personal health records (PHRs) are more person-centric, controlled by the individual or family member, and information is shared at the discretion of the individual. Both of these technology-mediated resources provide valuable tools for safe and efficient CCTM.

Care Coordination and Technology-Supported Interventions

Care coordination is arguably the most valuable in the setting of chronic disease management. Technology supporting personal health devices has promise for improving care coordination and the management of outcomes for individuals with chronic diseases, especially those related to behavior choices. For example, populations considered to be at high risk for cardiovascular disease (CVD) include those who use tobacco, have low physical activity levels, are obese, and have type 2 diabetes. Technology-supported interventions have resulted in positive results in these groups (Linke et al., 2016).

Smoking Cessation

Telephone technology to address smoking cessation, commonly referred to as "Quitlines," provides evidence-based support for smokers and maintains high utilization. Many Quitlines offer access to additional information and services, such as personalized plans and counseling, as well as social support. Although more technologically advanced methods are available, these Quitlines have continued to thrive. Other technology-based approaches include smartphone applications (apps), text messaging, social media platforms, and text-based support from trained counselors (Linke et al., 2016).

Obesity

Obesity represents a prevalent risk factor for multiple chronic diseases. In recent years, technology-based interventions have emerged as a promising strategy for supporting weight loss. Interactive computer or Web-based interventions are most common, and mobile technology, including text messaging and mobile telephone applications, is gaining popularity. These technologies integrate behavioral change strategies, health coaching, and wireless scales to support weight management (Linke et al., 2016).

Low Physical Activity

Insufficient physical activity is another prevalent risk factor for CVD and contributes significantly to health issues such as diabetes and metabolic syndrome. Technology-based assessments provided by self-tracking devices have increased in popularity and have the advantage of providing objective and accurate tracking of data. The technology supporting these applications is developing rapidly. These wearable technologies enable those who use them to better understand their needs and take control of their lives (Linke et al., 2016).

HIT Conclusion

Developing and improving HIT applications to manage chronic health issues is a growing field that offers significant support for CCTM in nursing. Improvements in technology will contribute to understanding, describing, and measuring structures, processes, and outcomes of care coordination. A positive downstream effect of this work will be improved recognition of the contributions of nursing toward improving healthcare in the United States, particularly in the areas of CCTM.

Summary

The changing state of healthcare delivery in the United States offers exciting opportunities for RNs in the practice of CCTM. The interplay of complex individual needs, new models of ambulatory care delivery, and technologic advances in communication and self-care creates an environment that allows for optimal use of nursing skills, knowledge, and competencies. The educational preparation for RNs provides the knowledge and skills needed to navigate this changing landscape of care and offers an opportunity for RNs to fully demonstrate the value of their contributions to quality and safe care for individuals, families, and populations.

Case Study

Tom Roberts is a 70-year-old White man, who receives primary care services at a practice near his home. Although Mr. Roberts has enjoyed good health for most of his adult life, he was diagnosed with hypertension at the age of 56 and hyperlipidemia at age 60. Mr. Roberts has become progressively less active since his retirement, steadily gaining weight. Last year he was told by his physician that he is "prediabetic," but he is unsure exactly what this means. At his annual visit last week, his body mass index (BMI) moved to 30.2, and annual lab results revealed a rise in A_{1c} levels to 6.8. Although Mr. Roberts' physician has mentioned the need for exercise, nutrition, and portion control, to date there has been no formalized plan for how to manage his health. The day after his annual visit, Mr. Roberts began to experience shortness of breath and mild chest pain. He presented to the emergency department, was admitted, and underwent an angioplasty, which he tolerated well.

Mr. Roberts has been married for 35 years. His wife is 65 years old and is limited by osteoarthritis in her hands, but otherwise in good health. They have two children, both of whom are married and live in another state. Mrs. Roberts is an active member of her church, but Mr. Roberts rarely attends. He does not have a strong support group of friends and does not socialize very often.

Jan has been an RN for 20 years, 17 of which she spent in an acute care setting, providing bedside nursing on a medical–surgical unit. Three years ago, Jan transitioned from acute care to a position in the primary care practice where Mr. Roberts is a patient. Jan attended an ambulatory nurse residency program to prepare her for her new role. She recently completed a year of study and successfully achieved professional certification as a CCTM-certified nurse. Jan has been appointed as an RN care coordinator with her practice and will now assume Mr. Roberts' care.

1. Use the nursing process to assess Mr. Roberts, and describe the steps, in order of priority, that Jan should take in managing Mr. Roberts' care.
2. What are the goals, immediate and long-term, for Mr. Roberts? How will Jan identify these goals, and who is involved in determining them?
3. What interventions will Jan use to accomplish the goals? Who will be involved in this implementation and how? What are the challenges to implementing her interventions?
4. What are examples of measurable outcomes for Mr. Roberts, and how will Jan evaluate those outcomes?

Key Points for Review

- The continuum of care is a concept that describes a system that guides and tracks individuals over time through a comprehensive array of health services spanning all levels and intensity of care. The continuum of care describes care across time and place, between and during care delivery encounters and care providers.
- The CCTM RN utilizes an evidence base to manage ongoing, longitudinal, individualized plans of care and follow-up plans of care for individuals, families, communities, and populations within the context of healthcare delivery across the care continuum.
- A care transition occurs when an individual moves from one setting of care to another. Transition management works in tandem with care coordination and describes the ongoing support of individuals, families, and populations as they navigate multiple systems of care delivery over time.
- Standardization of communication processes and discharge tools has been recognized as a key strategy for improvement of care transitions between hospital and home or next level of care.
- HIT supports care coordination activities by enabling the transfer of information and enhancing communication between individuals, families, and providers in different locations, as well as providing clinicians with tools for documenting and managing individual care using distance technology.

REFERENCES

Adams, J., Delengowski, A., & Robertson, B. (2019). Care coordination and transition management between acute care and ambulatory care. In S. Haas, B. A. Swan, & T. Haynes (Eds.), *Care coordination and transition management core curriculum* (2nd ed.). Anthony J. Jannetti Publications.

Agency for Healthcare Research and Quality. (2014). *Definition of care management.* https://www.ahrq.gov/professionals/prevention-chronic-care/improve/coordination/atlas2014/chapter3.html#definitions

Ahmed, O. I. (2016). Disease management, case management, care management, and care coordination: A framework and a brief manual for care programs and staff. *Professional Case Management,* 21(3), 137–146. https://doi.org/10.1097/NCM.0000000000000147

American Academy of Ambulatory Care Nursing. (2015). Joint statement: The role of the nurse leader in care coordination and transition management across the health care continuum. *Nursing Economics,* 33(5), 281–282.

American Academy of Ambulatory Care Nursing. (2016). *Scope and standards of practice for registered nurses in care coordination and transition management* (1st ed.). Anthony J. Jannetti Publications.

American Nurses Association. (2015). *Nursing: Scope and standards of practice* (3rd ed.). American Nurses Association.

American Nurses Association. (2017). *The nursing process.* https://www.nursingworld.org/practice-policy/workforce/what-is-nursing/the-nursing-process/

Austin, R., Mercier, N., Kennedy, R., Bouyer-Ferullo, S., Start, R., & Brown, D. (2019). Informatics competencies to support nursing practice. In S. Haas, B. A. Swan, & T. Haynes (Eds.), *Care coordination and transition management core curriculum* (2nd ed.). Anthony J. Jannetti Publications.

Bates, O., O'Connor, N., Dunn, D., & Hasenau, S. (2014). Applying STAAR interventions in incremental bundles: Improving post-CABG surgical patient care. *Worldviews on Evidence-Based Nursing,* 11(2), 89–97. https://doi.org/10.1111/wvn.12028

Bodenheimer, T., & Mason, D. (2017). *Nurses: Partners in transforming primary care.* Proceedings of a conference sponsored by the Josiah Macy Jr. Foundation in June 2016. http://macyfoundation.org/publications/publication/conference-summary-registered-nurses-partners-in-transforming-primary-care

Boutwell, A., Jencks, S., Nielsen, G. A., & Rutherford, P. (2009). *STate action on avoidable rehospitalizations (STAAR) initiative: Applying early evidence and experience in front-line process improvements to develop a state-based strategy.* Institute for Healthcare Improvement.

Bower, K. A. (2016). Nursing leadership and care coordination: Creating excellence in coordinating care across the continuum. *Nursing Administration Quarterly,* 40(2), 98–102. https://doi.org/10.1097/NAQ.0000000000000162

Camicia, M., Chamberlain, B., Finnie, R. R., Nalle, M., Lindeke, L. L., Lorenz, L., Hain, D., Haney, K. D., Campbell-Heider, N., Pecenka-Johnson, K., Jones, T., Parker-Guyton, N., Brydges, G., Briggs, W. T., Cisco, M. C., Haney, C., & McMenamin, P. (2013). The value of nursing care coordination: A white paper of the American Nurses Association. *Nursing Outlook,* 61(6), 490–501. https://doi.org/10.1016/j.outlook.2013.10.006

Cancino, R., Manasseh, C., Kwong, L., Mitchell, S., Martin, J., & Jack, B. (2017). Project RED impacts patient experience. *Journal of Patient Experience,* 4(4), 185–190. https://doi.org/10.1177/2374373517714454

Case Management Society of America. (2017). *Definition of case management.* http://www.cmsa.org/who-we-are/what-is-a-case-manager/

Cipriano, P. F. (2012). American Academy of Nursing on policy. The imperative for patient-, family-, and population-centered interprofessional approaches to care coordination and transitional care: A policy brief by the American Academy of Nursing's care coordination task force. *Nursing Outlook,* 60(5), 330–333. https://doi.org/10.1016/j.outlook.2012.06.021

Cronenwett, L., Sherwood, G., Barnsteiner, J., Disch, J., Johnson, J., Mitchell, P., Sullivan, T. D., & Warren, J. (2007). Quality and safety education for nurses. *Nursing Outlook,* 55(3), 122–131. https://doi.org/10.1016/j.outlook.2007.02.006

Davidson, G. H., Austin, E., Thornblade, L., Simpson, L., Ong, T. D., Pan, H., & Flum, D. R. (2017). Improving transitions of care across the spectrum of healthcare delivery: A multidisciplinary approach to understanding variability in outcomes across hospitals and skilled nursing facilities. *The American Journal of Surgery,* 213(5), 910–914. https://doi.org/10.1016/j.amjsurg.2017.04.002

Fernandes-Taylor, S., Berg, S., Gunter, R., Bennett, K., Smith, M. A., Rathouz, P. J., Greenberg, C. C., & Kent, K. C. (2018). Thirty-day readmission and mortality among Medicare beneficiaries discharged to skilled nursing facilities after vascular surgery. *Journal of Surgical Research,* 221, 196–203. https://doi.org/10.1016/j.jss.2017.08.041

Friedman, A., Howard, J., Shaw, E. K., Cohen, D. J., Shahidi, L., & Ferrante, J. M. (2016). Facilitators and barriers to care coordination in patient-centered medical homes (PCMHs) from coordinators' perspectives. *Journal of the American Board of Family Medicine,* 29(1), 90–101. https://doi.org/10.3122/jabfm.2016.01.150175

Haas, S., Swan, B. A., & Haynes, T. (2013). Developing ambulatory care registered nurse competencies for care coordination and transition management. *Nursing Economics,* 31(1), 44–49, 43.

Haas, S., Swan, B. A., & Haynes, T., (Eds.) (2019). *Care coordination and transition management core curriculum* (2nd ed.). Anthony J. Jannetti Publications.

Hansen, L., Greenwald, J., Budnitz, T., Howell, E., Halasyamani, L., Maynard, G., Vidyarthi, A., Coleman, E., & Williams, M. (2013). Project BOOST: Effectiveness of a multihospital effort to reduce rehospitlaization. *Journal of Hospital Medicine,* 8(8), 421–427. https://doi.org/10.1002/jhm.2054

Healthcare Information and Management Systems Society. (2018). *Continuum of care.* https://www.himss.org/news/advancing-continuum-care-delivery-analytics-adoption-models

Institute of Medicine. (2011). *The future of nursing: Leading change, advancing health.* The National Academies Press.

Jusela, C., Struble, L., Gallagher, N. A., Redman, R. W., & Ziemba, R. A. (2017). Communication between acute care hospitals and skilled nursing facilities during care transitions: A retrospective chart review. *Journal of Gerontological Nursing,* 43(3), 19–28. https://doi.org/10.3928/00989134-20161109-03

Lamb, G., & Newhouse, R. (2018). *Care coordination: A blueprint for action for RNs*. American Nurses Association.

Lamb, G., Newhouse, R., Beverly, C., Toney, D. A., Cropley, S., Weaver, C. A., Kurtzman, E., Zazworsky, D., Rantz, M., Zierler, B., Naylor, M., Reinhard, S., Sullivan, C., Czubaruk, K., Weston, M., Dailey, M., & Peterson, C. (2015). Policy agenda for nurse-led care coordination. *Nursing Outlook,* 63(4), 521–530. https://doi.org/10.1016/j.outlook.2015.06.003

Linke, S. E., Larsen, B. A., Marquez, B., Mendoza-Vasconez, A., & Marcus, B. H. (2016). Adapting technological interventions to meet the needs of priority populations. *Progress in Cardiovascular Diseases,* 58(6), 630–638. https://doi.org/10.1016/j.pcad.2016.03.001

Mehta, P. P., Santiago-Torres, J. E., Wisely, C. E., Hartmann, K., Makadia, F. A., Welker, M. J., & Habash, D. L. (2016). Primary care continuity improves diabetic health outcomes: From free clinics to federally qualified health centers. *Journal of the American Board of Family Medicine,* 29(3), 318–324. https://doi.org/10.3122/jabfm.2016.03.150256

National Quality Forum. (2017). *Care coordination endorsement maintenance project 2016–2017*. http://www.qualityforum.org/ProjectDescription.aspx?projectID=83375

Naylor, M. D., Aiken, L. H., Kurtzman, E. T., Olds, D. M., & Hirschman, K. B. (2011). The care span: The importance of transitional care in achieving health reform. *Health Affairs,* 30(4), 746–754. https://doi.org/10.1377/hlthaff.2011.0041

Norful, A., Martsolf, G., de Jacq, K., & Poghosyan, L. (2017). Utilization of registered nurses in primary care teams: A systematic review. *International Journal of Nursing Studies,* 74, 15–23. https://doi.org/10.1016/j.ijnurstu.2017.05.013

Oncology Nursing Society. (2017). *Oncology nurse navigator core competencies*. https://www.ons.org/sites/default/files/2017-05/2017_Oncology_Nurse_Navigator_Competencies.pdf

Rattray, N. A., Sico, J. J., Cox, L. M., Russ, A. L., Matthias, M. S., & Frankel, R. M. (2017). Crossing the communication chasm: Challenges and opportunities in transitions of care from the hospital to the primary care clinic. *The Joint Commission Journal on Quality and Patient Safety,* 43(3), 127–137. https://doi.org/10.1016/j.jcjq.2016.11.007

Robertson, D. A. (2017). Evaluation of a modified BOOST tool in the acute care setting: A retrospective analysis. *Journal of Nursing Care Quality,* 32(1), 62–70. https://doi.org/10.1097/ncq.0000000000000200

Samal, L., Dykes, P. C., Greenberg, J. O., Hasan, O., Venkatesh, A. K., Volk, L. A., & Bates, D. W. (2016). Care coordination gaps due to lack of interoperability in the United States: A qualitative study and literature review. *BMC Health Services Research,* 16(1), 143. https://doi.org/10.1186/s12913-016-1373-y

Sheikh, F., Gathecha, E., Bellantoni, M., Christmas, C., Lafreniere, J. P., & Arbaje, A. I. (2018). A call to bridge across silos during care transitions. *The Joint Commission Journal on Quality and Patient Safety,* 44(5), 270–278. https://doi.org/10.1016/j.jcjq.2017.10.006

Society of Hospital Medicine. (n.d.). *Transitions to improve outcomes.* https://www.hospitalmedicine.org/clinical-topics/care-transitions/

Spaulding, A., Harrison, D. A., & Harrison, J. P. (2016). Palliative care: A partnership across the continuum of care. *Health Care Management,* 35(3), 189–198. https://doi.org/10.1097/hcm.0000000000000115

Stubenrauch, J. (2015). Project RED reduces hospital readmissions. *American Journal of Nursing,* 115(10), 18–19. https://doi.org/10.1097/01.NAJ.0000471935.08676.ca

Swan, B.A., Haas, S., Haynes, T., & Murray, C. (2019a). Introduction. In S. Haas, B. A. Swan, & T. Haynes (Eds.), *Care coordination and transition management core curriculum* (2nd ed.). Anthony J. Jannetti Publications.

Swan, B. A., Haas, S., & Jessie, A. (2019b). Care coordination: Roles of registered nurses across the care continuum. *Nursing Economics,* 37(6), 317–323.

Toles, M., Colon-Emeric, C., Asafu-Adjei, J., Moreton, E., & Hanson, L. C. (2016). Transitional care of older adults in skilled nursing facilities: A systematic review. *Geriatric Nursing,* 37(4), 296–301. https://doi.org/10.1016/j.gerinurse.2016.04.012

Tomoaia-Cotisel, A., Farrell, T. W., Solberg, L. I., Berry, C. A., Calman, N. S., Cronholm, P. F., Donahue, K. E., Driscoll, D. L., Hauser, D., McAllister, J. W., Mehta, S. N., Reid, R. J., Tai-Seale, M., Wise, C. G., Fetters, M. D., Holtrop, J. S., Rodriguez, H. P., Brunker, C. P., McGinley, E. L., Day, R. L., & Magill, M. K. (2018). Implementation of care management: An analysis of recent AHRQ research. *Medical Care Research and Review,* 75(1), 46–65. https://doi.org/10.1177/1077558716673459

Wagner E. H. (1998). Chronic disease management: what will it take to improve care for chronic illness? *Effective Clinical Practice: ECP*, 1(1), 2–4.

Zazworsky, D., & Bower, K. (2016). Care coordination: Using the present to transform the future. *Nurse Leader,* 14(5), 324–328. https://doi.org/10.1016/j.mnl.2016.07.009

9

Telehealth and Virtual Care Nursing

Mary Elizabeth Greenberg and Carol Rutenberg

PERSPECTIVES

"... there are aspects of the professional expertise and reasoning of nurses that resist being transformed into rules that can be embodied in so-called experts systems ... ."

Greatbatch et al, 2005, p. 826–827.

LEARNING OBJECTIVES

Upon completion of this chapter, the reader will be able to:

1. Identify the key difference between telehealth triage and other telehealth nursing practices.
2. Discuss the real and potential impact of the enhanced Nurse Licensure Compact (eNLC) on telehealth nursing practices.
3. Explain three elements of telehealth nursing that help to ensure individual safety.
4. Identify four standards of practice that define and guide telehealth nursing practices.
5. Describe the role and proper use of decision support tools (DSTs) in telehealth triage.
6. Differentiate among the three types of telehealth nursing.
7. Delineate identified individuals' health needs that telehealth nursing services are suited to meet.

KEY TERMS

Care coordination
Care management
Decision support tools (DSTs)
Enhanced Nurse Licensure Compact (eNLC)
Telehealth nursing
Telehealth triage
Virtual care

Overview and Origins of Telehealth Nursing

Telehealth nursing services today are varied and ever growing, but that was not always the case. The earliest and still possibly the most recognized telehealth nursing service is telephone triage. Telephone triage initially arose out of the need for healthcare organizations to decrease costs in a capitated payment system in the 1980s. Telephone triage nurses were originally used as "gatekeepers," responsible for screening callers in order to reduce unnecessary emergency department (ED) visits.

From Telephone Triage to Telehealth

Initially, telephone triage, now known as **telehealth triage** (American Academy of Ambulatory Care Nursing [AAACN], 2018), took place entirely within the ambulatory care arena. After-hours telephone triage services were delivered from such settings as physician offices, ambulatory care clinics, call centers, and large healthcare organizations such as those in the Veterans Administration (VA). These settings and others remain active today in providing valuable telehealth nursing services.

Nursing practice over the telephone has been shown to make valuable contributions to healthcare. For example, telephone nursing has demonstrated safe care, reductions in unnecessary urgent care and ED visits, positive individual and provider satisfaction, and more efficient use of resources. For organizations providing telehealth nursing services, these outcomes have resulted in improved quality of care and reduced healthcare costs (Cox, 2016). With the success of telephone triage, telephonic services expanded to meet other individual needs including individual education, coaching, behavioral modification (such as smoking cessation or weight reduction), disease management, and postdischarge follow-up. The continually increasing reliance on mobile phones and other communication devices, coupled with frequent needs for immediate access to information, suggest that telephone nursing will continue to be the bedrock of telehealth nursing into the immediate and distant future.

Consider the following three examples:

Mrs. Adams' 6-month-old daughter is congested, fussy, having difficulty breastfeeding, and has a temperature of 101. Mrs. Adams does not know what to do and wonders if she should take the baby to see her pediatrician. Instead she calls the nurse line. During the call the nurse listens to Mrs. Adams describe her baby's symptoms and express her concerns. After an adequate discussion, the nurse assists Mrs. Adams in developing a plan to care for her baby at home. Mrs. Adams hangs up feeling reassured and confident that she can carry out the interventions discussed with the nurse. She is now feeling comfortable knowing signs of worsening condition and having the option of calling back if other questions or concerns arise.

Abby, a registered nurse (RN), sits at a bank of monitors. She notices that the weight and vital signs for Mr. Bennett, slightly elevated from the previous day, are now flagged on the screen to indicate they are outside of the set parameters. Aware that Mr. Bennett has a history of heart failure (HF) and was recently released from the hospital after a bout of pneumonia, Abby immediately calls Mr. Bennett. After a brief talk with Mr. Bennett, Abby determines that there was a mix-up with the pharmacy delivery and Mr. Bennett has been without his medication for 2 days. Per protocol, Abby instructs Mr. Bennett to take a diuretic and then is able to contact the pharmacy, get the appropriate medications delivered, and ensure that Mr. Bennett is back on schedule.

Ms. Marks had an appointment with her primary care physician earlier this week. This morning, Jeff noticed that Ms. Marks had sent a portal message in the middle of the night. She could not sleep because she was trying to remember what Dr. Dare had instructed her about her new medication regimen. She was taking warfarin and was accustomed to frequent changes, but this change eluded her and she wanted confirmation before she took her next dose. Jeff responded in the portal by first inquiring whether she was having any bleeding or other signs or symptoms. About 30 minutes later, Ms. Marks responded in the negative, reiterating the reason for her message. Jeff referred to the individual's record and sent Ms. Marks a message detailing her current regimen. He also reviewed the interactions of warfarin and leafy greens and then closed his note with an invitation for Ms. Marks to e-mail or call if she had any further questions or concerns.

What do these anecdotes have in common? They are all examples of telehealth nursing. Telehealth nursing is the delivery of nursing care and services over distance using some form of telehealth technology, also referred to as telecommunications technology (AAACN, 2018).

Telehealth nursing meets **care management**, access, education, or other health-related needs without requiring the individual to be physically present in the healthcare setting. Telehealth services are also referred to as "connected care" and "**virtual care**." Telehealth nursing services can vary from one-on-one care to population health; from a brief one-time interaction to an ongoing long-term relationship; and from technology as simple as the telephone to more sophisticated home or wearable monitoring devices and video conferencing. "The value of telehealth to the client is increased access to skilled, empathetic and effective nursing delivered through telecommunications technology" (National Council of State Boards of Nursing [NCSBN], 2014, para. 2).

The umbrella terms *telehealth* and *virtual care* include the concepts of telehealth nursing and telemedicine. The growth of telehealth services in recent years has been phenomenal. Outpatient telehealth encounters have grown 1,400% between 2014 and 2018 (FAIR Health, 2019). These telehealth encounters often include video visits or consults. Certainly, the RN has an important role in these encounters, often being present with the individual for on-site assessment, intervention, and coordination. This chapter addresses telehealth nursing roles designed to deliver nursing care that is more independent in nature and those that focus on connection and communication qualities necessary to ensure quality and safety in remote care delivery.

As various telehealth services become mainstream and continue to grow in depth, breadth, and significance, it is important to recognize that telehealth nursing still involves a nurse–individual relationship and embodies all that is nursing. Even though it is practiced by what was once considered nontraditional means, all types of telehealth nursing service, regardless of whether the recipient is the individual, family, or caregiver, is professional nursing. Once a nurse has responded to a call, a message, or other forms of communication with an individual, a nurse/individual relationship exists. Thus, the RN has a duty to provide individuals with the standard of care, defined as competent, prudent, and reasonable nursing practice. As with any form of professional nursing practice, telehealth nurses are held to the same legal, ethical, and professional standards of practice. Furthermore, like many specialty or subspecialty nursing practices, telehealth nurses are also guided by a scope and standards developed for and specific to the practice (AAACN, 2018).

Individuals living in rural areas with limited access to healthcare resources, homebound individuals with few options for transportation, individuals with multiple complex conditions, the busy working mother picking up her sick child from day care, and the individual needing migraine medication whose provider is on vacation are all potential beneficiaries of telehealth nursing services. Telehealth nursing facilitates access to the appropriate level of care, provides care to those without access to care, provides education and support to improve individual self-management, and assists individuals in navigating our complex healthcare system. As telehealth services expand throughout the healthcare system, it is important to recognize when the service belongs in the realm of professional nursing. This chapter discusses current practice, the standards of care, the nursing process, education, and preparation in telehealth nursing, practice models and settings, and future prospects.

Perception of Telehealth Nursing

It is important to note that there was a time telehealth nursing was not recognized as professional nursing. Healthcare administrators, providers, and even nurses failed to recognize the sophistication of practicing nursing remotely. In the 1990s, the professional and regulatory bodies the American Nurses Association (ANA, 1999) and the NCSBN (1997) both issued definitive statements declaring that telehealth nursing is indeed professional nursing practice. Telehealth nurses today must continually guard against the misconception that practicing nursing remotely using telehealth technology is not "real nursing." Perhaps this misconception arose because nursing is often recognized by tasks (eg, start IVs, give medicine, change dressings) rather than the cognitive nature of this practice. Telehealth nurses must often perform assessment without visual cues, provide advocacy and education, and coordinate care. The realization that the nurse is a knowledge worker is never more appropriate than in telehealth nursing.

Telehealth Nursing Today

Although telephone nursing remains the most utilized and visible form, telehealth nursing has expanded to include remote services such as individual monitoring, videoconferencing, information sharing, and complex chronic condition management. Telehealth nursing can be as varied as the technology utilized and the needs of each individual. The continued transition from inpatient to outpatient settings, the rapid evolution of technologic capabilities, the shrinking financial and human resources in the healthcare arena, and the influence of value-based reimbursement (pay for performance) have all contributed to the growth of telehealth nursing.

Telehealth nursing has outgrown the ambulatory care arena. With the rapid advancements in technology and the increasing ability to identify and meet individuals' needs, telehealth services are now being utilized throughout the healthcare system. For example, in acute care settings, Tele-ICUs provide surveillance, alerts, and support to the nursing staff. Discharge follow-up calls to facilitate self-care, bolster discharge teaching, and prevent readmission are utilized in both acute care and ambulatory care surgery centers.

Today, telehealth nursing is practiced within and across all settings in the healthcare environment. Telehealth nursing services may consist of a dedicated and formal service where many nurses are located in a call center and provide telehealth triage to a large defined population. In other settings, the nurses play a large role in telepresenting, or preparing individuals for videoconferencing with specialty providers. A provider office setting may have a dedicated nurse to manage symptom-based calls and/or coordinate care. Formal programs or services, ideally guided by organizational policies and procedures, provide orientation and training to the telehealth nursing staff and implement ongoing quality assessments of individual and program performance. However, often telehealth nursing services go unrecognized as being part of this larger specialty. For example, the ambulatory care RN who arranges for a direct individual hospital admission, a nurse in an outpatient surgery center who responds to a call from a post-op individual, and the interventional radiology nurse who contacts individuals to provide pre- or postprocedure instructions are all practicing telehealth nursing. Regardless of formal recognition or policy, it is in the nurse's best interest to be aware that interaction with any individual via telehealth technology (eg, telephone, portal, e-mail, text) is the practice of nursing.

Care management and **care coordination** are discussed in more detail in Chapter 8, but they are an essential component of telehealth nursing. Telehealth nursing uses assessment and collaborative planning by both the nurse and the individual to close all gaps (eg, knowledge, communication, medication, access, continuity) in an individual's healthcare journey. Care coordination often occurs in non-face-to-face settings and relies heavily on technology for interprofessional communication, collaboration, and information sharing. Care coordination illustrates how telehealth nursing spans acute care, ambulatory care, community, and home health.

Current Issues

No description or discussion of telehealth nursing would be complete without mention of issues that are central to the practice. In recent memory, no issue has had more impact on healthcare than COVID-19 (Box 9.1). Interstate practice, scope of practice, and individual safety are historic and current practice issues that may have bearing on any telehealth encounter. These topics are discussed in more detail later in this chapter.

BOX 9.1 Telehealth Nursing During and After the Coronavirus Pandemic

As the coronavirus (COVID-19) pandemic spread to the United States in early 2020, incredible efforts were made to prevent the healthcare system from being overwhelmed. Telehealth nursing played a major role in preserving resources and reducing demand on hospitals, emergency departments, and urgent care centers—a crucial need at that time. For close to 2 weeks, many organizations managed an up to tenfold increase in the demand for remote nursing. In addition to triaging callers to ensure they get the appropriate level of care, telehealth nurses helped to inform, advise, calm, and reassure often-panicked callers. Many organizations around the country provided communities with telephone triage, remote monitoring of COVID-19 patients at home, access to care and information via secure chats on patient portals, text messaging, and community call and chat services for those seeking COVID-19 information or guidance on testing, disinfecting, isolation, quarantine, masks, and other issues. Additional telehealth services initiated included outreach to vulnerable populations, monitoring employee health, and remote symptom management using mobile apps.

As the initial peak of the virus waned, nurses using telephone, video chats, and remote monitoring continued to play an important role in helping COVID-19 patients at home cope with and recover from the disease. Telehealth nursing also became increasingly valuable for slowing or stopping the spread via contact tracing. Furthermore, as hospitals, clinics, and providers became more available for nonemergency/non-COVID-19-related health problems and elective procedures, a key role of the telehealth nurse changed from managing COVID-19 and previously existing health-related concerns to patient outreach to ensure that essential cancelled procedures and surgeries were rescheduled. In the long-term wake of this pandemic experience, telehealth nurses will continue to be a crucial resource for coping with resurgences of the novel coronavirus and with other widespread health threats that may develop in the coming years.

Interstate Practice

The Board of Nursing (BON) in each state is the regulatory authority for nursing, and the scope of practice in each state is defined by the Nurse Practice Act (NPA). Because the practice transcends geographic boundaries, the locus of responsibility (ie, where the delivery of nursing services is taking place) is considered to be at the location of an individual and thus under the jurisdiction of the BON in that state. There are sometimes significant differences among the states, which can be problematic for telehealth nurses. Some important differences that affect telehealth nurses are the definition of nursing, the scope of practice for RNs and licensed practical nurses (LPNs), and the ability to recommend over-the-counter or prescription medications. Compliance with regulatory standards requires the nurse not only to be licensed in the state in which the care is being delivered but also to be practicing within the guidelines set out by the NPA for that state. Whether the nurse is answering a telephone call, facilitating a medication refill, or advising an individual about treatment of a fever, differences in the NPAs pose a challenge for nurses caring for individuals in multiple states.

In an effort to reduce the regulatory burden on nurses who are practicing in multiple states, in 2018 an **enhanced Nurse Licensure Compact (eNLC)** became effective. This potential legislation permits nurses in compact states to practice in other states that are members of the compact, effectively issuing these nurses a multistate license (NCSBN, n.d.). The eNLC is a solution for those nurses and individuals in compact states, but the dilemma still remains for nurses providing care in non-compact states.

Role and Scope of Practice

In many ambulatory care settings, especially in physician offices and outpatient clinics, the lines between scopes of practice for various roles are often blurred. In telehealth nursing, this is particularly problematic when unlicensed assistive personnel (UAP) are responding to individual calls or handling online requests. The ability to provide safe, efficient, and person-centered care is dependent on having the right level of personnel in each role, with every member of the staff working at the top of their license (Institute of Medicine, 2010). This means that RNs must be engaged in all elements of care that require assessment, critical thinking, clinical reasoning, and clinical judgment. This requires delegating everything that *does not* require an RN license to LPNs and UAP. In addition to having the right person in the right role, it is important that the RN have specialized training in telehealth nursing as well as other aspects of their job.

Individual Safety

Safety is always an issue in the delivery of individual care, but takes on added significance when the care is delivered with technology rather than in person. In telehealth nursing practices, awareness that nursing is taking place is critical. It is possible to be lulled into thinking that the nurse is merely collecting and transmitting information or scheduling individuals' appointments without recognizing the need for assessment and the critical thinking that is inherent in these tasks especially when dealing with a symptom-based encounter. For these encounters, **decision support tools (DSTs)** add an element of safety in that they provide a comprehensive list of assessment questions that are relevant to the primary symptom of the individual. The use of DSTs (discussed later in more detail) is a standard of practice for managing symptom-based calls. The use of DSTs does not ensure safety. Rather, they are a useful reference and act as a reminder and an aid, but it is the RN who must analyze, contextualize, and draw conclusions from the individual's responses.

An individual's safety is compromised the minute the telehealth nurse loses sight of the fact that telehealth nursing is professional nursing practice. In addition to practicing within identified standards of professional nursing, telehealth nurses also must keep in mind that any remote interaction with the individual, regardless of the original purpose of the contact, has the potential to be a triage encounter. Without exception, anytime an individual presents with a symptom, it is important that they be properly assessed by an RN. Even a chronic symptom, whether presenting by phone, e-mail, or online portal, deserves a close look because the individual perceives it as enough of a problem to contact the nurse about it. Furthermore, beyond the obvious, it is key to realize that if an individual does not need an appointment, they need *something*, and it is the responsibility of the RN to assess, recognize, and address that problem.

Telehealth Nursing Practice

Nursing is guided by regulatory/legal, professional, organizational, and ethical standards of practice. Standards that apply to professional nursing also apply to telehealth nursing. For example, hanging up on an individual who is being verbally abusive could be considered as individual abandonment. The rules and standards governing the practice of nursing are not mitigated because the nurse is not face to face with the individual. However, the same training, protection, and safety resources that are available for face-to-face encounters also should be available for telehealth nursing.

Standards of Professional Nursing Practice

The nursing process is the foundation of all nursing practice. However, utilizing the nursing process is not the only standard with which nurses must comply. The state's NPA, professional and specialty nursing standards, as well as organizational policies and procedures provide the standards by which nursing care is evaluated. These convey the minimum expectations of nursing and these standards are used to guide and determine the quality of care. In a legal matter involving a nurse, the experts and the legal team will first look to see whether the nurse was practicing outside of any of the relevant standards. Did the nurse comply with the existing standards? The prudent telehealth nurse will be well informed on standards of practice and make every effort to comply.

Nurse Practice Act

Standards of care that apply to telehealth nursing, as in all forms of professional nursing, include an NPA that is specified by each state's BON. It is the NPA in each state that defines the scope of nursing practice and grants licensure to those who meet the requirements. It is the responsibility of the telehealth nurse to be aware of where the individual is and thus in which state the care is being provided and to know the scope of nursing practice in that state.

Professional Organization Standards

The next set of standards that guide telehealth nursing practice is the ANA's *Nursing: Scope and Standards of Practice*, 3rd edition (2015a). These standards are based on the nursing process and provide a guide, a level of competence, and practice expectations for all nurses. The ANA also provides nurses with ethical standards. This Nursing Code of Ethics (ANA, 2015b) states the expectation of ethical behavior and decision-making in nursing.

Specialty Standards

In addition to the basic standards for professional nursing practice, there are specialty standards. Basic practice standards for the telehealth nurse are detailed in the Scope and Standards for Professional Telehealth Nursing developed and regularly updated by the AAACN since 1997.

Organizational Standards

The NPA, professional nursing, and specialty standards describe the competency level at which all nursing should be delivered. Accountability to the public and to the profession is demonstrated by adhering to these standards. Telehealth nurses are also accountable to their employers. Therefore, organizational standards in the form of policies and procedures also provide guidelines for professional practice. Policies and procedures are the guidelines for the specific organization or program in which the nurse is working. Organizational standards may be more stringent than professional or practice standards but should not be more lenient. For example, many telehealth programs today require DSTs as a standard of practice. It is the responsibility of the telehealth nurse to be knowledgeable of all the standards for practice, to practice within those guidelines, and to utilize the nursing process and relevant organizational tools in direct provision of care.

Nursing Process in Telehealth

The key platform for delivery of telehealth nursing is the nurse–individual interface. It is here that the nurse forms a relationship with the individual, identifies an individual's needs, and then finds ways to meet those needs while honoring the individual values and resources of the person. This nurse–individual interface occurs largely within the context of the **nursing process**, which is widely regarded as the basic standard of professional nursing practice. The next sections give a brief look at the nursing process in a symptom-based telehealth encounter.

Assessment

The individual assessment includes collection and interpretation of both subjective and objective findings. Distinguishing subjective and objective data is a bit more complicated for telehealth encounters than for face-to-face encounters. Many nurses have learned that "subjective" is what you *hear* and "objective" is what you *see*. Seeing, of course, is not an option in many forms of telehealth nursing, and hearing as well is not an option during online interactions with individuals or interpretation of physiologic monitoring parameters. In telehealth triage, the hearing is not only what the individual says, it is also what the nurse hears in the background; indeed, these background sounds may provide key data and insight into the care needs and context of the individual. Because of the critical thinking that is inherent in assessment, the data collection must always be conducted by an RN (Rutenberg & Greenberg, 2012).

Gathering Information

A good way to begin assessment is to listen carefully to the individuals as they describe their symptoms and the reason for contacting the nurse. As the individual tells their story, the nurse can identify symptoms, signs, and health concerns and look for relationships among the signs and symptoms. Assessment questions will then be based on the nurse analysis of the individual information. Verification and clarification with the individual are important to ensure accuracy and understanding of the problem. To ensure that something important is not missed, it is good practice to use a systematic process and a good documentation tool when assessing. The amount of time spent gathering information can be short and to the point as in an emergent situation or it can be comprehensive as in the case of a nonacute but complex healthcare need.

Subjective and Objective Findings

To understand the terms "subjective" and "objective" in a non-face-to-face (remote) encounter, we must change our thinking somewhat to realize that subjective data are what the individual reports and how the individual feels and cannot be confirmed with physical evidence. Reported symptoms and ongoing information being provided by the individual are subjective. Objective data are those pieces of information that can be measured and/or confirmed.

Measurement and confirmation of symptoms occur via responses to the nurse's inquiries and reports on the individual. It is also helpful to keep in mind that the individual, family, or caregiver can provide objective data by measuring such information as their blood pressure or their weight. The individual/family/caregiver also can be a participant in the collection of objective data by using their eyes, hands, or sense of smell to report findings such as pitting edema, discoloration, or the color and odor of drainage. Anything the nurse can assess using their visual, tactile, or olfactory senses can also be observed and reported by a well-coached individual or family member/caregiver.

Information gained from automatic remote monitoring of data is objective because it does not rely on a verbal report from the individual or family member. Remote monitoring may include the automatic gathering of data related to blood pressure, blood glucose, cardiac monitoring, as well as other physiologic parameters.

Some findings may be confirmed by both subjective and objective information. For example, if the individual *complains* of a cough, it is a subjective finding. If the nurse *hears* the individual cough, that finding would be objective. A fever (measured with a thermometer) is an objective finding, but feeling hot or feeling feverish is subjective. The data collected and documented during the assessment are useful in painting a clinical picture of the individual for anyone reviewing the notes.

Diagnosis

The telehealth RN uses critical thinking, clinical reasoning, and clinical judgment in the interpretation of the subjective and objective findings to develop a nursing diagnosis. The type of telehealth nursing will determine the elements of the nursing diagnosis. For example, in telehealth triage, the nursing diagnosis will identify the nature and urgency of the individual's problem, as well as any factors that might potentially confound the plan of care, such as individual reluctance to seek care. In care coordination, the nursing diagnosis is likely more traditional, such as "knowledge deficiency" or "self-care deficiency" regarding home care or the individual's medication regimen. In the case of monitoring physiologic individual parameters (such as remote monitoring of an individual's heart rhythm), the nursing diagnosis might be a definitive interpretation such as "asymptomatic tachycardia" or "atrial fibrillation with rapid ventricular response accompanied by dizziness and shortness of breath." In any case, the diagnosis should provide sufficient information to guide the nurse in identification of desired outcomes.

Desired Outcomes

In collaboration with the individual, the telehealth RN then identifies desired outcomes, or what they wish to accomplish in addressing the nursing diagnosis. In telehealth triage, the desired outcome in an individual with emergent chest pain might be to "reach definitive care prior to a catastrophic event." With an urgent abdominal pain, the desired outcome might be to "obtain evaluation prior to deterioration of the condition." The desired outcome in a nonurgent problem might be "individual/family/caregiver will comfortably and competently manage child's nausea and vomiting at home, promptly recognizing indications for medical evaluation."

Plan

The telehealth RN and the individual collaboratively develop a plan of care that outlines actions necessary to meet the desired outcomes. For example, in keeping with the examples given earlier, the plans might be (respectively), "to the ED now via emergency medical services (EMS)," "appointment today with primary care provider (PCP)," or "educate mother on home management of nausea and vomiting and identification of signs of dehydration that would prompt a call back."

Intervention

In the intervention, the telehealth RN outlines exact steps to accomplish the plan of care. Again, in keeping with the previous examples, interventions might be "advise individual to dial 911," "appointment made to see Dr. Jones at 1:30 pm today," or "mother instructed on rehydration of child and to call back if child is unable to retain liquids, develops signs of dehydration such as dry mouth, scant or concentrated urine, and/or dizziness upon standing."

Evaluation

Although there are multiple ways to evaluate a remote nurse–individual encounter, in the context of the nursing process, evaluation specifically assesses whether the interventions accomplished the desired outcomes. This differs from evaluation of the telehealth program, which assesses whether the overall service accomplished the expected outcomes.

Evaluating an Encounter

Evaluation in telehealth nursing encounters focuses on the quality of the encounter. Quality measures for each encounter include use of the nursing process, adequate assessment, and a disposition that is consistent with the assessment information. The basic question to be answered is, was the individual's need accurately identified and addressed? In a telehealth encounter, evaluation of the outcome of the call focuses on whether the needs of the individual have been met. One important way to assess this is to ensure that the disposition (eg, final advice to individual) is consistent with the assessment data and diagnosis.

Evaluation also includes confirmation of individual understanding of, and agreement with, the plan. Are they comfortable with the information provided? Do they intend to carry out the plan? Are there any additional questions or concerns? Does the individual know whom to contact if the need arises? If the individual is hesitant, uncomfortable, or unwilling to implement the plan, then it is the nurse's responsibility to acknowledge and explore the reluctance and address the unidentified individual needs. When necessary to ensure safe care and/or individual comfort and satisfaction, a recheck or follow-up with the individual may be initiated by either the individual or the telehealth RN.

Evaluating a Program

It is important to note that evaluation of the telehealth encounter is different from evaluation of the telehealth service program. As noted earlier, each telehealth triage encounter is evaluated according to how well the individual nurse met the needs of the individual. Evaluation of the program will assess outcomes such as overall safety (eg, were dispositions accurate and consistent with assessment data), satisfaction (eg, individual survey), and cost savings (eg, appropriate use of resources).

Documentation

In telehealth nursing, the medical record serves primarily as a communication tool among all members of the healthcare team. Documentation of the telehealth encounter informs and updates the health team members and thus contributes to the continuity and coordination of care for the individual. It is also, of course, a legal document and serves to help the RN organize their thinking. This takes on special importance when there is no physical individual present and the medical record is often the only tangible source the nurse has during the encounter. The old adage that "if it's not written, it didn't happen" may not be true, but what is almost indisputably true is, "if it's not written, you can't prove it happened." For this and other reasons, it is important for the nurse to document pertinent negatives (what the individual doesn't have) as well as pertinent positives (signs or symptoms that are present).

A good format for documentation that is basic and easy to follow is found in the SOAPIE format. This format is familiar to many (it is an expansion of the traditional SOAP format) and it provides comprehensive evidence of use of the nursing process. The addition of implementation and evaluation to the traditional SOAP note allows the RN to fully determine the success of the care plan.

- **S**ubjective: Assessment findings that reflect information reported by the individual that is not subject to validation.
- **O**bjective: Assessment findings reflecting information that is subject to validation.
- **A**ssessment or Diagnosis: The nursing diagnosis or conclusion the nurse reaches based on the subjective and objective findings.
- **P**lan: The plan developed collaboratively with the individual to address the nursing diagnosis and achieve desired outcomes.
- **I**mplementation: Steps taken to operationalize the plan of care.
- **E**valuation: The strategy the nurse will use to determine whether the interventions were effective.

Decision Support Tools

In telehealth triage, the nurse's inability to see or touch the individual creates the potential for ambiguity in the process of individual assessment and decision-making, most notably in triage encounters. This potential for uncertainty, coupled with the largely independent nature of telehealth triage nursing, has prompted development of different types of tools to support and guide telehealth triage and other forms of telehealth nursing. Variously regarded as protocols, guidelines, and algorithms, they are collectively referred to as DSTs. These tools help guide the process and supplement the nurse's knowledge, experience, and intuition.

DSTs play an important role in the delivery of care using telehealth technologies and their use is widely regarded as the standard of care (AAACN, 2018). DSTs provide significant support for telehealth triage by serving as a checklist to ensure adequate assessment and they help to standardize decision-making within an organization; however, they must be used appropriately, or their use can become a hindrance to quality care delivery (Tariq et al., 2017).

DSTs are available in the form of books or manuals and as software applications. Those imbedded in software applications provide additional assistance with documentation and report generation to track workload. Either way, it is critical that the telehealth triage nurse be aware that these DSTs exist only to supplement the nurse's own knowledge base (AAACN, 2018; Ernesater et al., 2009) and serve as a checklist to minimize the likelihood that something of importance is overlooked.

DSTs are not specific to telehealth triage. In remote monitoring and other ongoing individual services (eg, chronic disease management), computerized decision support systems (CDSSs) are often integrated into the electronic health record and used by nurses. CDSSs in nontriage telehealth nursing not only help with decision-making but also provide prompts, alerts, and guidelines for interventions based on recorded data.

Use of Decision Support Tools

DSTs provide many advantages. They serve as a safety net by providing a list of questions or factors to minimize the potential for the nurse to forget or overlook a critical element of the assessment. This is especially important for relatively inexperienced nurses and even for expert nurses when they are rushed or fatigued. They supplement the RN's own knowledge base because it is impossible for even an experienced RN to have all-inclusive and comprehensive knowledge about all symptoms for which the individual might consult the nurse. DSTs simplify the nurse's work by providing a searchable database. They also improve professional security and increase credibility (Ernesater et al., 2009).

Likewise, there are disadvantages to the use of DSTs. They have been perceived as interfering with decision making by imposing unnecessary control. They may obstruct independent thinking and occasionally result in recommendation of a disposition that the nurse disagrees with, resulting in advice that is "irrational and unnecessary" (Ernesater et al., 2009, p. 1079).

Efforts are ongoing to develop artificial-intelligence-based DSTs, but the nurse must keep in mind that many individual care considerations are, at present, beyond the scope of existing DSTs. Many of these considerations are those that support individualization of care, examples of which are listed as follows:

- Chronic illnesses: Although DSTs do incorporate mitigating factors such as diabetes or immunosuppression, other chronic illnesses that may impact decision-making are often not included in the logic of the DST itself.
- Age and gender: Age and gender may not always be addressed in a specific DST but still may be factors to address in addition to criteria included in the DST.
- Accessibility: Influences such as time of day, distance from care, and prevailing weather or traffic conditions are not included in DSTs, but also must often be considered.
- Socioeconomic determinants: Variables such as available resources, health literacy, and cultural considerations must be addressed outside the scope of the DST.

Whereas some degree of standardization is desirable and has the potential to decrease error, the nurse must be ever alert to the importance of individualizing care. Regardless of the quality or construct of the DSTs, the telehealth triage nurse must regard these as decision *support* tools rather than decision-making tools.

It is important that all nurses use, but not rely on, DSTs to be sure nothing has been overlooked. It also is critical that the RN not lose sight of the fact that DSTs are checklists and are not intended to override or replace the critical thinking, clinical reasoning, or clinical judgment of the telehealth RN.

Telehealth Skills, Competencies, and Certification

Traditionally, most telehealth education has been in the form of on-the-job training. However, there is a growing need for formal education to keep up with technology and the growth of the nursing profession. Traditionally, ambulatory care nursing in general has received little attention in undergraduate education, and telehealth nursing in particular often received no attention at all. Thus, nurses engaging in telehealth nursing either acquired postgraduation education or not at all, perhaps never realizing that talking with an individual over the phone or interacting via e-mail did indeed represent the practice of nursing and thus required all the attention afforded to any form of nursing.

Necessary education about telehealth nursing should be both deep and broad, with attention required to many dissimilar elements. First, higher level critical thinking skills must be taught and cultivated. Second, baseline general nursing knowledge and knowledge of diseases is important and must represent lifelong learning. Third, the nurse must have specialized knowledge specific to telehealth nursing (eg, assessment and communication that is not in a face-to-face setting). Fourth, technical knowledge surrounding use of telehealth technology is critical and generally organization specific. And finally, nurses who provide virtual or remote care must have knowledge of local resources that are available and suitable for the individual in distant locations.

In addition to orientation or education in the workplace, the requisite knowledge, skills, and attitude about telehealth nursing should be formally acquired either through undergraduate or graduate nursing education, with online or external courses or certification.

Reasoning Skills

Critical thinking, clinical reasoning, and **clinical judgment** are necessary for the management of almost every telehealth encounter. Thus, education on these important concepts is needed in the context of virtual care and telehealth. A fourth element, **clinical competence**, is acquired through experience and application of the previous three skills.

Critical thinking has been defined as "reasonable reflective thinking focused on deciding what to believe or do" (Ennis, 2015, p. 32). Elements of critical thinking roughly correlate with steps of the nursing process, emphasizing all the more why the nurse must consciously follow the nursing process faithfully.

Clinical reasoning is a challenging element of nursing, in part because of the ambiguity encountered in defining it. A conceptual analysis of clinical reasoning resulted in the following definition: "Clinical reasoning in nursing is defined as a complex cognitive process that uses formal and informal thinking strategies to gather and analyze individual information, evaluate the significance of this information, and determine the value of alternative actions" (Simmons, 2010, p. 1156). The concept of clinical reasoning is also embedded in Benner's skill acquisition model (Benner et al., 1996). It is an important element of telehealth triage nursing incorporating "experience, knowledge, skills, and caring" (Simmons, 2010, p. 1156).

Clinical judgment is the conclusion reached as a result of the critical thinking and clinical reasoning conducted by the nurse. The telehealth nurse seeks to address deficits in the individual's ability to provide self-care and advocate for themselves and to detect real or potential gaps in care.

Clinical competence combines all of the accumulated skills and knowledge described earlier. The RN needs a robust clinical knowledge base, because in telehealth nursing there is little if any opportunity to control the nature of the individual encounter. For instance, in follow-up or management of HF, the individual might present with worsening shortness of breath. Although the shortness of breath might be related to the individual's baseline HF, it might also represent an unexpected pathology such as pneumonia or a pulmonary embolus. The nurse must be vigilant to identify and promptly triage any symptom-based encounters. Given that the nurse cannot predict unexpected presentations, an extensive knowledge base is an important part of individual care. DSTs, as previously discussed, are helpful tools to supplement the nurse's own knowledge base.

Telehealth nurses must possess knowledge specific to telehealth triage, because potentially any encounter could present a need for triage. Identification of any potential symptoms must always be the first step of the telehealth process. This specific knowledge includes attitudinal skills such as to avoid accepting individual self-diagnosis or jumping to a conclusion, speaking directly with the individual whenever possible, and always erring on the side of caution. These and other telephone triage/telehealth practice principles will be discussed at greater length later in this chapter.

Technical Skills

Technical skill in manipulating the telehealth technology is essential. This knowledge may be as simple and general as typing proficiency or as specific and complex as being able to expertly navigate the telehealth software. Because of the wide variability of telehealth technology, this facet of education and training must generally be conducted on-site within the specific organization.

Certification

Certification is a professional credential that recognizes knowledge and expertise in the specialty area of certification. Certification in Telephone Nursing Practice (C-TNP) was available from 2001 to 2007 through the National Certification Corporation. The certification examination was discontinued due in part to flagging interest. However, nurses who achieved this certification prior to its discontinuation may maintain the certification by meeting continuing education (CE) requirements.

At present, the American Nurses' Credentialing Center (ANCC) supports board certification in Ambulatory Care Nursing (RN-BC), which has incorporated a significant amount of telehealth nursing content. Today, telehealth nurses are encouraged to acquire ambulatory care certification in recognition of their content knowledge in this area of practice. Another certification offered by the ANCC is the Informatics Nursing Certification. Nursing informatics is highly valued in telehealth nursing as the focus is technology, information management, and nursing practice. The informatics nurse is perfectly situated to bridge the gap between technology and clinical practice.

Telehealth Nursing Practice Models

Most practicing nurses engage in telehealth nursing as part of their regular duties. However, nurses, providers, and administrators often fail to recognize that common nurse–individual interactions over the telephone, Skype, portal, e-mail, video, and other technologies constitute nursing practice. The nurse is the first person responsible for recognizing that the remote activities in which they engage constitute nursing practice. This section will provide an overview of three notable roles that involve substantial telehealth nursing.

Telehealth Triage

Telehealth triage nurses assist callers to access the appropriate level of care according to their symptoms or healthcare concerns. A telehealth triage encounter may begin with, "I have a toothache," and end in an emergency call for a 58-year-old male caller with jaw pain, shortness of breath, and diaphoresis. Or, a telehealth triage encounter may begin with a panicked, "Something is wrong with my baby," and end in a lengthy coaching session about breastfeeding when the baby is congested. Navigating these and other individual concerns safely required in-depth knowledge and skill.

Purpose

The purpose of telehealth triage is to identify the nature and urgency of an individual's problem and assist the individual in getting the appropriate level of care. Individuals who present with a symptom-based concern must be triaged. If the contact is via an inbound telephone call, ideally the call is routed directly to the RN who has the skills and knowledge to assess the individual, prioritize the immediate healthcare needs, and direct the individual to the appropriate level of care. If a symptom-based contact comes over the computer via the individual portal or e-mail, the RN must be notified promptly and must then contact the individual by telephone to assess the individual.

Triage is a dynamic real-time process that is not amenable to asynchronous written interaction such as is found in portal or e-mail messages. Any telehealth encounter has the potential to require triage, although that need may not always be immediately evident. Thus, a careful inquiry of the individual regarding the presence of any symptoms is critical to identification of triage encounters that might present under another guise. The following case provides an example of this process (Box 9.2).

BOX 9.2 Importance of Careful Triage

A 70-year-old woman, Mrs. Lewis, contacted her primary care provider's office with "one quick question" which was "Is nitroglycerin still good after 10 years?" Of course, a registered nurse (RN) and even many unlicensed personnel know that the answer to that is "no."

However, when the cautious RN asked her, "Why do you ask?", wanting to be sure the individual was not experiencing chest pain, Mrs. Lewis replied that she was asking because she had been cleaning out her medicine cabinet and throwing her expired medications in the trash can. Sheila, the nurse, continued to probe and discovered that the real reason for the call was that Mrs. Lewis was babysitting for her 18-month-old grandson who had gotten into the trash can and was found sitting on the floor playing with a nitroglycerin bottle with the lid open and several tablets on the floor next to him.

This example illustrates the fact that not all individuals will be forthcoming with the *real* reason for their contact unless asked. They often request the information they *think* they need in order to make a decision about the health of themselves or a loved one. For this reason, all telehealth encounters require investigation and accurate identification of the problem. There is some reason or unmet need motivating the individual to reach out.

Practice Principles

Because of the complexity of managing an individual using primarily verbal clues, it is critical that all triage encounters be managed by RNs. The authors believe "there is no other form of nursing in any setting that requires more critical thinking and independent clinical judgment than telephone triage" (Rutenberg & Greenberg, 2012, p. xi). Because opportunities for telehealth nursing are integrated throughout the healthcare system, most ambulatory care nurses will likely be providing telehealth triage during their practice. Because of this likelihood, all nurses should be aware of the basic principles necessary to provide safe and effective triage using telehealth technology.

BOX 9.3 Key Principles of Telehealth Triage

- Avoid accepting individual self-diagnosis. Although individuals often know what is wrong with them, there are times that they do not. The telehealth triage nurse must keep an open mind and go through a systematic assessment process.
- Avoid jumping to a conclusion or stereotyping the individual.
- Avoid assumptions regarding frequent contacts from the same individual. Because problems do change and evolve, the nurse must adequately reassess the individual with each new encounter.
- Speak directly to the individual, whenever possible. Not only does the individual have first-hand knowledge of their problem, but this contact gives the registered nurse the opportunity to directly assess the situation.
- Consider every call life-threatening until proven otherwise, and err on the side of caution. If the nurse is unsure or unable to confidently assess, plan, or address the concerns of the caller, referral for assessment by a provider is necessary.
- Use, but do not overdepend on the decision support tools. These are checklists to be sure nothing important has been overlooked; they augment but do not replace nursing skills and judgment.
- Provide timely and thorough documentation. Thorough documentation provides evidence of the nursing process, supplies an important form of healthcare communication, and assures continuity of care.
- Remember individual advocacy. Often individuals (especially those who are very sick) already know the right disposition and are most in need of acknowledgment, support, and collaboration in carrying out the plan of care.

Note. American Academy of Ambulatory Care Nursing. (2018). *Scope & standards of practice for professional telehealth nursing* (6th ed.). Author.

Telehealth triage is primarily conducted over the telephone, although some organizations are introducing a visual component that may be conducted over the computer using an application such as Skype or FaceTime. Communication with the individual when triage is necessary must be direct and real time. The key principles of telehealth triage are summarized in Box 9.3.

Design Challenges

Some elements of program or service design can be problematic and should be addressed or compensated for by the telehealth triage nurse. For example, failure to formalize the telehealth triage service within an organization may result in nurses who are multitasked, simultaneously dealing with in-person and telehealth nursing priorities. Multitasking often results in the fatigued, rushed, and distracted RN. To ensure safe practice, measures should be taken to insulate the telehealth triage nurse from other pressing responsibilities. Ideally, the triage nurse should have a dedicated role and workspace.

Additionally, attention should be paid to routing protocols. Poor call routing may result in triage by unqualified personnel, in which case the chief complaint as identified by the initial responder may not correspond to the real reason for the encounter, sometimes resulting in an unnecessary delay in care.

Settings

Telehealth triage can be and is practiced in any setting where an individual has a telephone or other communication device and access to a nurse. Telehealth triage services (eg, telephone triage, nurse advice lines) are offered by individual and provider group practices, by insurance companies, and by healthcare organizations. The most formalized and possibly recognized setting is call centers, some with nurses working virtually from home. Telehealth triage also takes place in primary care and specialty doctors' offices and clinics of all varieties.

Specialty areas such as College Health Centers, Departments of Corrections, and a number of federal agencies such as the Department of Defense, the VA, and Indian Health Service often have robust telehealth triage services, as do Home Health and Hospice agencies.

Same-day surgery centers contact individuals post-op to assess their status, so those contacts often will result in triage encounters. Telehealth triage also takes place in inpatient settings when recently discharged individuals contact the inpatient nurse who cared for them in the hospital or discharged them home, or when inpatient nurses make discharge follow-up calls.

Remote Monitoring/Telemonitoring

Remote monitoring is another service that plays an important part in telehealth nursing. It allows the individual to remain in the home or the community knowing that not only is their health data being reviewed and monitored but they also are connected to a nurse. The nurse role in remote monitoring is to interpret the data, intervene when appropriate, and provide individualized education and support. Remote monitoring is no longer confined to the home or health center. Mobile health devices now allow individuals to monitor or manage their own condition. They also permit data transmission, which provides an option for the nurse to access real-time data.

Mobile health devices can be as simple as reminders, alerts, text data, and image sharing. However, they also can be sufficiently complex to measure, store, and transmit physiologic data such as blood pressure, oxygen level, heart rate, and even blood glucose levels. Mobile health devices have also been developed to share text data and images. The capabilities of the particular mobile health device can often be customized according to the needs of the individual. In this way, they assist with individual and family self-management and allow for timely nursing interventions to prevent more severe health problems. A provider referral is required for coverage of remote monitoring by most insurers. Conditions commonly referred for remote monitoring include HF, diabetes, hypertension, high-risk pregnancy, and mental illness.

Purpose

The purpose of remote monitoring is to identify trends or events in the data and intervene early enough to prevent a healthcare crisis or hospitalization. Remote monitoring is popular with most recipients because it takes the place of traveling to see the provider but still preserves provider contact.

Changes in the individual's condition are recognized and managed remotely by the nurse, thereby averting an urgent or inconvenient visit to a healthcare facility. Remote monitoring and the associated ongoing and supportive connection with a nurse can be a particularly valuable option for individuals with conditions that are newly diagnosed or difficult to manage.

Practice Principles

Telehealth practice principles for remote monitoring are based on nursing knowledge of the individual and the particular condition. This type of nursing practice uses data transmitted via the monitors to ensure that the individual remains within set parameters and to intervene appropriately if the individual data are outside of set parameters. Ongoing communication, education, and support facilitate self-care and help to identify issues and intervene early. Nurses are perfectly positioned to provide ongoing individualized education and support for individuals. Interventions when needed can consist of a brief consult with the individual; an education or review session; a change in medication, diet, or activity; or even a provider appointment or EMS call.

Deviation from preestablished parameters may be monitored by technicians or unlicensed personnel. However, changes in the parameters must be interpreted and addressed by the RN. In autonomous nursing practice, DSTs and nursing judgment guide decision-making and actions taken in response to changes in the individual condition. In collaborative nursing practice, standard orders or protocols equip the nurse with provider directives and the parameters guiding their implementation. Based on the information transmitted to the nurse, the role of the nurse likely requires assessment, appropriate intervention, communication and coordination with the provider and other members of the team, documentation, and follow-up to ensure continuity of care.

Settings

Telemonitoring or remote monitoring has historically been conducted in the home with nurses being housed in a monitoring center in a large healthcare organization. For example, the VA has an impressive telemonitoring presence that provides services to homebound veterans.

Home health agencies and smaller health systems also provide remote monitoring services for high-risk populations. With the capability of new wearable technology, individuals are able to monitor themselves (ie, blood pressure, blood glucose), store the data, and report at a later time, thus bringing telemonitoring into everyday life.

Remote Care Management

Although much of this discussion on telehealth and remote monitoring has focused on single encounters, ongoing care management also is maintained through telemonitoring and telehealth. Care management, individual engagement and education, once limited to face-to-face encounters, can now be initiated, reinforced, or augmented remotely. It is important to note that the management and coordination of individual care is a responsibility of, and a standard of practice for, all RNs. In fact, "Engaging the patient and the family to participate in determining the needs and preferences surrounding their care and providing education and securing essential equipment, supplies and community resources to manage their care has long been part of the scope of the practicing registered nurse (RN)" (Haas et al., 2014, p. 141).

Coordinating care involves communication and the exchange of information within and across the healthcare system. Care management and coordination often involves multiple healthcare providers and services, and has been done primarily via telehealth technology (eg, telephone, fax, electronic health record). Nursing care coordination activities, while an expectation and responsibility of the nurse, have historically gone unrecognized (AAACN, 2016). As a result, the nursing contributions in this arena have not been visible, even though care coordination improves individual engagement, decreases costs by more effective use of resources (reduces missed appointments and unnecessary ED use), educates individuals, helps prevent errors, and improves safety and quality (DeBlois & Millefoglie, 2015). The remote management and coordination of individual care is primarily a role for RNs, although other personnel may sometimes assist with this role under the supervision of the RN.

Purpose

The purpose of remote care management is to develop and/or continue implementation of a plan for continuity of care, identify and address any gaps in care, and ensure individual and family understanding of and ability to participate in the individual care plan. Care management helps the individual navigate the complex healthcare system, access appropriate resources, and identify real or potential gaps in care and close those gaps. The nurse works closely with the individual and family to determine the needs and expectations, resources, and options available.

Practice Principles

Care management activities are integral in ensuring continuity of care for the individual and it is likely that every nurse will have the opportunity, and the responsibility, to provide remote care management. Therefore, it is very important that all nurses possess telehealth competencies (Haas et al., 2014), including knowledge of telehealth principles such as the Health Insurance Portability and Accountability Act, privacy and confidentiality, the need to adapt communication style depending on the recipient, and expertise with the technology used. Consider the following example in Box 9.4.

BOX 9.4 Telehealth Care Coordination After an Acute Myocardial Infarction

Mr. Gonzales, a 63-year-old widower, was hospitalized in an acute care facility following an acute myocardial infarction. He is now being discharged home after a short stay in a skilled nursing rehabilitation facility. John, the care coordination and transition management nurse, assesses Mr. Gonzales by telephone to determine his current status and his needs. He calls the office of Mr. Gonzales' cardiologist and coordinates appointments between the cardiologist and his primary care provider (PCP). John arranges for an initial Home Health visit. He calls the pharmacy to confirm Mr. Gonzales' medications and makes arrangements with a neighbor to help Mr. Gonzales administer his medications on a weekly basis.

Practice principles in planning and coordinating Mr. Gonzales' care would include individual-centered care, advocacy, education, and support. Care management begins during his transition from rehabilitation to home, but it will be a long-term process, and the majority of care management activities take place remotely. Because the nursing interventions often involve other professionals and settings, care management activities most often take place in the virtual environment, using telephone, fax, e-mail, and/or online portal. The practice is highly collaborative and good communication skills are of vital importance in providing accurate and safe individual-centered care.

Care management activities (telehealth nursing activities that do not involve triage or remote monitoring) require oversight by and participation of RNs. Any act of assessment or evaluation (such as individual understanding), planning, or revision of the plan of care are within the exclusive domain of the RN. Other telehealth activities, such as communicating uncomplicated test results, facilitating straightforward medication renewals, or reinforcing previous teaching, may be delegated, consistent with the five Rights of Delegation (NCSBN, 2016).

In the process of coordinating care for an individual remotely, the RN must be on guard for individual complaints or reports of symptoms. Symptoms must be assessed, identified for urgency and acuity, and followed by appropriate nursing interventions and documentation.

Settings

Remote nursing care management, care coordination, and care coordination and transition management occur throughout the entire healthcare system, in the community, and in the homes of the individuals. Nurses use technology to communicate and collaborate with individuals and providers; share, store, update, and manage information; and arrange services. These activities can take place entirely in a virtual environment.

Future Challenges and Opportunities

Telehealth nursing provides nurses with an opportunity to practice autonomously but collaboratively with the interprofessional team. Telehealth nurses are in a position to be strong advocates for individuals, helping them find their way among the disparate elements of our healthcare system. Nurses will continue to be the individual's bedrock. In addition to advocating for them, nurses will be their coaches, educators, and supporters and will be improving the health of our population by developing strong relationships with individuals they have possibly never met face to face.

Although telehealth nursing has come a long way, it still has much opportunity to expand. Multiple influences suggest that telehealth nursing practice will continue to grow. Elders are living longer and living with chronic illnesses, often with limited resources, which is placing a growing demand on our healthcare system. In addition, the aging of America has impacted the healthcare professions directly. Not only are individuals aging, but healthcare professionals are likewise finding their way to the path of retirement, leaving behind significant shortages in nurses and other healthcare professions. This will result in shrinking human resources occurring simultaneously with growing demand.

Telehealth nursing will likely be a major contributor to handling this major problem for the healthcare system. Telehealth nursing focused on prevention, wellness, education, care coordination, and triage can help streamline the healthcare journey and ensure efficient use of resources.

Telehealth technology also can help ease the healthcare burden through a focus on health and wellness rather than disease management. Technologic advances are enabling nurses to virtually transport themselves to the individual's side, allowing them to deliver care to the individuals where they live. The continued technologic explosion in our society has made Americans more comfortable with and even increasingly dependent on technology than ever before. In a time of social media and a desire for information at one's fingertips, telehealth nursing is well suited for the tech-savvy generations to come.

Aside from issues related to access to healthcare, external challenges also exist in the form of natural disasters that cause displaced populations and new or evolving diseases that may have a far-flung impact. Telehealth nursing is ideally positioned to address these challenges. Telehealth allows for nursing resources to be mobilized and delivered remotely. Provided there is telephone and/or Internet service, nurses in other states can do much to triage, advise, direct, and respond to victims in need. Individuals, whether displaced or simply needy, will be able to depend on telehealth nurses to provide support, coaching, and advocacy more than ever before.

Telehealth and virtual care might be considered the new frontier in healthcare. Having to do more with less and provide quality in the bargain will be the nurse's challenge, but nurses are ideally positioned to make a significant impact in the world of telehealth. Telehealth spans both the ambulatory care setting and select aspects of the inpatient setting. It is a complex practice addressing almost every element of healthcare in the United States and allows nurses to meet individuals where they are and meet the needs as the individuals perceive them.

Summary

The purpose of this chapter has been to convey both the challenges of quality telehealth nursing and the opportunity it provides to apply the core principles of nursing in practice. The focus of each telehealth nursing encounter must be on the individual, not the technology. In the telehealth setting, where few variables can be controlled by the nurse, individualization of care is of utmost importance. Individuals are generally in their own environment, dealing with factors that might impact their immediate healthcare need.

It has been noted that "connecting" with the individual might be the key to an effective encounter (Rutenberg & Greenberg, 2012). However, professional demeanor and methods of connecting with the individual take on different considerations in the practice of telehealth nursing. Although empathy, listening skills, paraphrasing, and other common communication techniques taught in nursing school are also important in the telehealth setting, variables such as eye contact, touch, and therapeutic silence are not options when communicating with the individual through most telehealth technology. Therefore, the telehealth nurse may need to use other techniques when connecting with an individual. Tone of voice, active listening, responses of encouragement, support, and interest are important in ensuring that the individual feels heard and is not being judged. In providing individual-centered care via technology, the nurse must listen for and confirm the health information as well as the values and wishes of the individual.

Without visual and tactile information regarding the caller, the nurse is unable to factor in some elements of the individual's reality. Although DSTs and other types of protocols are often a mainstay in telehealth nursing practice, care should be given to the individual's individual circumstances in assessing the individual and developing a plan of care.

Myriad factors beyond the healthcare issue at hand may directly impact the situation. For example, many individuals are reluctant to seek care that might pose an undue financial burden on them. Others might be afraid of losing control if they follow the recommendations of the nurse. Additionally, life responsibilities such as family, job, recreation, faith commitment, clubs, and other elements such as availability of resources (ie, transportation or family support) might significantly impact the individual's ability to agree or comply with an otherwise acceptable plan of care. Individualized care requires the nurse to explore values and options with the person, collaborating with the individual in developing a plan of care that is not only acceptable to the individual but also ensuring their safety. Coaching, education, and advocacy are more critical than ever before in the realm of telehealth nursing.

Case Study

RN Maria works in a family medicine practice, where her primary responsibility is giving advice and handling sick calls from patients. That morning, Mrs. Elliott had called regarding her 10-week-old baby, Carolina. Mrs. Elliott thinks the baby might be teething early and is seeking advice about how to make her feel better. She specifically asks if an over-the-counter numbing gel is ok to use, explaining that she's getting mixed messages from the Internet.

When asked to describe Carolina's symptoms and behavior, Mrs. Elliott replied, "Just the usual teething symptoms, fussy, not eating, fever." When asked to elaborate, Mrs. Elliott stated, "She's not sick. I just need some simple advice and don't have time to answer a bunch of questions." Maria expressed empathy and patiently explained to Mrs. Elliott that she was definitely going to help her make the right decision for her baby, but because all babies are different, she just needed to know a little more about her first.

Specifically, Maria asked how Carolina was nursing, how often she was having wet or dirty diapers, and how she was acting in general. Her mother replied that she wasn't very interested in nursing and was not latching well, but "I'm sure that's to be expected with a sore mouth." Carolina wasn't having as many wet diapers as usual, nor had she had a bowel movement today, which the mother also attributed to her apparent poor appetite. Also, she seemed to be sleeping almost all of the time that she wasn't crying, was "spitting up a lot," and didn't seem to want to be held. Mrs. Elliott reported an axillary temperature of 100.8. When asked about a rash, she acknowledged that her skin looked a little "blotchy" and that she had just begun noticing some tiny dark purplish spots on Carolina's palms.

Recognizing that, especially in a newborn, these were troubling signs and symptoms that required an urgent evaluation, Maria told Mrs. Elliott that she should have Carolina seen right away. Supported by her DST, Maria advised Mrs. Elliott to take her baby directly to the ED for evaluation. Mrs. Elliott began to protest that her daughter was "just teething," to which Maria replied that babies this young, whose behavior was different than usual, were not eating well, and were running a temperature over 100.8°F, needed to be evaluated to be sure they were not actually sick.

1. Which parts of the case study illustrate the components of the nursing process: assessment, diagnosis, plan, intervention?
2. Which parts of the assessment are subjective? Which are objective?
3. Why did Maria advise the mother to take her baby to the ED instead of coming into the clinic?

Key Points for Review

- Quality and safety in telehealth nursing practice depend upon well-educated and informed nurses, use of nursing standards of practice and DSTs, and an awareness that nursing care (with all attendant responsibility and accountability) is being delivered remotely.
- Professional nursing practice takes place and is regulated by the BON in the state where the individual is located, rather than where the RN is located.
- Telehealth triage is required any time an individual presents with new or different symptoms and requires the specific RN competency of assessment.
- Remote monitoring allows the RN to provide ongoing care for chronic conditions as well as to monitor for physiologic changes in short-term or acute need episodes.
- Telehealth nursing is ideal in meeting individuals' needs for access to care, triage, care coordination and continuity, education, and support.

REFERENCES

American Academy of Ambulatory Care Nursing. (2016). *Scope and standards of practice for RNs in care coordination and transition management*. Author.

American Academy of Ambulatory Care Nursing. (2018). *Scope & standards of practice for professional telehealth nursing* (6th ed.). Author.

American Nurses Association. (1999). *Core principles on telehealth: Report of the interdisciplinary telehealth standards working group*. Author.

American Nurses Association. (2015a). *Nursing scope and standards of practice* (3rd ed.). Author.

American Nurses Association. (2015b). *Code of ethics for nurses with interpretive statements*. Author.

Benner, P., Tanner, C., & Chesla, C. (1996). *Expertise in nursing practice: Caring, clinical judgement, and ethics*. Springer Pub.

Cox, D. (2016, April). *Impacting primary care access and client satisfaction through 24/7 centralized nurse triage and treatment across a large health care system* [presentation]. American Organization of Nurse Executives Annual Meeting, 2016, Fort Worth, USA.

DeBlois, D., & Millefoglie, M. (2015). Telehealth: Enhancing collaboration, improving care coordination. *Nursing Management,* 46(6), 10–12. https://doi.org/10.1097/01.NUMA.0000465402.45956.99

Ennis R. H. (2015) Critical thinking: A streamlined conception. In M. Davies & R. Barnett (Eds.), *The Palgrave handbook of critical thinking in higher education.* Palgrave Macmillan.

Ernesater, A., Holmstrom, I., & Engstrom, M. (2009). Telenurses' experiences of working with computerized decision support: Supporting, inhibiting, and quality improving. *Journal of Advanced Nursing,* 65(5), 1074–1083. https://doi.org/10.1111/j.1365-2648.2009.04966.x

FAIR Health. (2019). *A multilayered analysis of telehealth (White Paper).* https://mma.prnewswire.com/media/947336/A_Multilayered_Analysis_of_Telehealth___A_FAIR_Health_White_Paper.pdf?p=pdf

Greatbatch, D., Hanlon, G., Goode, J., O'Cathain, A., Strangleman, T., and Luff, D. (2005). *Telephone triage, expert systems and clinical expertise. Sociology of Health & Illness*, 27, 802–830. https://doi.org/10.1111/j.1467-9566.2005.00475.x

Haas, S. A., Swan, B. A., & Haynes, T. S. (Eds.). (2014). *Care coordination and transition management core curriculum.* American Academy of Ambulatory Care Nursing.

Institute of Medicine. (2010). *The future of nursing: Leading change, advancing health.* National Academies Press.

National Council of State Boards of Nursing. (1997). *Telenursing: A challenge to regulation. National Council,* Position Paper. Author.

National Council of State Boards of Nursing. (2014). *The NCSBN position paper on telehealth nursing practice.* https://www.ncsbn.org/3847.htm

National Council of State Boards of Nursing. (2016). *National guidelines for nursing delegation.* https://www.ncsbn.org/NCSBN_Delegation_Guidelines.pdf

National Council of State Boards of Nursing (n.d.). *Nurse Licensure Compact (NLC).* https://www.ncsbn.org/nurse-licensure-compact.htm

Rutenberg, C., & Greenberg, M. E. (2012). *The art and science of telephone triage: How to practice nursing over the phone*. Telephone Triage Consulting, Inc.

Simmons, B. (2010). Clinical reasoning: Concept analysis. *Journal of Advanced Nursing,* 66(5), 1151–1158. https://doi.org/10.1111/j.1365-2648.2010.05262.x

Tariq, A., Westbrook, J., Byrne, M., Robinson, M., & Baysari, M. (2017). Applying a human factors approach to improve usability of a decision support system in tele-nursing. *Collegian,* 24, 227–236. https://doi.org/10.1016/j.colegn.2016.02.001

UNIT 4

Ambulatory Settings: Roles and Competencies

10

Primary Care

Mary Blankson

PERSPECTIVES

"When someone thinks about nurses, I don't want them to just be thinking about someone wearing a nursing cap and doing bedside care at the hospital. I hope the general public sees the role we're playing in the community, and that it becomes well understood and seen."

Anonymous quote. (2019). *In their own words: Nurse insights on unmet needs of individuals.* Robert Woods Johnson Foundation.

LEARNING OBJECTIVES

Upon completion of this chapter, the reader will be able to:

1. Describe the historical basis of primary care nursing and why it is an essential element of the care continuum.
2. Understand the defining elements of the patient-centered medical home (PCMH) model.
3. Describe the elements of the role of the primary care registered nurse (PCRN), including an understanding of this role within the context of the larger interprofessional collaborative practice team.
4. Explain the various social determinants of health that contribute to overall individual complexity and therefore to the developed role of the primary care nurse as complex care manager.
5. Understand how the shift in payment models from fee-for-service to value-based reimbursement is further developing the role of the primary care nurse.

KEY TERMS

Complex care management
Patient-centered medical home (PCMH)
Primary care nursing
Primary care registered nurse (PCRN)
Social determinants of health
Value-based care

History and Definitions

Primary care nursing has had a complex beginning. Traditionally, the medical field focused on the individual clinician, namely the generalist physician, and it was in the discussion surrounding this role that the terminology of "primary care" was formalized. Public outcry about issues that are struggles even today—ranging from the shortage of physicians, high cost and fragmentation of care, and lack of accessibility—drove the American Medical Association to request an evaluation of family medicine.

The Millis Commission Report (1966) clearly identified the role of the primary physician as one that focused not only on diagnosis and treatment but also on prevention and health promotion as the primary "resource and counselor" to individuals and their families. The Willard Committee took place around the same time and stated similarly that medical school education should emphasize the role of the primary family physician in order to ensure coordination and continuity of care and to better balance the trend toward specialization (Willard, 1966). Finally, the Folsom Commission Report of 1967 outlined the need to define the primary care team and work toward integration of services while also focusing on communities to further promote health by linking it to a more holistic view including the social, emotional, and environmental factors that contribute to overall health (Folsom, 1967).

As time went on, new voices continued to describe and further develop what we now use as a working definition of primary care. In 1978, the Institute of Medicine (IOM, now known as the National Academy of Medicine) submitted a report on primary care that attempted to give a formal definition and that was updated in 1984 with the term "community-oriented" primary care. This was then refined in 1996 as an amalgam of both the 1978 and 1984 concepts, which combined the ideas of both family and community care: "Primary care is the provision of *integrated, accessible healthcare services* by *clinicians* who are *accountable* for addressing a large majority of *personal health care needs*, developing a *sustained partnership* with *patients*, and practicing in the *context of family and community*" (IOM, 1996).

In her 1992 book *Primary Care: Concept, Evaluation and Policy*, Dr. Barbara Starfield describes primary care as: "the point of entry into the health services system and the locus of responsibility for organizing care for patients and populations over time" (Starfield, 1992). In her 1994 article in *The Lancet*, Dr. Starfield asserts that primary care ensures that care is less costly because providers not only order fewer tests and procedures but also work toward preventing the development and progression of chronic illness. She uses examples from 11 developing countries that have implemented primary care and where communities were generally healthier, took fewer medications, and were happier with their overall medical care (Starfield, 1994).

Ultimately, the concept of primary care became the foundation of modern care delivery. Primary care was designed to be the gatekeeper and coordinator of care for all individuals. Secondary, tertiary, and emergency care encompass all care delivered in consultation to support primary care either as outpatient specialty services (short-term/acute consultation: secondary, or long-term/chronic consultation: tertiary) or as care to manage issues that require emergent inpatient management (emergency) (Starfield, 1994). As Dr. Starfield described it best, based on the original 1978 IOM committee report, primary care is not just a stand-alone discipline. Rather, it is actually the context or practice environment in which individuals receive care.

Although the early terminology of primary care focused on the role of the primary care physician, the concept of delivering disease prevention healthcare services in the community was not a new one to nursing. From the establishment of the Henry Street Settlement in the late 1800s by nursing leader Lillian Wald to the development of the Public Health Nurses system, nurses focused on that concept well before the conversation of the terminology began. Nurses were embedded in the community and mostly focused on health promotion, education, prevention, population management, care coordination, and the like. Their established roles made them a perfect fit on the care team delivering primary care. However, over the course of the last century, roles were shifted into acute care settings to better support the higher level of acuity there, with a recent workforce study showing that roughly 56% of nurses are still working in the hospital setting (Budden et al., 2013). In recent years, the national focus has shifted toward preventive care and keeping individuals out of the hospital, as discussed further.

Workforce

The focus of the primary care workforce used to be directly on the role of the primary care provider (PCP). However, in 2015, the Association of American Medical Colleges (AAMC) predicted a physician shortage of 12,500 to 31,100 in primary care by 2025 and stated that addressing this shortage will require innovation and embracing team-based care (AAMC, 2015). Given the aging of the population, increasing complexity of care, and rapid pace of changes in primary care delivery and payment models, there has been increasing focus not only on other provider types such as advanced practice registered nurses (APRNs) and physician assistants (PAs) but also—as the AAMC press release states—on other members of the extended care team through team-based care (AAMC, 2015). This long-known strategy has reinforced the need for developed primary care teams where every member has a defined role and practices at the top of their license, certification, or training. Typical team members include the PCP (Doctor of Medicine [MD], Doctor of Osteopathic Medicine [DO], APRN, or PA), medical assistants (MAs), registered nurses and/or licensed vocational or practical nurses, clinical team members from other disciplines such as behavioral health, and finally nonclinical team members such as community health workers (CHWs), health coaches, and centralized operation teams that manage referrals, medical records, and other functions. It is within this team context that innovation in primary care delivery is found, including the role of the **primary care registered nurse (PCRN)**.

Part of the challenge in primary care is that the care delivery model is becoming more complex with greater focus on and movement toward **value-based care**. Although these changes will be discussed later in this chapter, it is in this context that the role of the PCRN is seen to be growing steadily in the workforce. As the demand for PCRNs increases, training for the nursing workforce must also shift to better prepare RNs for roles that rely heavily on refined communication skills, advanced critical thinking, and skill sets in chronic illness care management. This includes training the PCRN to manage an individual's complexity, including a robust knowledge of **social determinants of health** and how they impact individuals' daily struggles to self-manage their chronic illnesses and achieve or maintain health.

The Bureau of Labor Statistics states that the role of the RN is likely to grow by 15% from 2016 to 2026 (U.S. Department of Labor, 2017). This projection is attributable to enhanced roles in the management of chronic conditions as well as other ambulatory roles, given the push to attain shorter hospital stays not only to reduce cost but also to accommodate individuals' preference for care in their homes and on an outpatient basis (U.S. Department of Labor, 2017). So, although 56% of nurses worked in hospital settings (Budden et al., 2013) in 2013, the shift is beginning, and this number is likely to change radically as the priority becomes preparing nurses to fill the growing number of roles in primary care to support chronic disease management and the workflow shifts to support value-based payment models.

Patient-Centered Medical Home and High-Functioning Primary Care

The **patient-centered medical home (PCMH)** model is another key driver of the expansion of the PCRN role. The American Academy of Pediatrics (AAP) developed the concept for the PCMH model in 1967 in an effort to improve care for children and youth with special healthcare needs by focusing on having a central health record to better support coordination of care for these children. In a statement 30 years later, the AAP went on to better describe the elements of the model to include improved access to care, continuity of care, coordinated care, culturally sensitive care, and compassionate and family-centered care (AAP, 1999b).

As the definition was broadened, the PCMH model grew to incorporate additional concepts such as:

- partnership with the individual as an engaged member of the team
- health promotion
- education and goal setting, including an integrated, individual-specific care plan (with a full assessment of health literacy with regard to their specific conditions)
- enhanced support for transitions of care
- an enhanced description of how to address culturally sensitive care to include care delivered in the native language of the individual as well as by the appropriate method an individual prefers (oral, written, etc.)
- consideration for relevant community resources and connection to nonclinical services that address social determinants of health
- access to 24-hour care to ensure more cost-effective care, including access to after-hours advice

Given that the model has specific deliverables associated with it, national organizations began to look toward formal recognition to identify practices that were successfully embracing these ideals. Between 2008 and 2009, the Accreditation Association for Ambulatory Health Care began offering accreditation, which included aspects of the PCMH model, but later offered only a certification for PCMH, which ensured organizations incorporated all of their PCMH standards into their programs. The National Committee on Quality Assurance (NCQA), The Joint Commission (TJC), and the Utilization Review Accreditation Commission (URAC) also established programs during the same time frame.

Recognition as a certified PCMH includes specific steps and requirements; in order to gain recognition as a PCMH through NCQA, a clinical organization must demonstrate adherence to PCMH standards and guidelines. However, the concepts, competencies, and criteria for recognition as a PCMH, listed in Box 10.1, include comprehensive, integrated care, as well as community connections.

BOX 10.1 NCQA's Six Core Concepts

- *Team-based care and practice organization* focuses on communicating roles and responsibilities around the PCMH model of care to each team member as well as the patient and their family or caretaker(s). This includes ensuring appropriate, role-specific training, workflows, policies and support, as well as patient brochures, campaigns, and other patient education materials.
- *Knowing and managing your patients* refers to using patient information to deliver evidence-based care. This includes medication reconciliation, clinical decision support, and responding to social determinants of health through connection to community resources.
- *Patient-centered access and continuity* focuses on ensuring 24-hour access to support and advice for all patients as well as defining empanelment at the organization.
- *Care management and support* outlines the expected collaboration between the patient, their family or caretaker(s), and the care team to define and implement care plans.
- *Care coordination and care transitions* describes the support patients should get as they transition between levels of medical care, as well as how the organization tracks patient results and referral consults as care is delivered outside of the PCMH.
- *Performance measurement and quality improvement* ensures that the organization focuses on ongoing improvement to enhance the patient experience. NCQA has included three specific areas of distinction that can also be achieved: patient experience reporting, behavioral health integration, and electronic measure reporting (NCQA, 2017).

Note. NCQA = National Committee for Quality Assurance; PCMH = Patient-centered medical home. National Committee for Quality Assurance. (2017). *NCQA PCMH standards and guidelines (2017 edition)*. http://store.ncqa.org/index.php/catalog/product/view/id/2776/s/2017-pcmh-standards-and-guidelines-epub/

TJC has similar criteria to support its PCMH certification process, with a particular focus on team roles; integration of services; enhanced access; comprehensive, evidence-based, coordinated care; and a systems approach to performance improvement and safety (TJC, 2018). Although all of these competencies are specific to recognition as a PCMH, they also describe the components of what has been called high-functioning primary care practice, incorporating the importance of interprofessional teamwork in that context (Sullivan et al., 2016).

There are several barriers to full acceptance and implementation of the PCMH model as well as other models for high-functioning primary care. Often additional staffing is required to coordinate care and implement various other aspects of the model, which includes the central role of the PCRN. It is rare that the additional services delivered are directly reimbursed, which contributes to the barriers of full acceptance and implementation of the model, as it increases the overall cost per visit. This is likely to change as the payment model for primary care transforms to one based on value, where PCMH concepts are often required as a part of such contracts or agreements.

Another barrier is that staff are challenged to embrace ongoing change and additional work burden, which may lead to staff dissatisfaction, particularly when they do not fully understand their specific role on the care team and in the PCMH. This also makes it challenging for smaller organizations or practices to implement, as they sometimes have fewer roles represented on their teams. By continuing to address such barriers to acceptance and implementation, and as value-based payment models are developed and implemented throughout the United States, the PCMH movement has laid the groundwork for the transformation of primary care practice and the ongoing conversation about components of high-functioning primary care.

Team-Based Care

Team-based care is defined as: "the provision of health services to individuals, families and/or their communities by at least two health providers who work collaboratively with patients and their caregivers to the extent preferred by each patient to accomplish shared goals within and across settings to achieve coordinated, high-quality care" (Mitchell et al., 2012, p. 5). The concepts of team-based care apply to effective delivery of healthcare in all settings; however, in this context teams are discussed as an essential component of high-functioning primary care.

The definition of team-based care set forth by the IOM focuses on describing how different healthcare providers and teams involved in the care of an individual across the continuum should work together for the benefit of the individual. In 2014, the IOM published an additional report expanding on that description of the healthcare team. That report focused on the role of the patient as a member of the team and also identified other care team members such as MAs, nurses, receptionists, and social workers (Okun et al., 2014). In so doing, the report acknowledged that successful team-based care requires an engaged patient and a fully activated team.

Primary Care Medical Teamlet

In discussing the team in team-based care, it is important to acknowledge those who make up the team. The first component of the team is, of course, the individual patient. Patient engagement is critical to the success of the team, and ideally all team members are working toward achieving that end. The focus on the PCMH model has supported the standardization of team-based care as the "gold standard" or best practice for delivering primary care not only to manage the burden of work in primary care by drawing on the talents and training of all team members but also to focus a significant amount of energy on the patient. This approach promotes coordination of care, efficiency, effectiveness, value, and improved satisfaction for both the patient and the members of the care team (Mitchell et al., 2012; Schottenfeld et al., 2016).

The medical *teamlet* (meaning "little team") focuses on the dyad relationship most often composed of a PCP and an MA (Bodenheimer & Laing, 2007). This is a smaller component of the overall team-based care model but one that is critical to enhancing care delivery and increasing overall quality and throughput for the patient in primary care (Bodenheimer & Laing, 2007). There typically is an additional connection to a PCRN, whether for direct visit support or for other support such as ongoing care management, along with additional connections to all of the other various care team members. The core teamlet, however, focuses directly on quality and efficiency in the PCP schedule and works to utilize roles like MAs to the fullest of their training, education, and certification to manage the majority of downstream tasks that do not require licensed staff. It is important as a PCRN to recognize the value and importance of such nonlicensed roles in ensuring that the PCRN practice is truly top-of-license.

Team Roles

Team-based care models vary as to which roles are centralized and which are decentralized. Typically, the MA role is responsible for rooming patients, administering planned care, and supporting the provider directly. As the core member of the teamlet, they are most successful when there is continuity in the teamlet (Bodenheimer & Laing, 2007). When it comes to the PCRN role, some are centralized and some are not. Telephone triage and some elements of care management—particularly transition management—are at times addressed centrally.

Complex care management (CCM), which is discussed more fully below, can be delivered in a decentralized manner as well. PCRNs that are decentralized are likely assigned, or empaneled, to the PCP's patient panel to support CCM functions along with more advanced visit support. PCRNs in a decentralized role also are typically engaged in direct patient care through their own appointment schedule for independent nursing visits delivered via standing or delegated order, along with participating in overall population management, again focused on the assigned panel of patients.

"Empanelment is the act of assigning individual patients to individual primary care providers (PCP) and care teams with sensitivity to patient and family preference. Empanelment is the basis for population health management and the key to continuity of care" (Safety Net Medical Home Initiative, 2013).

Each healthcare organization defines a typical staffing ratio determined by how many support staff members are required to address the typical provider panel. Ratios are therefore derived from a detailed review of an organization's role descriptions, overall volume of responsibilities per staff member, and the specific state's scope of practice regulations for PCRNs, MAs, and other team roles as applicable. Staffing ratios should be reviewed regularly as new workflows, tasks, and competencies are added to ensure the model continues to support the quality of care being delivered. This is particularly important as primary care delivery changes related to overall payment reform in a value-based environment.

This overall team concept is vital to the development and acceptance of the PCRN role as it emphasizes all team members practicing at the top of their license, education, training, or certification. This model requires that PCRNs relinquish some tasks in order to opt for higher level responsibilities such as those required in CCM and independent nursing visits by standing or delegated orders (Flinter et al., 2016). Care must be taken to measure each team member's contribution to the whole whenever possible to better understand the overall impact of each team member to the overall care of the patient. For example, elevating the role of the MA often leads to a higher functioning PCRN that can accomplish more in the way of panel review and CCM.

It is important to note that team-based care is required to fully implement the PCMH or high-functioning primary care model. It requires every team member to be leveraged to deliver on the concepts and criteria set forth in the model. Colocation is a fundamental concept in team-based care, meaning that staff are located and sit together as they deliver care to a PCP's panel (Flinter et al., 2016).

Integration of Care

As the care team grows to include other disciplines, it is important to consider how integration prevents practice from remaining in silos. Care delivered in silos typically results in more value being placed on the team and discipline rather than on the patient and their actual experience. Comprehensive integrated care is an essential concept of the PCMH model and is most often used to describe behavioral health involvement on-site in the care of individuals. It can, however, include other disciplines, for example, dental and other ancillary medical team providers such as chiropractors or registered dietitians. Integrated care at its core describes when care providers deliver care together (Flinter et al., 2016). The patient's visit is no longer just a medical visit, but perhaps they receive fluoride varnish from the dental hygienist and a warm handoff to a behavioral health provider to address their positive depression screening within their medical visit (Baird et al., 2014; Flinter et al., 2016).

This increases overall access to the patient, given that whichever evidence-based services they may need that day can be delivered by various care team members in the context of a single visit. By virtue of teams being colocated, it is easy to utilize the patient's examination room to address any and all aspects of care. Often the MA who rooms the patient will choreograph the visit to ensure that the medical provider schedule and overall throughput is not negatively affected by the other team members delivering other aspects of care.

A shared electronic health record (EHR) and plan of care are important to ensure all care team members are working together on the same issues and supporting the patient to success. When care is in silos, there is no integrated approach to problem solving, and it is challenging to ensure the patient is not overwhelmed because the specific plans of care developed by each provider, when put together, are not achievable for that individual.

The advent of integrated practice allows for the fluid support of individuals seeking both medical and behavioral healthcare. Behavioral health issues are extremely common and have often gone unaddressed in primary care. Even when staffed with behavioral health clinicians, it is important for the PCRN to assist in identifying individuals who would benefit from this care and to spend time supporting behavioral health as a routine intervention for change support and coaching, along with routine treatment of behavioral health diagnoses. PCRNs must advocate for individuals and proactively support them to care with behavioral health when risk factors are identified. This may take several encounters, but it is imperative that PCRNs continue to support, review benefits, and make themselves available for behavioral health triage when symptoms exacerbate.

PCRNs also should be empowered to work on behalf of their patients to take advantage of integrated resources to address barriers to care. This could be done by allowing PCRNs, by standing order, to initiate care from other team members such as behavioral health or the registered dietitian. They should also be empowered to review the ongoing care plan with a patient regardless of who aided the individual in setting the specified goals and outcomes. The PCRN can ensure individuals with a dental issue are seen the same day by dental or that individuals being seen in dental who are due for medical services are able to receive them alongside their dental visit. The PCRN should be activated to assist the patient to take advantage of all relevant, evidence-based services that will help that individual reach their goals and maintain or move toward health. Box 10.2 provides an example of a center that takes a proactive approach to care coordination in its practice.

BOX 10.2 Proactive Warm Handoff

The CHCI, a large, statewide FQHC, headquartered in Middletown, CT, implemented the proactive warm-handoff process in 2016. CHCI had previously implemented the standard warm-handoff process, where medical team members could leverage colocated behavioral support should they identify a specific need for a patient. This could arise from their general observation or from routine depression screening, etc. In this model, the team also would leverage a behavioral health provider to come into the patient's room and spend time connecting with the patient. This is not typically a very long encounter, but enough to establish a therapeutic connection and to coordinate care to additional services for behavioral health either at CHCI or outside of CHCI should it require a higher level of care (or based on the patient's preference).

The proactive version leverages blocked time in the behavioral health provider's schedule for warm handoff to identify patients who may be at risk for a behavioral health condition. CHCI currently reviews data from the EHR to identify individuals who have a behavioral health condition but have not been engaged in care with CHCI's behavioral health team, as well as individuals with a prior positive screening for depression or a diagnosis of chronic pain with chronic opioid use. These individuals are identified on a dashboard for the behavioral health providers to coordinate with the team's MA as to when they can see the patient and introduce themselves and their services. The majority of individuals are either engaged in care elsewhere or are not interested in services at this time, but they often share that they are glad to know that behavioral health services are delivered at CHCI should they ever need them.

Note. CHCI = Community Health Center, Inc.; EHR = electronic health record; FQHC = Federally Qualified Health Center; MA = medical assistant.

Nonclinical Roles

Nonclinical team members are critical to the success of team-based care and the PCMH model. These team members support significant facets of the administrative and logistic coordination of care and navigation for individuals and the teams that serve them. Examples of role types that represent this group include CHWs, patient navigators, case managers or logistic care coordination support, referral teams, medical records staff, reception staff, and call center service associates. These roles are critical to ensuring that PCRNs and other clinical team members are truly able to practice at the top of their license, education, training, or certification. All team members need to understand each other's roles so as to best leverage the varying strengths offered and responsibilities carried out by each team member.

Interprofessional/Intraprofessional Communication

Communication among the various care team members is key as individuals travel along the full continuum of care. Concepts of both inter- and intraprofessional communication are important for the PCRN to grasp to be successful in their role. Interprofessional communication refers to the communication with care team members of other professions or disciplines, whereas intraprofessional communication refers to communication within the same profession, in this case nursing. Both are challenging at times but translate to a higher quality of care, better individual outcomes, and a better patient experience overall if done well. PCRNs must be able to clarify PCP orders, present cases and questions to PCPs for support, deliver care by standing order when applicable, delegate activities to MAs where scope allows, and work to include other nonclinical team members in aspects of care coordination. PCRNs must also communicate with specialty providers, homecare nurses, discharge planners, and other staff outside of the actual setting where they deliver care.

Ensuring that communication is clear and comprehensive, yet succinct, is a skill that requires development and ongoing feedback. PCRNs must be committed not only to understanding all roles on the care team (clinical and nonclinical) but also ensuring that they value them and know exactly how to leverage them appropriately for the benefit of the individual.

In a discussion in the 2014 IOM report, patients were cited as noticing when a team worked well together and communicated versus when they did not (Okun et al., 2014). Ensuring the patient experience is protected in a way that improves engagement is critical to encouraging them to actually become a part of the care team, which in turn is critical to the overall success of the team.

Registered Nurse Roles in Primary Care

Larger primary care practices are increasingly identifying a chief nursing officer (CNO) to lead the medical support teams that work directly with PCPs. This role ensures that there is someone responsible not only to set the vision for the discipline of nursing in primary care but also to create the tools needed to equip and develop PCRNs in all areas of required competency. The CNO is responsible for overseeing and supporting nursing advancement, along with further defining nurse-sensitive indicators and nursing data models to better quantify the impact of PCRNs. The CNO is also at times responsible for MAs and other clinical support team members, which ensures an interprofessional approach and a valuing of all team members in contributing toward the goal of high-quality care delivery and ultimately improved individual outcomes.

The role of the CNO in primary care requires a significant depth and breadth of knowledge given that sites may not have the same resources as their hospital counterparts, such as laboratory services or a pharmacy to support and lead their medication management program. Also, nurses in primary care often have significant responsibility for issues related to infection control, with oversight by the CNO. The CNO must have knowledge of all regulatory requirements and must work to ensure that each one of these program domains supports individual and employee safety as well as meets the demands of a busy primary care practice. It is beneficial for the CNO to have doctoral-level education to better support collaboration in research and translation, quality improvement, and even to address challenges in informatics.

The CNO works in direct collaboration with other clinical and operational leaders in the practice to ensure full acceptance and reinforcement of the team-based model of care. The CNO should dedicate significant time to developing support team members to see the value of their own role in the overall care team as well as the roles of others and to support the development of their sense of responsibility for the measures and interventions driven by each of their roles.

The role of the PCRN has been studied in a number of formats. The Robert Wood Johnson Foundation funded a program in 2012 to identify highly effective team-based care models at health centers across the country. The Primary Care Team: Learning from Effective Ambulatory Practices (LEAP) program led by Drs. Ed Wagner and Margaret Flinter began reviewing a group of 227 practices and after 45-minute interviews were able to thin the group to 30 high-performing sites that represented a diverse group based on geographic location, health center type, and population served. The researchers conducted three day-long site visits with the final 30 centers and then reviewed the findings of the visits to identify and highlight innovative practices and common threads that distinguish a high-performing site (Flinter et al., 2017). In terms of the role of the PCRN, the researchers noted much diversity, ranging from PCRNs completing standing order visits to performing the role of a central care manager. Most LEAP sites did have nurses as a part of their care teams, reinforcing that this is one of the hallmarks of high-performing teams.

The role of the PCRN is likely to continue to expand given the decrease in the PCP population (MDs/DOs, APRNs, and PAs) relative to the U.S. population (Bauer & Bodenheimer, 2017). The challenges that need to be addressed to support this expansion involve overall healthcare payment reform, education reform, and a review of scope of practice to ensure that all states are able to support PCRNs to practice at the top of their license (Bauer & Bodenheimer, 2017).

A systematic literature review done in 2017 described the most common PCRN roles that are likely to be fully embraced as primary care continues to integrate team-based care and the transition to a value-based payment model. The described roles include renewing routine chronic medication refills, answering individuals' questions, delivering patient education with regard to both acute and chronic illnesses (including home care instructions), and finally care management work (including self-management goal [SMG] setting and motivational interviewing [MI]) (Norful et al., 2017). This review notes that in order for PCRNs to take on these roles, it will be important for nonlicensed roles to be high functioning. It also requires nursing leaders such as CNOs to collaborate with other clinical leaders to develop clear policies and protocols to support this work (Norful et al., 2017).

Primary Care Registered Nurse Competencies

Defined competencies are vital to ensure the greatest impact of the PCRN role on both team-based care and ultimately on overall individual outcomes. Although a universal set of PCRN competencies has not been adopted, general competencies for the PCRN include critical thinking, flexibility, triage, care coordination and care management, education and coaching, focusing on areas ensuring health literacy, goal setting, adherence support, and behavioral change management, highlighted by competencies in self-management support and MI.

Age-specific competencies also may be required in practices that see the full age range. Although there certainly are population-specific practices that focus on pediatrics, adolescent care, geriatrics, women's health, and others, PCRNs in family practice must be prepared for the possibility that they may be expected to have experience and expertise for individuals across the life span. PCRNs also should be comfortable with change as guidelines are updated regularly by national bodies such as the United States Preventive Services Task Force (USPSTF) and the American Diabetes Association.

As of this publication, a certification in primary care nursing is not available; however, this specialty may lend itself well to that type of recognition in the future.

Education and Behavior Change

Behavior change and patient education is covered more fully in Chapter 7. However, the PCRN plays the essential role of delivering patient education and addressing health literacy, and some of these areas will be discussed further.

Providing education is fundamental to support behavioral change through ensuring individual-centered techniques and approaches (written, audio, visual, and other educational methods), along with confirming individuals' understanding and health literacy with regard to chronic illnesses or other patient-specific challenges. Utilizing techniques such as the Teach-Back and Show-Me methods will ensure that PCRNs confirm individuals' understanding and therefore contribute to overall adherence, establishment of a therapeutic partnership, improved individual experience, and ultimately improved patient clinical outcomes and self-perception of health (Brega et al., 2015).

Behavior change techniques such as MI and SMG setting are related general competencies that specifically distinguish PCRNs. Other staff members may engage in MI and SMG setting to varying degrees, including MAs, CHWs, and behavioral health providers, but PCRNs should ensure that every encounter for chronic illness follow-up involves encouraging such individuals to achieve particular goals and therefore work toward having greater control over their own health. PCRNs support individuals to think about what is most important to them and to identify ways they could improve their situation or support their ability to achieve and/or maintain progress toward that specific goal.

Triage and Telehealth

A detailed discussion of telehealth is provided in Chapter 8, but certainly telehealth is well utilized in primary care and is a focus of much of the innovation in the role of the PCRN, including aspects of telephonic care management, triage, portal messaging, virtual visits, and others. Some of these roles are centralized, and others are disseminated to the local medical teamlets. They are evidence of work to enhance individual engagement by delivering care through a variety of methods, many of which take into account the individual's ability to come to the clinical site. Many PCRNs prefer to be in the room with individuals, so it is imperative that telehealth roles be properly recruited in terms of job description and competency, to ensure they are attracting the right audience. It also takes a different skill set to be able to interact with individuals through portals, telephonically, and through other virtual means. These are skills and competencies that are newly being integrated into organizational onboarding and, in some academic institutions, in the training and education for RNs.

PCRN telehealth care management roles can assist with transitions of care by connecting with newly discharged individuals, as well as managing callers who may not have a specific complaint but are flagged in the system as having significant clinical risk. The goal is to ensure that individuals who are at highest risk get the immediate attention of a clinically skilled workforce to manage their appointments and to review their needs in order to avoid future admissions and exacerbations that are more likely in this population. A significant challenge to this role is that often there are not dedicated PCRNs for these roles, in which case it is an add-on responsibility to already busy PCRNs delivering direct clinical services.

For in-person triage, the PCRN must be able to ask questions based on the complaint and then collect relevant clinical information through their assessment to help make the final decision about which level of care is suitable for the individual and the timing of that care. Sometimes this requires the PCRN to collaborate with other care team members such as the PCP, behavioral health provider, dental provider, and others. However, because the PCRN is able to take the full history and also assess and collect necessary data, the burden to the provider-level staff is minimal for these visits.

Documenting data on in-person triage aids in determining whether a provider is needed to see such individuals, given how often PCRNs have walk-in triages and how frequently those are found to be primary care appropriate issues.

Preventive Care and Screening

Primary prevention delivered by the PCRN is the work done to prevent illness before it happens, mainly through interventions such as health promotion education and immunization support. Secondary prevention for the PCRN involves screening interventions and any other tools that support identifying current risk. Tertiary prevention for the PCRN focuses on intervening to avoid or minimize deterioration of an ongoing chronic illness. All levels of prevention can involve other team members as well, but the PCRN often plays a leading role to address evidence-based care that goes beyond data collection and requires patient-specific education or additional assessment.

PCRNs are not only involved in delivering preventive services at individual patient encounters. They also participate in systems-level decision-making through their involvement in committee work to support organizational performance improvement in areas such as infection control, or related to clinical measures such as immunization rates, or adherence to evidence-based guidelines, for instance, with depression or intimate partner violence (IPV) screening. Health promotion involves a wide range of strategies, including sharing educational resources or programming, which often includes work from PCRNs in developing materials that are targeted to meet the needs of the specific population served.

Health promotion can also be addressed through evaluation of social determinants of health. All team members should be familiar with the items assessed and be able to recommend appropriate organizational or community resources as needed. At times, this may include connecting an individual to a higher level clinical or even a nonclinical team member for additional assistance. One screening tool is the Protocol for Responding to and Assessing Patients' Assets, Risks, and Experiences (PRAPARE) created by the National Association of Community Health Centers (NACHC, 2016). This initiative was developed in an effort to support community health centers across the United States that are responsible for the healthcare of more than 27 million individuals, the majority of whom are considered uninsured, underinsured, at risk for and/or living in poverty, and those impacted most by challenges in their social determinants of health.

As stated earlier, PCRNs typically assist with immunizations and routine screenings. PCRNs can order and administer immunizations via standing order, even though in many states nonlicensed staff such as MAs may be allowed to complete the administration portion. Some children are on "catch-up" schedules and benefit from having the support of a PCRN to ensure delayed immunizations are properly tracked for appropriate follow-up intervals. MAs complete many screenings in primary care, but they often rely on PCRNs to assist with any screens that are positive and require further history or assessment to better understand and appropriately respond.

IPV is another preventable public health problem that impacts millions of individuals in the United States every year. IPV is described as physical or sexual violence or stalking or psychological aggression (including coercive acts) by a current or former intimate partner (Breiding et al., 2014). More than one in three women and one in four men will experience IPV during their lifetime (Centers for Disease Control and Prevention, 2010). Screening for IPV in primary care is needed to ensure individuals can be proactively identified.

The PCRN is often a team member that an individual may disclose to, and therefore, they must be ready to support regardless of what level of intervention the individual is looking for. The PCRN must be prepared to ensure individual safety by not giving materials that are inappropriate or that could put the individual in harm's way if found. PCRNs must also know the appropriate hotlines and other local, state, and national resources to assist in locating shelter housing for those seeking support from IPV or to report issues such as child or elder abuse as applicable. Although both child and elder abuse must be reported under the PCRN's mandated reporter status, reporting is not required with regard to IPV. Therefore, reporting of IPV should be at the discretion of the individual involved in the IPV situation.

Trauma is more challenging in that it can be caused not only by personal experience or witnessing physical or emotional violence but also by witnessing natural disasters, accidents, and other incidents that may have caused harm to the person or another person. There is growing evidence for screening both adults and children for trauma in primary care to ensure proactive identification and support to limit some of the possible long-term impacts. The PCRN needs to create an environment in which individuals feel safe to disclose such information in order to access the care required to address the particular concern. This can be challenging as it often requires consistent demonstration over time to build a safe environment.

PCRNs also support much of the care management being conducted, including routine chronic illness health maintenance, such as foot checks and retinal screens for individuals with diabetes and ongoing SMG setting, health literacy, and education support as recommended. Even though PCRNs may leverage other care team members for ongoing follow-up and coaching support for individuals, they often are the ones who oversee the care management process to prevent the status of an individual's chronic illness from becoming more severe.

Screening guidelines can be found in specialty organizations such as the American Cancer Society, as well as the National Guidelines Clearinghouse (http://www.guideline.gov/) for practice recommendations. The United States Preventive Services Task Force (USPSTF) has a comprehensive list of recommendations for screening and prevention; the screening recommendations for primary care can be found in Table 10.1.

TABLE 10.1 USPSTF A AND B SCREENING RECOMMENDATIONS

Screening Test	Grade[a]
Abdominal Aortic Aneurysm: men aged 65–75 years who have ever smoked	B
Abnormal Blood Glucose and Type 2 Diabetes Mellitus: Screening: adults aged 40–70 years who are overweight or obese	B
Asymptomatic Bacteriuria in Adults: Screening: pregnant persons, adolescents, adults, seniors	B
Breast Cancer: Screening: women aged 50–74 years	B
Cervical Cancer: Screening: women aged 21–65 years	A
Chlamydia and Gonorrhea: Screening: sexually active women	B
Depression in Adults: Screening: general adult population, including pregnant and postpartum women	B
Depression in Children and Adolescents: Screening: adolescents aged 12–18 years	B
Gestational Diabetes Mellitus: Screening: asymptomatic pregnant women, after 24 weeks of gestation	B
Hepatitis B Virus Infection: Screening, 2014: persons at high risk for infection	B
Hepatitis C Virus Infection in Adolescents and Adults: Screening: adults aged 18–79 years	B
Hepatitis B Virus Infection in Pregnant Women: Screening: pregnant women	A
HIV Infection: Screening: pregnant persons	A
HIV Infection: Screening: adolescents and adults aged 15–65 years	A
High Blood Pressure in Adults: Screening: adults aged 18 years or older	A
Intimate Partner Violence, Elder Abuse, and Abuse of Vulnerable Adults: Screening: women of reproductive age, adolescents, adults, seniors	B
Latent Tuberculosis Infection: Screening: asymptomatic adults at increased risk for infection	B
Obesity in Children and Adolescents: Screening: children and adolescents 6 years and older	
Osteoporosis to Prevent Fractures: Screening: women 65 years and older; postmenopausal women younger than 65 years at increased risk for osteoporosis	B
Rh(D) Incompatibility: Screening: pregnant women, during the first pregnancy-related care visit	A
Syphilis Infection in Nonpregnant Adults and Adolescents: Screening: asymptomatic, nonpregnant adults and adolescents who are at increased risk for syphilis infection	A
Syphilis Infection in Pregnant Women: Screening: pregnant women	A

Note. HIV = human immunodeficiency virus; USPSTF = United States Preventive Services Task Force. From U.S. Preventive Services Task Force. 2020. www.uspreventiveservicestaskforce.org

[a] A Grade recommendations: The USPSTF recommends the service. There is high certainty that the net benefit is substantial. B Grade recommendations: The USPSTF recommends the service. There is high certainty that the net benefit is moderate or there is moderate certainty that the net benefit is moderate to substantial.

Protocols and Standing or Delegated Orders

PCRNs are able to complete nursing visits that impact a large group of individuals through standing orders. A standing order is one that allows PCRNs to use an algorithm or other written instructions to carry out clinical care on a provider's behalf for individuals who meet specific criteria. Standing orders can be used to address a variety of acute and chronic issues such as uncomplicated urinary tract infections for women, sexually transmitted infection screening and treatment, pregnancy testing and contraceptive counseling, basal insulin titration for individuals with diabetes, asthma well care and in-house spirometry, or directly observed therapy for the treatment of latent tuberculosis. Each of these would specify to whom the standing order applies and define what the PCRN should assess, along with a prescribed treatment algorithm based on the assessment being carried out (Flinter et al., 2016). Should an individual not meet the criteria, the PCRN would then elicit support from the PCP. Standing orders must be well developed and must cover many if not all potential scenarios, as they apply to a broad base of individuals.

Providers may also create delegated orders for a specific individual, which should include all relevant information and specific treatment guidelines for the PCRN to follow for that particular person (Flinter et al., 2016). Delegated orders differ from standing orders in their focus; a standing order may apply to any individual who fits the population covered by that standing order, as described earlier. A delegated order is employed for a specific individual, either for a one-time event or for an ongoing medical need for that individual.

In contrast to delegated or standing orders, protocols are sets of actions that generally fall within the scope of RN practice. They allow the RN to implement care based on best practices, without requiring provider orders.

It is most effective for standing orders, delegated orders, and protocols to be developed with considerable input from both the providers and the PCRNs in the organization, as well as ensuring a full review by a legal consultant who can ensure the applicable state scope of practice act fully supports the standing or delegation of orders. Full PCP support of these and other team-based care workflows allows team members to maximize their contributions, potentially avoid or reduce provider burnout, and ensure an individual-centered experience for the individuals receiving care. In order to successfully carry out either standing or delegated orders, PCRNs must be competent and understand their role on the primary care team, be confident in their assessment abilities, and have access to a broad base of knowledge.

Behavioral Health in Primary Care

The purpose of interprofessional collaboration is to support relationships between the PCRN and other members of the care team, such as the behavioral health team members. Particularly in the realm of CCM, many individuals have comorbid behavioral health conditions. Uncontrolled or exacerbating behavioral health conditions can also exacerbate already poorly controlled medical conditions. Additionally, some medications used to treat behavioral health conditions impact medical conditions, particularly those with metabolic side effects.

Even when individuals may actually benefit from behavioral health intervention and support, often they do not proactively seek it. The PCRN can play a direct role in all of these examples by: (1) actively reviewing individuals for risk factors and for potential benefit from behavioral health services, including but not limited to routine screening, suicide risk assessment and others, (2) proactively utilizing warm handoffs to ensure direct and immediate connection to behavioral health services, (3) supporting routine screening for medication-related or condition-specific issues, and (4) supporting individuals with multiple chronic conditions to achieve self-management over time (Flinter et al., 2016). PCRNs also expand the opportunities to encourage individuals to receive evidence-based care by ensuring this care can be delivered in the context of other visit types, for example, during behavioral health or dental appointments.

Substance Use Disorder and Harm Reduction

Because there are many key populations seeking primary care services, the PCRN must be prepared to work on behalf of all individuals and to be as supportive and nonjudgmental as possible. For example, harm reduction principles should be used in the implementation of screening and treatment for drug and alcohol abuse in primary care. This ensures support and positive reinforcement of even incremental progress toward minimizing the harmful effects of substance use (Harm Reduction Coalition, 2019). The Substance Abuse and Mental Health Services Administration published a white paper in 2011 that outlined the underlying evidence supporting screening, brief intervention, and referral to treatment, its overall impact, and successful model implementations. Many team members, including the PCRN, can deliver brief interventions that support individuals to move toward treatment for their substance use. Interventions are most effective when they are brief and when they are delivered more than once, all with a supportive approach (Substance Abuse and Mental Health Services Administration, 2011).

PCRNs also play a significant role with this population in terms of delivering routine follow-up and in-between care for medication-assisted treatment (MAT) involving monitoring of buprenorphine or other regimens by standing order, or through routine care management services. In this way, PCRNs can share responsibility and support PCPs while ensuring an integrated approach where the behavioral health and medical team collaborate to deliver MAT services, which ensures full realization of their identity within the primary care setting (Haddad et al., 2013).

Population Health

The concept of population health was well developed by the Institute for Healthcare Improvement in a white paper entitled *A Guide to Measuring the Triple Aim: Population Health, Experience of Care, and Per Capita Cost* (Stiefel & Nolan, 2012). The aim is to ensure that all subpopulations receive quality clinical care to better address their specific disease burden. This includes a comprehensive understanding of health—not just medical well-being but health in terms of behavioral health, social determinants of health, and overall health literacy. In the end, quality clinical care should translate into an improved experience for an individual and therefore hopefully lower overall healthcare cost, which is the third element of the original Triple Aim (Stiefel & Nolan, 2012).

The PCRN can identify subpopulations at risk or groups of individuals requiring specific intervention, complete the work required to mitigate the risk, and aid an individual to maintain or move toward health. For example, the PCRN can be responsible for tracking abnormal cancer screening results that may have multiple steps for follow-up. In this example, the PCRN may be described as a case finder who can best look at population metrics for individuals with cancer to define a needed outreach and then can assist in the planning and implementation of that specific outreach. In this way, the PCRN can lead quality improvement efforts and look at larger issues impacting the communities served by their organizations.

The PCRN can also assist with appropriate referrals to other team members such as behavioral health or even to outside organizations including cardiac rehabilitation, the wound clinic, and others. This ensures both that the individuals' care is fully coordinated and that they are receiving the appropriate treatment from the most appropriate care team member (both within and outside of the PCRN's organization) given their particular training and expertise. A more complete discussion of vulnerable populations and socioeconomic determinants of health can be found in Chapters 13 and 14.

Complex Care Management

Care coordination and CCM are not synonymous. CCM usually describes the specific role of the PCRN in the overall process of care coordination, which typically involves every member of the team. The extent of the care coordination delivered depends on both the specific needs of the individual and the level of training, education, and licensure of the specific staff delivering the service. All organizations should work to define the particular competencies associated with each role on the care team with regard to care coordination or CCM. This ensures that the entire care team remains meaningfully engaged in the overall process.

CCM is one of the largest domains of the PCRN role, in that it encompasses all of the efforts required to support individuals to self-management of their chronic illness. In a 2016 Health Resources and Services Administration (HRSA) National Cooperative Agreement webinar focused on workforce transformation (hosted by the Community Health Center, Inc. in Middletown, CT), Ed Wagner, MD, MPH, of the MacColl Center for Healthcare Innovation described CCM as the most complex end of a spectrum of services delivered by the clinical care team to promote care coordination activities. Dr. Wagner described activities associated with low-level care coordination such as logistic support, which could be completed by non-licensed staff such as patient navigators, MAs, and the like. As activities move toward greater complexity—involving things like transitions of care, medication reconciliation, medication titration, chronic illness management, and self-management support—PCRNs become CCM team leaders to guide the way in collaboration with the PCP (Community Health Center, Inc. [CHCI] & the MacColl Center, 2016).

Skills for Complex Care Management

PCRNs need additional experience in many areas to ensure their success in caring for individuals, particularly in the realm of CCM. These RNs need education in MI and SMG setting, especially with regard to individuals with behavioral health, substance use, and multiple chronic issues. Additional support is also needed to manage the challenges that may be identified as affecting an individual's social determinants of health. PCRNs must build their capacity to confidently tackle complexity one step at a time, while honing their skills in identifying individuals ready to engage while motivating others toward engagement. In so doing, PCRNs may take the lead on the care team, a role that fully uses the knowledge and skills inherent to nursing education.

Care Continuum and Community Resources

The care continuum in its entirety is important to consider when working to effect change for individuals that qualify for CCM services. These individuals often receive care in multiple settings, including the emergency department, inpatient hospital, home care, hospice and palliative care, school systems, and others. Systems at times have access to additional data including claims data, adjusted clinical group scores, and other information that better defines an individual's risk based on diagnoses, cost, and other factors. These individuals often benefit from additional care coordination, which can be challenging given the number of agencies and clinicians already involved in their care, each holding their own important piece of the puzzle that is the individual's plan of care.

PCRNs can lead in this area by enhancing care team communication through interventions such as coordinating an interprofessional case conference. This involves coordinating all main players on the patient's care team (both internally and externally to the PCRN's organization) to review the plan of care and to address barriers to care for that specific individual. After discussing solutions, the team comes away with a comprehensive plan that all organizations will use to support a consistent approach to the care they deliver to that individual.

In addition to the various care providers along the care continuum, individuals typically are engaged with various community resources. Social determinants of health screening is an important aspect of primary care delivery that should be considered when reviewing current or identifying needed community resources. This topic is covered in more detail in Chapter 14, but examples include individuals who experience homelessness (those without housing), housing instability (those at risk of losing their housing or those that have frequent moves), or unhealthy homes (homes with insect or rodent infestations, mold, lead paint, carbon monoxide, radon, or other hazards) (U.S. Department of Housing and Urban Development, 2014). It is important that the PCRN knows how to screen for ways these and other conditions impact the population in the community where they serve, particularly the individuals they are serving in CCM.

PCRNs must not only serve individuals who may be impacted by these issues but also consider the role they themselves can play in health policy, social policy, and community engagement and partnerships to support change in this area. This important area of RN involvement is more fully discussed in Chapter 3.

Pediatric Primary Care

Although there are several specialties that may incorporate or fall under the umbrella of primary care, it may be appropriate specifically to address the specialty of pediatrics. The PCRN has multiple responsibilities with regard to caring for pediatric patients, ranging from preventive roles with immunization support, caregiver education on developmental milestones, response to abnormal screening results such as developmental, depression, or pediatric trauma screening, adolescent contraceptive counseling, to roles focused on CCM of children with ongoing complex chronic health needs. Safety, nutrition, proper medication use, and even home care instructions for caregivers to navigate minor illness and injury are frequent topics for counseling supported by the PCRN role. PCRNs must be comfortable with common holds used to prevent movement and therefore potential injury or blood-borne pathogen exposure during immunizations and other procedures.

Communication is extremely important for the PCRN to master as part of their role in supporting pediatric patients. Ensuring age-specific competencies for the various age groups in pediatrics is important to ensure age-appropriate instructions for specimen collection, procedures, and other information regarding specific care actions delivered during the child's visit. There are also times the PCRN acts as the child's advocate to aid in expressing their thoughts and feelings about their care, as well as to identify potential abuse or neglect covered by the PCRN's status as a mandated reporter.

Transition planning is another core competency for PCRNs to ensure that adolescents are well supported with a structured yet individualized approach to prepare for transitioning to an adult care provider. This involves growing the adolescent's self-efficacy with relation to managing their own health and developing their own relationship with their various healthcare providers. This process should start well in advance of their actual transition to adult care to ensure there is time to develop these skills.

Healthcare for children also can be complicated by medical, social, or behavioral issues. They may already have care delivered by many members of the healthcare team ranging from medical specialists to other disciplines such as behavioral health, but there may also be various caretakers involved in the care of the child, including daycare or school, parent(s), grandparent(s), and others. The PCRN can leverage their competencies in CCM to not only deliver needed coordination but also support the caretakers as they ensure the safety and well-being of the child being treated.

At times this may include managing new durable medical equipment orders, leveraging an MA to coordinate transportation for appointments, or even setting SMGs with the child to support engagement with their own healthcare. Coordination can involve ensuring not only that the child's needs are met in terms of timely access to equipment and specialty consults but also that the PCP has all of the information needed to individualize the care delivered based on all of the other members of the extended care team and their various additions to the child's plan of care. Coordination could also involve addressing body image issues related to the child's condition or supporting periodic respite for caretakers (which includes assessing and addressing their need for additional support even in terms of their own health and well-being). As with all CCM care delivery, PCRNs should review the child's social determinants of health and make referrals to organizational or community partners when applicable.

Insurance and Economic Issues

Access to insurance and healthcare benefits is extremely important for any individual. From routine screenings and management of acute issues to care required for ongoing chronic illness, healthcare benefits make it possible for individuals to access care without having to cover the total expense. Healthcare finance can be very challenging for many because it often requires some level of health literacy: knowing both what to access and how. Dealing with insurance, even aside from the challenges of understanding the communications from insurers such as explanation of benefits forms and concepts such as in-network care versus out-of-network care, insurance companies may require completing applications or other forms to secure access to benefits.

Medication issues are a significant part of primary care, both for the individual and for the PCRN assisting in prescription coverage. For the individual, it requires an understanding of concepts such as brand name versus generic name and the impact to overall cost when choosing between the two. The PCRN can assist the individual to find programs for medication cost relief, such as discount pharmacy programs and medication assistance programs offered by individual pharmaceutical companies.

Most individuals access insurance either through their employment or through government programs (either state or federal). Whether an individual has insurance or not, the care delivered and the medications prescribed typically come with some amount of cost. It is important for the PCRN to ask relevant questions to ensure that individuals can actually afford the regimens they are on and can afford to get to specialty or other appointments scheduled on their behalf.

At times, individuals must fill out complex forms (particularly for state or federal program applications and renewals) that are difficult to complete without some assistance. PCRNs should also ensure that the organization or practice for which they work is monitoring benefits to ensure quick referral to patient navigators or other similar positions to assist in application completion or other routine support to improve an individual's ability to maintain or attain insurance coverage as well as gain an understanding of how to best utilize that coverage for their overall benefit.

The PCRN should be aware of other economic issues that affect overall health, such as utilities, food access, and transportation. All individuals receiving CCM services should be assessed for access to the appropriate resources needed to support their specific chronic illness. For utilities, this could include ensuring access to electricity to cook food, refrigerate medications, supply power as needed for medical equipment, or even cool their living spaces during the warmest months so as to not exacerbate their respiratory condition. PCRNs should perform a diet recall to assess an individual's access to nutrition appropriate for their chronic illness. It is also important to assess whether additional medication may be needed to address various deficiencies that contribute to suboptimal health.

Last, the PCRN should review the individual's access to transportation. Lack of transportation can often impact an individual's ability to pick up prescriptions from the pharmacy on time, see their various healthcare providers (both primary care and specialists), and maintain employment, thereby further jeopardizing their economic status as well as their access to health insurance. All of these variables can lead to regimen nonadherence, overdue chronic illness surveillance or screening (such as routine laboratory testing), or general lack of access to care. Strategies to address these barriers include using pharmacies that mail or deliver medications to the home and coordinating medical transportation through the individual's current insurance carrier. Virtual visits present additional innovative solutions that will increasingly be utilized as payment for such services becomes available.

Health Information Technology, Data Tracking, and Clinical Decision Support Systems

Health information technology (HIT) is a term used to describe the creation and use of data and other electronic tools to support care teams and patients as they interact to work toward the mutual goal of improving health (Health Information Technology Advisory Committee, 2018). This term includes the EHR and even the way an individual may communicate with a provider or care team via an online portal. Health data tracking tools also fall into this category, including any systems giving clinical decision support.

The term "clinical decision support systems" (CDSSs) is used to describe data tools that assist a care team member in making a decision about an individual's care whether it is planned care such as routine cancer screening or something that is condition specific such as foot checks or retinal screening for all individuals with diabetes. CDSSs also include tools such as data dashboards and care gap reports. Most organizations have defined policies and procedures to support both the creation and use of CDSSs. Primary care continues to change rapidly with the focus moving to value-based payment models, so a focus on HIT and CDSS tools is important to ensure that all members of the care team are considering new and evolving ways clinical teams and individuals communicate and interact regarding health.

Structured Data

Structured data is one important component of HIT. For individual outcomes or other clinical markers to be measured, the organization must collect structured data. Whether it is ensuring that a depression screening is completed on every individual every year or ensuring that all individuals who have diabetes receive a hemoglobin A_{1c} test at least every 6 months, every measure must involve some aspect of structured data to show whether in fact each action was completed. In most value-based programs, it is also important to ensure that appropriate coding be addressed with structured data to support accurate claims reporting of items, such as completed screenings and in-house laboratory tests.

Structured data may also be used to answer a question. For example, how many individuals screen positive for depression? Or how many individuals with diabetes have a hemoglobin A_{1c} that is greater than 9.0%? This information not only helps a practice or clinical team understand the level of risk for the community they serve based on actual trends but also helps to review the relative quality of the care being delivered to their specific panel of individuals. Identifying areas where additional resources or interventions may need to be implemented can aid in supporting a particular community.

Structured data also supports teams to not only make individual-specific decisions but also utilize algorithms or checklists to ensure a more accurate and therefore higher quality patient encounter. This includes visit templates, which are created to ensure that a team member asks all expected evidence-based questions and addresses all specific areas of concern for a specific visit type. An example of this could be a well-child visit template, which is designed for a particular age group. This template would include all developmentally appropriate questions to ask caregivers, as well as all expected areas of anticipatory guidance to support caregiver education.

Structured data also may be used to remind the PCRN or the PCP to implement evidence-based screening and intervention for a variety of health issues. For instance, a pop-up reminder may appear in the EHR to obtain osteoporosis screening for an older female patient, or to discuss colonoscopy with a individual who falls in the appropriate age range.

In addition to the examples just mentioned, structured data also may be used to develop an order set for standing orders. This allows a team member to access a grouping of particular clinical orders that may apply to a specific situation. For example, an order set designed to support a PCRN to treat an uncomplicated urinary tract infection for an adult female may include specific lab orders for urinalysis and culture, specific education materials, as well as medication orders that could be chosen as a part of a set algorithm for the visit. As with all other HIT tools, organizations typically have defined policies and procedures to support both the creation and use of such templates and order sets in the form of standing orders or other policies describing job expectations.

Dashboards

Dashboards are useful tools to support teams with CDSSs, including population-based care reviews as well as at the point of care when an individual is presenting for a face-to-face visit. Patient visit dashboards are typically used to organize routine planned care, including routine cancer screening, depression screening, IPV screening, and many other evidence-based, quality-of-care measures. This dashboard type also includes condition-specific care such as foot checks, retinal screening, and screening for microalbuminuria for individuals who have diabetes. It also may include care items to support the evidence-based treatment of individuals with chronic pain such as routine functional assessment. Each item must include structured data to ensure that the dashboard can effectively determine whether this care has been delivered in the expected time frame. The dashboard also knows when the time frame resets. For example, many organizations reset depression screening yearly, whereas hemoglobin A_{1c} may reset every 3 or 6 months, depending on the result of the prior laboratory test.

Dashboards are often created to support tracking of care gaps or individuals who may be lost to follow-up. For example, a dashboard created to focus on diabetes may identify individuals who have diabetes by provider panel and then drill down further to list all quality-of-care metrics that are measured for these individuals, including last blood pressure reading, retinal screening, foot check, hemoglobin A_{1c} level, and last dental or behavioral health visit (should the team want to capture oral health or know who has accessed behavioral health for support in this population). Dashboards can often be sorted by column so that team members can review and identify individuals who need to be recalled to the office, as they may be overdue for expected care. Organizations need to consider how to provide dedicated time to care teams to utilize this data to close care gaps and reestablish those that have been lost to follow-up.

Scorecards and Accountability

Scorecards are an expected extension of clinical dashboards as they summarize overall quality metrics to support a care team's understanding of overall performance. Measures that are addressed in dashboards have defined denominators (the group of individuals that the measure applies to) and numerators (the group of individuals that successfully had the care item delivered). For example, the denominator for foot checks for individuals with diabetes would be all individuals who have a diagnosis of diabetes captured through the diagnosis code being added to the person's problem list in the EHR. The numerator would then be defined as individuals with diabetes who had a foot check within the last 12 months possibly as captured with structured fields within the examination section of the EHR. To ensure appropriate metrics,

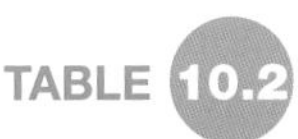

USE OF CLINICAL DECISION SUPPORT SYSTEM TOOLS

CDSS Tool	Example(s)
Structured data	Incorporate pop-up EHR reminders: depression screening for all individuals
	Answer quality improvement question: How many individuals have a hemoglobin A_{1c} greater than 9%?
	Develop a visit template: appropriate questions for a well-child visit
	Create standing orders: RN care for uncomplicated urinary tract infection
Dashboard	Find individuals who are overdue for an office visit for diabetes follow-up
	Compare clinic results on hypertension management with recommended guidelines
Scorecard	Identify patients with diabetes who have had a foot check in the past 12 months

Note. CDSS = clinical decision support system; EHR = electronic health record; RN = registered nurse.

for example, only individuals seen within the last 12 months may be included, particularly if the data are meant to describe how successful the care team is at delivering the prescribed care when it is noted as due on the dashboard. These data can then be used to inform an ongoing performance improvement process to ensure appropriate accountability for the applicable team member. For example, if it is the PCRN's responsibility to ensure all individuals with diabetes have a discussion documented at least every 6 months around self-management, then this should appear on their performance scorecard.

Some metrics may show up on more than one team member's scorecard. For example, hypertension control could be seen as the responsibility of both the PCP and the PCRN because they both can effect change for individuals with elevated blood pressure. Each organization should determine which team member is responsible for each care item or step in the care item. As another example, overall depression screening rates may be attributed to an MA, but responding to a positive screen may be the PCP, behavioral health team member, or the PCRN. Responsibility is typically assigned based on state scope of practice, training, and a commitment to ensuring that all team members are practicing to the top of their license and education, with appropriate policies and procedures to support each expected workflow and intervention.

Table 10.2 provides examples of the CDSS tools described earlier.

Economic Impact of the Primary Care Registered Nurse Role

The role of the PCP has continued to change over the years as the team has continued to grow and as role delineation has become a direct focus in team-based care. The role of the PCRN has been a part of this transformation. As individual complexity and the volume of individuals needing care have increased, all roles have been better leveraged to provide comprehensive care. Incident-to provider visit care is one example of this, where the PCRN supports the PCP's encounter with an individual during their clinical day. Incident-to service means that, even though the PCRN may be delivering or contributing to the service, only the provider is identified in the billing. This topic is covered in more detail in Chapter 2. However, in the primary care setting, incident-to service activities could be a request to give education regarding a new medication, to address a lab abnormality, or even to show an individual how to apply dressing materials to a wound on an ongoing basis. At times, it is to help individuals set SMGs or continue to work on an existing care plan for their chronic illness.

This is an important aspect of team-based care as it requires that the various team members accomplish as much as possible for the individual in the most efficient way without requiring that the provider be the one to organize it or do it all. This approach increases individual access because the provider can do a portion of the visit and move on to the next individual while the team completes all other care that needs to be delivered. However, incident-to billing means that the role of the PCRN and others in providing this more efficient care is often not identified, making it more challenging to effectively quantify the direct impact to the healthcare system. Ongoing research will be important in measuring the impact in terms of shared savings and overall value, as the payment model in primary care continues to transition, further supporting the business case for the PCRN role.

Value-based care is one of the main drivers for continued expansion of the role of PCRNs, who are now able to work in collaboration with PCPs to review and track care for the highest risk individuals in a provider's panel, including those with uncontrolled chronic illness, those transitioning from hospital or skilled nursing facility to home, and those who are high emergency department utilizers. PCRNs are unique in that they can more easily deliver care by standing order utilizing defined algorithms that take advantage of their critical thinking and assessment skills, or through delegated provider order, including medication titration if required. The main focus is on the PCRN as complex care manager and leader to support the process of care coordination for high-risk/high-need individuals in hopes of reducing overall healthcare cost and therefore risk.

There are several ways that payers reimburse PCRN care delivery, and more are in development as the transition to value-based payment models continues. In some states, PCRNs in some practices can bill incident-to services. Some states directly reimburse PCRN care delivered by standing or delegated order without the direct involvement of a provider (MD/DO, APRN, or PA). Other opportunities for reimbursement include CCM-related services for care delivered by a PCRN or other clinical care team members between visits. Reimbursement can also be made from shared savings or other value-based payments that are related to achievement of quality-of-care benchmarks such as lower cost of care or improvement in specific clinical outcome measures. At least one service, the Annual Wellness Visit, is billable as an RN visit and reimbursed by the Centers for Medicare and Medicaid (CMS) funding.

Performance Data Reporting

As value-based payment models become more common, it will be important to have an identified role or department own the responsibility of performance data reporting. Team members with formal informatics training are also beneficial given that they typically have a greater understanding of how data are used to ensure performance measurement. This also supports communication between the data team and the clinical team members by having a common language or understanding as to the goal of the implementation. If data reporting is claims based, then the data or business intelligence (BI) team should be utilizing visit coding as structured data to pull projected performance. This may also give an organization greater reason to ensure the presence of certified billers and coders to support the clinical teams in capturing all of the delivered care with correct coding.

If performance measurement is based on the organization submitting data reports, this allows for greater flexibility in the collection of structured data. This in turn allows the organization which in turn allows the organization to capture care delivered in multiple ways to address the same measure, such as when smoking cessation counseling is required for any individual who identifies as an active smoker and each team member chooses to utilize an alternate section of the EHR to document this counseling. The data or BI team could capture this data in any of the locations and count it toward the numerator of the measure.

Regardless of how the data are measured, the organization should acknowledge teams' efforts with regard to the additional work of proper coding or completing additional structured data. This added burden of data entry may require attention to the fourth aim of the quadruple aim: focusing on improving the work life of providers and clinical teams (Bodenheimer & Sinsky, 2014). To address this problem, one strategy has been to move additional structured data entry downstream to nonclinical team members such as scribes or MAs.

Summary

The role of the PCRN is extremely important in the overall continuum of care. In addition to increased knowledge of basic PCRN competencies, nursing students now have greater access to training that emphasizes patient centeredness, value-based care, complexity, and social determinants of health. When they are better prepared for the challenges they will face, more nurses are likely to choose primary care as their entry point to the nursing workforce, especially as they find more opportunities to receive training that addresses the rapidly changing primary care practice environment.

With the workforce continuing to grow as projected, academic preparation and clinical placements (and preceptors) must be further enhanced to ensure appropriate reinforcement of PCRN competencies. As this happens, residencies and demonstrations of PCRN impact will facilitate formal documentation of the importance of this critical role. Advanced roles will continue to develop, reinforcing the natural pathways for academic progression that already exist but are currently underutilized both for enhanced roles as PCRN leaders and for those wishing to advance their clinical scope of practice. Organizations that have well-developed roles should be identified as best practices and used to support model spread just as in the LEAP project sites, which described many innovative roles along with that of the PCRN (Flinter et al., 2017). Multidisciplinary collaboration and strong academic–clinical partnerships will ensure this transformation gains momentum to meet the growing demand for this vital role.

Case Study

Tara is a 45-year-old woman with uncontrolled hypertension. She reports that she does not take her blood pressure medication every day because of cost concerns. At today's medical visit the MA completed a screening for intimate partner violence (IPV) as part of routine planned care. This screening was positive, and Tara began to tear up as she was answering the questions. The MA reached out to the PCRN because the provider was in the next room with another individual. As the complex care manager at this PCMH, the PCRN is prepared to go into the room to discuss Tara's uncontrolled hypertension and to work to hopefully enroll her in a care management program for ongoing support. After being notified of the individual's emotional reaction to the IPV screen, the PCRN goes in to check on her and offer a warm handoff or other applicable services. Tara is still upset when the PCRN enters the room and states she does not "know what to do."

Consider the following questions:

1. How should the PCRN approach this discussion with Tara about her uncontrolled hypertension and positive screen for IPV? Would one issue or the other take priority? Why, or why not?
2. What is the specific role of the PCRN in this encounter? What could the ongoing role of the PCRN be for Tara?
3. What other team members might the PCRN pull in to address the various aspects of Tara's care?

Key Points for Review

- The role of the PCRN is an important aspect of high-functioning primary care practices, and it will continue to grow and expand as practices and clinics adopt the patient-centered medical home model and the move toward value-based care.
- The role of the PCRN involves core competencies in chronic illness management and CCM, where the nurse is identified as a leader on the care team and is activated toward proactive identification and management of individuals in need of additional support.
- PCRNs need additional knowledge and experience in order to be successful in this role postlicensure. This includes a working knowledge of key populations such as those who struggle with substance use, individuals with impacted social determinants of health, and those with comorbid behavioral health conditions.
- Performance measures and clinical outcome measures should be identified to ensure the impact of the PCRN can be better measured and understood. This includes ensuring shared responsibility between the PCP and their PCRN, which will ensure a more engaged care team.
- Training the next generation will be critical as the role of the PCRN continues to develop. Academic–clinical practice partnerships should be developed to better support and integrate this role into the larger landscape of baccalaureate nursing training.

REFERENCES

American Academy of Pediatrics, Committee on Children with Disabilities. (1999a). Care coordination: Integrating health and related systems of care for children with special health care needs. *Pediatrics, 104*, 978–981. https://doi.org/10.1542/peds.104.4.978

American Academy of Pediatrics, Committee on Pediatric Workforce. (1999b). Culturally effective pediatric care: Education and training issues. *Pediatrics, 103*, 167–170. https://doi.org/10.1542/peds.103.1.167

Association of American Medical Colleges. (2015). *New physician workforce projections show the doctor shortage remains significant.* https://www.aamc.org/newsroom/newsreleases/426166/20150303.html

Bauer, L., & Bodenheimer, T. (2017). Expanded roles of registered nurses in primary care delivery of the future. *Nursing Outlook, 65*(5), 624–632. https://doi.org/10.1016/j.outlook.2017.03.011

Bodenheimer, T., & Laing, B. (2007). The teamlet model of primary care. *Annals of Family Medicine, 5*, 457–461. https://doi.org/10.1370/afm.731

Bodenheimer, T., & Sinsky, C. (2014). From triple to quadruple aim: Care of the patient requires care of the provider. *Annals of Family Medicine, 12*, 573–576. https://doi.org/10.1370/afm.1713

Brega, A., Barnard, J., Mabachi, N., Weiss, B., DeWalt, D., Brach, C., & West, D. (2015). *AHRQ health literacy universal precautions toolkit, second edition. (Prepared by Colorado Health Outcomes Program, University of Colorado Anschutz Medical Campus under Contract No. HHSA290200710008, TO#10.) AHRQ Publication No. 15-0023-EF*. Agency for Healthcare Research and Quality.

Breiding, M. J., & Chen, J., & Black, M. C. (2014). *Intimate partner violence in the United States—2010*. National Center for Injury Prevention and Control, Centers for Disease Control and Prevention.

Budden, J., Zhong, E., Moulton, P., & Cimiotti, J. (2013). Highlights of the national workforce survey of registered nurses. *Journal of Nursing Regulation, 4*(2), 5–14. https://doi.org/10.1016/S2155-8256(15)30151-4

Bureau of Labor Statistics, U.S. Department of Labor. (2017). *Occupational outlook handbook, registered nurses*. https://www.bls.gov/ooh/healthcare/registered-nurses.htm

Centers for Disease Control and Prevention: National Center for Injury Prevention and Control, Division of Violence Prevention. (2010). *National intimate partner and sexual violence survey: 2010 summary report.* https://www.cdc.gov/violenceprevention/pdf/NISVS_Executive_Summary-a.pdf

Flinter, M., Blankson, M., & Ladden, M. J. (2016). Registered nurses in primary care: Strategies that support practice at the full scope of the registered nurse license. In *Registered nurses: Partners in transforming primary care. Recommendations from the Macy Foundation Conference on Preparing Registered Nurses for Enhanced Roles in Primary Care*. Macy Foundation.

Flinter, M., Hsu, C., Cromp, D., Ladden, M., & Wagner, E. (2017). Registered nurses in primary care: Emerging new roles and contributions to team-based care in high-performing practices. *Journal of Ambulatory Care Management, 40*(4), 287–296. https://doi.org/10.1097/JAC.0000000000000193

Folsom, M. (1967). *Health is a community affair: The report of the National Commission on Community Health Services.* Harvard University Press.

Haddad, M., Zelenev, A., & Altice, F. (2013). Integrating buprenorphine maintenance therapy into federally qualified health centers: Real world substance abuse treatment outcomes. *Drug and Alcohol Dependence, 131*(0), 127–135. https://doi.org/10.1016/j.drugalcdep.2012.12.008

Harm Reduction Coalition. (2019). *Principles of harm reduction.* https://harmreduction.org/about-us/principles-of-harm-reduction/

Health Information Technology Advisory Committee. (2018). *Health IT: Advancing America's health care.* https://www.healthit.gov/sites/default/files/pdf/health-information-technology-fact-sheet.pdf

Institute of Medicine. (1978). *A manpower policy for primary health care: Report of a study.* National Academy Press.

Institute of Medicine. (1984). *Community-oriented primary care: A practical assessment, volume I. The Committee Report.* National Academy Press.

Institute of Medicine. (1996). *Primary care: America's health in a new era.* The National Academies Press.

Millis, J. (1966). *The graduate education of physicians: The report of the citizen's commission of graduate medical education (Millis Commission).* American Medical Association.

Mitchell, P., Wynia, M., Golden, R., McNellis, B., Okun, S., Webb, C., Rohrbach, V., & Von Kohorn, I. (2012). *Core principles & values of effective team-based health care.* Discussion Paper, Institute of Medicine.

National Association of Community Health Centers. (2016). *PRAPARE implementation and action toolkit.* http://www.nachc.org/research-and-data/prapare/toolkit/

National Committee for Quality Assurance. (2017). *NCQA PCMH standards and guidelines (2017 edition).* http://store.ncqa.org/index.php/catalog/product/view/id/2776/s/2017-pcmh-standards-and-guidelines-epub/

Norful, A., Martsolf, G., de Jacq, K., & Poghosyan, L. (2017). Utilization of registered nurses in primary care teams: A systematic review. *International Journal of Nursing Studies, 74,* 15–23. https://doi.org/10.1016/j.ijnurstu.2017.05.013

Okun, S., Schoenbaum, S., Andrews, D., Chidambaran, P., Chollette, V., Gruman, J., Leal, S., Lown, B. A., Mitchell, P. H., Parry, C., Prins, W., Ricciardi, R., Simon, M. A., Stock, R., Strasser, D. C., Webb, C. E., Wynia, M. K., & Henderson, D. (2014). *Patients and health care teams forging effective partnerships (discussion paper).* Institute of Medicine.

Safety Net Medical Home Initiative. (2013). *Empanelment: Establishing patient provider relationships, executive summary.* http://www.safetynetmedicalhome.org/sites/default/files/Executive-Summary-Empanelment.pdf

Schottenfeld, L., Petersen, D., Peikes, D., Ricciardi, R., Burak, H., McNellis, R., & Genevro, J. (2016). *Creating patient-centered team-based primary care (AHRQ Pub. No. 16-0002-EF).* Agency for Healthcare Research and Quality.

Starfield, B. (1992). *Primary care: Concept, evaluation and policy.* Oxford University Press.

Starfield, B. (1994). Is primary care essential? *The Lancet, 344*(8930), 1129–1133. https://doi.org/10.1016/S0140-6736(94)90634-3

Stiefel, M., & Nolan, K. (2012). *A guide to measuring the Triple Aim: Population health, experience of care, and per capita cost. IHI Innovation Series white paper.* Institute for Healthcare Improvement.

Substance Abuse and Mental Health Services Administration. (2011). *Screening, brief intervention and referral to treatment (SBIRT) in behavioral healthcare.* https://www.samhsa.gov/sites/default/files/sbirtwhitepaper_0.pdf

Sullivan, E. E., Ibrahim, Z., Ellner, A. L., & Giesen, L. J. (2016). Management lessons for high-functioning primary care teams. *Journal of Healthcare Management, 61*(6), 449–466. https://doi.org/10.1097/00115514-201611000-00011

The Joint Commission (nd). Primary care medical home certification program. https://www.jointcommission.org/accreditation-and-certification/certification/certifications-by-setting/hospital-certifications/primary-care-medical-home-certification/

The Working Party Group on Integrated Behavioral Healthcare; Baird, M., Blount, A., Brungardt, S., Dickinson, P., Dietrich, A., Epperly, T., & deGruy, F. (2014). Joint principles: Integrating behavioral health care into the patient-centered medical home. *Annals of Family Medicine, 12*(2), 183–185. https://doi.org/10.1370/afm.1633

U.S. Department of Housing and Urban Development. (2014). *Protecting children from unhealthy homes and housing instability.* https://www.huduser.gov/portal/periodicals/em/fall14/highlight3.html

Willard, W. (1966). *Meeting the challenge of family practice: The report of the ad hoc Committee on Education for Family Practice.* American Medical Association.

11

Episodic Care

Stephanie G. Witwer and Beckie Kronebusch

PERSPECTIVES

"The health care system is undergoing rapid changes that put new emphasis on population health, quality of care, and the value of the services delivered. ...nurses, by sheer numbers, will play a significant role in this transformation, and will themselves be transformed in the process."

Fraher, E, Spetz, J, Naylor, M. (2015). Nursing in a transformed health care system: New roles, new rules. (Research Brief). Penn LDI, Interdisciplinary Nursing Quality Research Initiative. http://ldihealtheconomist.com/media/inqri-ldi-brief-nursing.pdf

LEARNING OBJECTIVES

Upon completion of this chapter, the reader will be able to:

1. Apply elements of the Standards of Professional Clinical Practice to ambulatory care settings.
2. Identify opportunities to advance professional nursing practice in ambulatory care settings.
3. Compare and contrast select episodic ambulatory care settings.
4. Understand the key role of the registered nurse (RN) in episodic ambulatory care settings.

KEY TERMS

Ambulatory surgery
Diagnostic and therapeutic centers
Home-based services
Infusion centers
Nursing process
Palliative home care
Standards of Professional Clinical Practice
Transitional care services
Urgent care centers

Introduction

This chapter is designed to help the reader understand how standards of practice build the foundation of nursing care regardless of the episodic ambulatory setting. Chapter 11 identifies examples of challenges found in episodic environments and describes implementation of ambulatory care nursing practice in select specialized ambulatory settings and populations.

Episodic care is a term that describes a broad range of problem-focused services. These services may be designed to address acute symptoms (eg, urgent care), be a step in comprehensive diagnosis and treatment (eg, diagnostic imaging centers), or provide definitive care (eg, surgery centers). Individuals may be able to directly access episodic services or require licensed provider referral. Services provided in episodic care settings are distinct from primary care, designed to be either one-time or limited series, with limited or no ongoing relationship between healthcare provider and individual.

Guiding Principles for Episodic Ambulatory Care

Ambulatory care environments may appear to be a confusing patchwork of services that lack common infrastructure and coordination. Services are varied and occur in multiple settings such as hospital-based outpatient departments, medical group practices, individual provider offices, community health settings, schools, specialized surgical or diagnostic centers, homes, and other residential settings. Care settings and services continue to transform with evolving individual needs and breakthroughs in technology and medical treatment. Regardless of setting, however, nursing practice is guided by the **Standards of Professional Clinical Practice** as defined by the American Nurses Association (ANA, 2015), the American Academy of Ambulatory Care Nursing (AAACN, 2017), and the clinical specialty of the practice setting and population.

Ambulatory care nursing practice supports this ever-increasing array of episodic settings that are characterized by the following:

- high-volume, rapid patient throughput, usually from a few minutes to less than 24 hours
- rapidly increasing patient acuity
- increasingly technical interventional procedures
- unpredictability
- incorporation of diagnostic and therapeutic services for patients of all ages with acute, chronic, palliative, and end-of-life needs
- highly specialized interprofessional teams
- strong patient/family involvement
- a growing need for effective patient transitions to and from the episodic care site (Mastal & Paschke, 2019)

Individual-Centered Care

One of the hallmarks of ambulatory care nursing is the partnership between nurses and individuals/families. AAACN (2017) states that "[a]mbulatory care RNs, acting as partners, advocates, and advisors, assist and support individuals/families in the optimal management of their health care, respecting their culture and values, individual needs, health goals, and treatment preferences" (p. 6). Although many definitions of client-centered care exist, it is considered a dimension of quality in which individuals and families, rather than clinicians, have control over healthcare decisions (Hughes, 2011). Principles of client-centered care (in this text, synonymous with individual-centered care) were promoted by Cronenwett et al. (2007) in their recommended curricula for quality and safety education for prelicensure nurses and continue today through the efforts of the Institute for Quality and Safety Education (QSEN) for nurses.

Individual and family involvement is of paramount importance in episodic ambulatory care. In these fast-paced environments, encounters are short, and clinicians are often seeing an individual for the first time. Because individuals and families bear primary responsibility for pre-encounter preparation and providing information about current and continuing care needs, the **nursing process** provides an effective system for planning, organizing, and providing care. Effective partnership with individuals and families enhances care outcomes, quality, safety, and individual experience (Patient- and Family-Centered Care, 2018), and nurses are uniquely positioned for this partnership.

Standards of Professional Clinical Practice for Ambulatory Care Nursing

The AAACN has identified Standards of Practice for Professional Ambulatory Care Nursing (AAACN, 2017). These standards are organized into two domains: Standards of Professional Clinical Practice and Standards of Nursing Organizational and Professional Performance. Regardless of role, setting, population, or specialty, registered nurses (RNs) are expected to competently perform standards of practice. Practice setting and population needs drive the specific competencies required for each standard.

The terms "nursing process" and "Standards of Professional Clinical Practice" reflect the nurse's clinical reasoning process. This well-established process is used by the nurse to exercise clinical judgment. Tanner (2006) describes clinical judgment as an "interpretation or conclusion about a patient's needs, concerns, or health problems, and/or the decision to take action (or not), use or modify standard approaches, or improvise new ones as deemed appropriate by the patient's response" (p. 204). Utilization of the Clinical Standards is the model from which the RN is able to exercise clinical judgment. The following sections describe components of the Clinical Standards and examples of how they are used in episodic ambulatory care practice.

In ambulatory practice settings, some aspects of the nursing process may be implicit. Nursing process steps may be encompassed in standardized forms and processes and expert knowledge of the planned care or procedure. It is important to note that even well-designed processes do not consider unique individual needs and challenges. Part of the value that an RN brings to ambulatory care practice is the ability to exercise clinical reasoning and judgment, anticipating both potential and actual problems and implementing plans designed to prevent harm and improve quality and individuals' experience.

Assessment

Assessment of the individual's health status is a crucial first step for the ambulatory care nurse. It is through this exchange that the nurse can garner key insights into physical, psychological, or social issues that impact the individual's current and continuing care. This early step in the individual's care encounter is critical for the development of a therapeutic relationship, allaying anxiety, and setting the tone for a positive individual experience.

It is important that the RN systematically collect data, both through physical exam and interview to prepare the individual for the upcoming encounter. In ambulatory care environments, assessment may also include reviewing pertinent health history in the electronic health record or as supplied by the individual, family members, and caregivers with specific additional information for the episodic care setting.

In episodic care, this assessment should include questions designed to determine the following:

- preparedness for the current care episode
- completion of preparatory instructions
- medication reconciliation, including medications recently taken
- current status of chronic conditions that could impact treatment, including urgent or emergent symptoms
- understanding of treatment plan and anticipated outcome of care
- continuing care concerns

In ambulatory care environments, assessment may occur face to face and/or through a combination of telecommunication strategies (eg, telephone, video, web-based tools, remote monitoring, electronic communication, survey completion). Face-to-face assessment allows the nurse to incorporate verbal and nonverbal communication, as well as other sensory information into the assessment. Assessment utilizing telecommunications requires a keen focus on verbal and emotional cues, empathic communication, and active listening (Smith, 2013). Information collected is validated with the individual/family, and significant findings are identified.

Assessment quality can be impacted by anxiety, time pressures, and the experience of the RN; it is also important to recognize that unconscious biases, stereotypes, and prejudices may influence the quality of the assessment process (Levett-Jones et al., 2010). Given the nature of the ambulatory care environment, several disciplines may be involved in the initial assessment, including licensed and nonlicensed staff. It is critical that the design of the assessment process consider the elements necessary for safe, high-quality care, the scope of practice of individuals participating in assessment, and that the output is synthesized and supports needs of the interdisciplinary team, and that pertinent findings are shared.

Nursing Diagnosis

Diagnosing occurs as the nurse reviews and analyzes relevant data to make a clinical judgment about the health and well-being of the individual and risks and benefits of the ambulatory encounter. AAACN (2017) describes nursing diagnosis as a "professional RN statement that represents the RN's clinical judgment about the patient's response to actual or potential health conditions or needs" (p. 17).

Alfaro-LeFevre (2009) highlights four areas of diagnostic responsibility for nurses:

1. **Recognizing signs and symptoms.** In this responsibility, ambulatory care nurses consider the individual-specific, expected, and unexpected symptoms that may impact planned treatment. For instance, if the individual is presenting for planned **ambulatory surgery**, but is currently having an exacerbation of chronic obstructive pulmonary disease (COPD), additional evaluation will be necessary to determine whether the surgery can occur.
2. **Predicting problems for those at risk.** In this responsibility, ambulatory care nurses identify potential risks or complications with an eye toward prevention. An example of how this occurs in episodic ambulatory environments is an elderly individual with limited mobility presenting for symptoms of urinary tract infection (UTI) in an urgent care setting. This individual may be at risk for falls. If risk is assessed, additional interventions are designed to prevent a fall.
3. **Identifying human responses to illness or symptoms.** An individual-centered approach considers how the current condition is impacting the individual's life, or, potentially, how the individual's life is impacting the current condition. An astute ambulatory care nurse will recognize that a 30-year-old woman presenting to urgent care with UTI symptoms but exhibiting signs of fear, other unexplained injuries, weeping, or other unexpected illness responses warrants additional assessment and planning.
4. **Initiating actions and referrals.** In this responsibility, the ambulatory care nurse may initiate urgent or emergent care if assessments indicate that level of care. Less urgent needs may also require referrals or postepisodic care services, such as referral to a pharmacist to help the individual identify ways to obtain prescribed medications at a lower cost.

In the ambulatory care environment, it is important that actual and potential problems are identified and strategies to prevent and mitigate risk and address issues are shared with the interdisciplinary team and individual/family to provide optimal care.

Outcome Identification

The next step in the process of implementing professional clinical standards is identification of expected outcomes/goals and care planning. AAACN (2017) describes this step as one in which the RN "identifies and specifies the expected outcomes of an individual plan of therapies and/or treatment(s) using input from the client/family, other health professionals, and current scientific evidence" (p. 17).

Identification of expected outcomes/goals provides a vehicle for communication among individual/family, nurse, and interdisciplinary team to discuss the expected course and planned benefits of the episode of care, individualized to the individual or situation. In the episodic ambulatory care environment, particular procedures or services may have predetermined expected outcomes. For instance, it would be expected that an individual presenting for diagnostic radiology would not have significant complications and be able to return to their pre-exam state soon after completion of the procedure.

Expected outcomes/goals help direct nursing interventions and become a measure of success or quality by evaluating instances in which outcomes were not met. Including the individual/family in discussions regarding expected outcomes helps to allay anxiety, identify learning needs, and pinpoint continuing care challenges. Although challenging in fast-paced ambulatory care environments, it is important to identify and plan for transitional or continuing care needs.

Planning

In the planning phase, the RN "outlines a set of written statements that identify specific needed services and interventions with measurable and achievable short and long-term goals that meet expected outcomes" (AAACN, 2017, p. 17). To perform this step competently, the nurse applies information and knowledge obtained from a variety of sources, such as the following:

- assessment information gleaned from individual/family, past and current medical history
- knowledge about the planned procedure, treatment, or care needed
- input from the interdisciplinary team
- regulatory standards such as The Joint Commission (TJC) and state requirements
- institutional standards and guidelines
- specialty practice standards

In many instances, computer-supported standard plans or care algorithms provide the basis for the initial plan of care (Alfaro-LeFevre, 2009). Individuals, families, and caregivers play a critical role in the continuing care of the individual, and their input must be incorporated into the plan. For example, some individuals have extreme anxiety or claustrophobia during enclosed space-imaging procedures. The plan of care should consider nursing and medical interventions designed to reduce anxiety, such as music, aromatherapy, distraction, and premedication. The RN plays a pivotal role in the integration of medical needs, standards, and expected outcomes with the wishes of individuals and families. In the fast-paced, high-acuity ambulatory care environment, transitions of care require careful planning. Ideally, special needs are identified during the initial assessment.

Implementation

Implementation of planned interventions is the most visible part of the nursing process. AAACN (2017) describes implementation in the ambulatory care environment as one in which the RN "provides nursing care services to meet the client's needs and goals and documents all activities" (p. 17).

Thorough implementation of care that the RN truly practices is at the intersection of art and science. One way to think about expert ambulatory care practice is through the lens of Bloom's domains of learning. Bloom describes the learning process across three domains—cognitive, psychomotor, and affective. These domains also describe aspects of ambulatory care nursing practice. First, in the cognitive domain the nurse must have a strong knowledge base regarding human responses to illness and injury, the procedure/treatment planned, and outcomes expected. Cognitive knowledge in a specialty is integral to the nursing process. Second, in the psychomotor domain, the nurse must provide competent care, integrating and synthesizing assessment and planning, and exercising skilled technical care and judgment. Lastly, nurses must demonstrate caring, compassion, and creativity in the affective domain. This is where skills such as individual engagement, empathic communication, and motivational interviewing provide key opportunities to inform, teach, and support individuals and families as they engage in care processes. The experienced nurse simultaneously integrates all domains. The example in Box 11.1 illustrates how the experienced RN seamlessly integrates all domains.

Nursing interventions are key actions performed by the nurse to assess and monitor health status; reduce risk; resolve, prevent, or manage problems; facilitate independence and the return home or to their current residence; and support a positive individual experience (Alfaro-LeFevre, 2009). Assessing and monitoring health status includes pre-, during-, and posttreatment and may involve call-back later to check health status. A frequent nursing intervention is to provide education and self-management support. Active involvement of individuals and family members can be encouraged through demonstration/return demonstration, teach back, and decision-support tools. As with any other care transition, the return to home should be well planned with clear after-visit care instructions, expected course of recovery, concerning complications to report, and how and when to seek help.

A key differentiator between ambulatory and inpatient environments is the strong interdisciplinary nature of ambulatory practice. RNs work closely with team members to deliver needed care. RNs perform independent and collaborative interventions that often include delegation and referral of care activities to licensed and unlicensed team members. In order to do this effectively, the RN must be familiar with the scope and responsibilities of all team members.

RNs must be skilled communicators, synthesizers, and coordinators of care to ensure the individual has a high-quality, safe, efficient experience and that they are well prepared to return home.

Evaluation

Evaluation of care is a key step in maintaining and improving care quality. As discussed by Alfaro-LeFevre (2009), critical evaluation "can make the difference between care practices that are doomed to repeat errors and care practices that are safe, efficient, and constantly getting better" (p. 228). AAACN (2017) describes evaluation as the "Professional RN's continual appraisal of the client's status and the effectiveness of the care received, revising the care plan and interventions as appropriate" (p. 17). To be effective, evaluation should occur on multiple levels, considering outcomes of individual patients, populations, and the healthcare delivery system.

Evaluation of the outcomes of individual patients often centers on the achievement of expected outcomes. An example might include determining whether safety interventions were effective in preventing a fall for a high-fall risk individual receiving care in an infusion center. Evaluation of care at the population level may involve looking at outcomes achieved from a large

BOX 11.1 Application of Bloom's Domains

Shawna is an RN who is providing intravenous antibiotic care in an individual's home subsequent to a hospitalization. When she arrives at the person's home, she finds the individual to be very anxious and is hesitant about continuing. The nurse assesses the individual, with special regard to her concerns. She finds the person does not understand the reason for these treatments and why she continues to have so much fatigue.

Shawna listens intently, providing empathy and support (**affective domain**). She then provides information about the purpose of the medication, potential side effects, and the length of treatment and reinforces the hospital discharge instructions (**cognitive domain**).

When the individual agrees to the medication, Shawna skillfully administers the medication (**psychomotor domain**). Before leaving, she again assesses the individual for any continuing needs or concerns.

BOX 11.2 Population-Level Care Evaluation

The outpatient breast surgery center currently has a standard pain control regimen prescribed at discharge for every individual undergoing routine lumpectomy. This regimen includes both opioid and nonopioid medications, giving individuals the maximum choice in how to achieve the desired pain control. At discharge, the nurse discusses pain control regimens and how to alternate and taper opioid and nonopioid medications with individuals.

In light of national concerns about overprescription of opioid medications, surgery center staff questioned the current pain control regimen and decided to conduct a postdischarge pain control assessment. A survey was developed, and nurses called individuals within 2 weeks of discharge with specific questions about which prescriptions were filled, the pattern of use, and satisfaction with pain control. Information from 25 individuals was compiled, reviewed by the team, and, as a result, the number of opioid pills dispensed at discharge was reduced from 25 to 5.

group of individuals with similar diagnoses or needs. For instance, pain control is an important outcome for individuals having outpatient surgery. These concepts are summarized in Box 11.2.

Evaluation at the health system level seeks to improve quality, safety, and service, while reducing overall cost. This is often described as improvement in value, and many organizations have identified key indicators of overall value. These data are continually collected and may be available to staff and leaders in a quality dashboard. Components of a dashboard are variable, but may include individual satisfaction data, adverse events, service volume and cost, and institutionally defined quality measures.

As an ambulatory care nurse, you should note the importance of reflecting and thinking analytically about the care provided as a nurse or as part of a team. What are the problems or challenges that occur? Are there knowledge deficits that you identify in yourself or the team? Are there ideas you have for improvement in processes or flow? Have you recently read a research study that successfully used a different approach? Are there safety issues you have observed? A healthy team environment welcomes ideas for improvement. RNs have the knowledge, skills, and abilities to make significant quality improvements in ambulatory care settings.

Professional Nursing Practice in Episodic Care Settings

Professional nursing practice describes behaviors and activities expected of nurses practicing in all settings. In addition to clinical standards, AAACN has identified Standards of Practice for Professional Ambulatory Care Nursing (AAACN, 2017), as noted in Box 11.3.

BOX 11.3 Standards of Nursing Organization and Professional Performance

- Ethics
- Education
- Research and Evidence-Based Practice
- Performance Improvement
- Communication
- Leadership
- Professional Practice Evaluation
- Resource Utilization
- Environment

Note. American Academy of Ambulatory Care Nursing. (2017). In C. Murray (Ed.), *Scope and standards of practice for professional ambulatory care nursing* (9th ed., p. 17). Author. Used with permission of American Academy of Ambulatory Care Nursing (AAACN), aaacn.org

These standards identify many areas in which RNs can contribute strongly to ambulatory practice settings.

Professional nursing practice in ambulatory care settings is still young. As a result, the nursing role is less well defined and continually evolving. Nurses may practice in settings in which there are few or no other RNs. This section will describe examples of challenges and opportunities to implement professional performance standards and illuminate the unique strengths that the professional nurse brings to the ambulatory care setting.

Professional Image and Strength

The nursing profession has devoted considerable effort to advancing the professional image of nurses over many years. Although continued effort is needed, improvements have been made, particularly in inpatient settings in which the nursing role is well defined. This work has not been undertaken to the same degree in ambulatory care settings and needs to occur. The work environment and work values have a strong impact on professional image and identity (Hoeve et al., 2013). Thus, as nurses assume these roles, it is important for them to help define the professional role, highlight nursing strengths, and implement professional nursing standards.

One of the strengths of the nursing profession is the therapeutic relationships nurses establish with individuals and families. This is critically important in episodic ambulatory care environments in which encounters with team members tend to be short and targeted at specific interventions. Nurses provide the thread of continuity and address the needs of the individual both before and after the ambulatory encounter. They help individuals understand what they will experience during the encounter, anticipate challenges, and prepare to go home. They provide expert care, proactively identify safety risks, and plan for discharge. This work is important—nurses and nurse leaders need to acknowledge, articulate, and demonstrate the worth of this unique contribution. The nurse–individual relationship is a professional strength.

Another component of professional nursing practice is a commitment to continuous learning, skill development, and implementation of evidence-based practice. This is especially true in ambulatory care settings. Care is continually evolving, individual acuity is increasing, and new technologies and medications are frequently introduced. Procedures previously performed in hospitals with multiday stays are now performed in ambulatory centers. A commitment to lifelong learning is important in order to be able to maintain currency in this environment.

Professional comportment is not often discussed as part of professional performance; however, it does influence power and perception. How nurses perceive themselves, refer to themselves, and use language impacts their professional image. Expressions of self-confidence, optimism, and compassion elicit enhanced respect from both colleagues and individuals. The image a nurse projects impacts their ability to positively influence unit decisions.

Much of the work of ambulatory care practice is based in an interdisciplinary team. The role of the nurse is enhanced when they value collaboration and partnership with all team members. The nurse must understand the unique value that nursing contributes to team goals and be prepared to articulate that proposition with data. This includes participating in groups and teams that are making decisions that affect practice and resource allocation.

Another area of professional strength for RNs in ambulatory care practice is their ability to create and manage a safe environment of care for individuals and staff. Regulatory and specialty specific standards such as those promoted by state health departments, TJC, and the Occupational Safety and Health Administration (OSHA) are often familiar terrain for nurses. Environment of care standards are numerous and diverse, with examples including infection control, equipment disinfection, medication management and storage, inventory control, and point-of-care testing requirements. Nurses' expertise in this area is critical to ambulatory practices, and this expertise can be a significant source of nursing power and influence.

Nursing Leadership

All nurses working in ambulatory settings have both the opportunity and the responsibility to exercise positive leadership. Nurses exercise this opportunity by demonstrating the following:

- a receptive attitude and open mind to the opinions of all team members
- a focus on continuous improvement, system safety, and efficiency
- a commitment to creative solutions and positive outcomes
- a willingness to train and mentor new staff and students
- participation and leadership of teams, committees, and groups related to the work unit, nursing, the institution, and community
- advocacy for individuals and the profession through institutional, community, and public policy venues
- active participation in professional organizations and other groups defining, advancing, and advocating for the professional nursing role in ambulatory practice

Considerations in Select Episodic Care Settings

Episodic care is the most frequent type of care provided in ambulatory practice. In this section, several types of episodic care will be highlighted: ambulatory surgery, **infusion centers**, **diagnostic and therapeutic centers**, urgent care, and evolving **home-based services**. Each of these settings has unique characteristics and standards, setting-specific assessment and care considerations, collaboration and support services, population considerations, individual care risks, and legal and regulatory considerations.

These specialty care settings generally have a high volume of individual encounters in short periods of time (Laughlin & Witwer, 2019). This section will demonstrate how nurses working in these environments implement the Standards of Clinical Practice as well as applicable specialty standards, work collaboratively with other healthcare professionals to address acute illnesses, chronic diseases, health promotion, and provide education.

Overview and Characteristics: Ambulatory Surgery

According to the National Health Statistics Report, an increasing number of procedures are being performed in ambulatory settings, particularly as medical innovation has, and will continue, to advance and allow for procedures to be performed safely in the outpatient setting (Hall et al., 2017). It is estimated that outpatient procedures represent more than 80% of all surgeries as derived from the 2013 American Hospital Association reported data (Munnich & Parente, 2018). Ambulatory surgery settings include freestanding ambulatory surgery centers (ASCs) or procedural settings aligned with a hospital outpatient department.

Individuals in these settings may move from admission to discharge quickly or require additional levels of care considerations. "The perioperative nurse is a nurse who specializes in perioperative practice and who provides nursing care to the surgical client throughout the continuum of care" (Goodman & Spry, 2014, p. 2). Nurses play a critical role in the individual's surgical or procedural experience and must be proficient in perioperative care, which includes three phases: preoperative, intraoperative, and postoperative care.

Standards: Ambulatory Surgery

Standards for nursing distinguish what a reasonable and prudent nurse would do in similar circumstances and determine a model for measuring quality. Aside from accreditation and other regulatory standards that have been discussed, the American Society of Perianesthesia Nurses (ASPAN) and the Association of Perioperative Registered Nurses (AORN) are leaders in perioperative practice standards. These standards address provision of nursing care, safety, ethics, and the professional nursing role.

The perianesthesia standards from the ASPAN (2017–18) address evidence-based practice, regulatory requirements, technology, and nursing practice. The standards from both ASPAN and AORN specifically address ethics, maintenance of a safe environment, quality improvement, research, coordination of care, a plan of care for optimal individual outcomes, assessment, health teaching and promotion, and collaboration with members of the healthcare team (ASPAN, 2017–18).

Workplace safety is addressed through various organizations. The Occupational Safety and Health Administration (OSHA) publishes and enforces workplace safety applicable to ASCs (www.osha.gov). Also, the National Institute for Occupational Safety and Health focuses on worker safety and health, including standards on biologic hazards (www.cdc.gov/niosh). TJC standards focus on the promotion of safety (www.jointcommission.org). TJC's focus on safety includes equipment and building safety, disaster preparedness plans, fire safety specifically addressing a response plan, and employee competence through fire drills (Goodman & Spry, 2014). Additional fire safety measures are considered with the performance of a fire risk assessment to provide guidance to personnel in preventing fires during procedures and responding appropriately if a fire should occur.

Assessment and Care: Ambulatory Surgery

Individuals preparing for a procedure or surgery generally undergo a risk assessment, often called a preanesthetic medical evaluation, to determine whether they are medically acceptable for the planned procedure. This may be completed days to weeks before the scheduled procedure or on the day of the procedure. As more procedures are performed in ambulatory settings and the number of complex individuals increases, the preprocedure assessment is key to gauging risk and directing care. The American Society of Anesthesiologists (ASA) guidelines require anyone needing an anesthetic to be given a history and physical evaluation including previous anesthesia, appropriate diagnostic testing, an ASA-physical status score, and a discussion with the individual or responsible party before obtaining informed consent (ASA, 2013).

The nursing assessment of the ambulatory surgical individual includes gathering and reviewing additional information as part of the perioperative team. Verification of the individual, the planned procedure, last oral intake, and informed consent are performed by the preoperative nurse upon individual admission to the area. Subjective data assessment includes review of the individual's health history including allergies, previous surgical experience, a review of systems, verification of the individual's current medications, family and social history if appropriate, and the individual and family/caregiver learning needs assessment. Any current or history of drug, tobacco, or alcohol use should also be discussed. Objective data collected should include the individual's physical status, vital sign measurements, systems assessment, and review of any applicable diagnostic testing results.

Roles of the nurse in the procedural/operating room vary in ambulatory settings. The circulating nurse is often the first face the individual sees on entry into the procedural room and the nurse greets the individual to help them feel as comfortable as possible and address anxieties. First and foremost among the many activities performed by the perioperative nurse is serving as the client advocate (Goodman & Spry, 2014). The scrub nurse or assistant has specific roles related to the planned procedure and also interacts with the individuals to ease distress. Table 11.1 discusses these roles.

Postoperative nursing care involves continued assessment of the individual and providing emotional support to the individual and/or family/caregivers present. Vital sign monitoring; system assessment compared with baseline; appearance of the procedural/surgical site; and

TABLE 11.1 NURSING ROLES IN SAME-DAY SURGERY

Circulating nurse	• Coordinates care of the individual • Serves as the individual advocate • Assists in activities outside of the sterile field • Works with the scrub nurse or scrub assistant to prepare instruments, equipment, and other supplies • Verifies instrument count before, during, and after the procedure with the team • May initiate surgical checklists and procedural pause/"time out" • Performs ongoing patient assessment and documents relevant data • Collaborates with the anesthesia and surgical team to ensure patient safety and comfort
Scrub nurse	• Prepares instruments, equipment, and other supplies • Verifies instrument counts before, during, and after the procedure • Participates in the procedural pause • Hands the procedural team instruments and supplies and maintains a clean and organized instrument tray/sterile field • Relays needs to the circulating nurse throughout the procedure

level of pain, sedation, and nausea should occur throughout the postoperative period. The nurse tailors therapy and comfort measures based on their assessment.

If an individual has had an anesthetic, a postanesthetic recovery screening tool, for example, the Modified Aldrete, is used. Items assessed are activity, respiration, circulation, consciousness, oxygenation, pain, ambulation, feeding, urinary status, and status of any dressing(s)/drainage. This scoring helps the nurse determine the individual's readiness for discharge to home or the need for a continued acute phase of care in a higher care setting, such as an intensive care unit. Transfers and dismissals are coordinated by the postoperative care team.

On the basis of the preoperative learning needs assessment and the nurse's determination of whether the individual is ready, discharge instructions and teaching are done, ensuring the individual and family or caregivers understand and have the resources needed on dismissal.

Collaboration and Support Services: Ambulatory Surgery

The periprocedural/perioperative team involves many roles and varies according to location and the needs of the procedure and individual. If the individual will be given an anesthetic, an anesthesiologist and/or a certified registered nurse anesthetist will be involved in the individual's care. Premedication for pain and nausea should be discussed with the anesthetic and surgical teams. Technicians that collect blood samples for labs or other diagnostic data such as an electrocardiogram may interact with the individual as well.

Operating and procedural rooms are busy settings, involving many personnel, including the surgical/procedural team, which may include consultants, fellows, residents, and nurses. Surgical technicians may be the assisting personnel, and anesthesia technicians ensure equipment is sterilized and safe. Desk and scheduling staff are also integral to the individual's surgical/procedural experience. Certain populations may need additional support staff, and, in particular, collaboration with child life specialists, where available, enhances the pediatric individual experience.

The perioperative nurse coordinates the individual's care throughout the perioperative period. The plan of care requires collaboration with others and coordination of services needed.

The importance of the nurse's assessment cannot be overstated, but is not completed in a vacuum, forming instead a piece of the individual's encounter ensuring safe and quality care.

Population Considerations: Ambulatory Surgery

Considerations of specific populations' needs are vital for safe and quality care in ambulatory surgery. Although there are many individual populations for which special considerations may be needed, in this section pediatrics, geriatrics, and individuals with health issues will be discussed.

Pediatric Individual

The perioperative experience can be especially stressful for children and their families/caregivers. Consideration of the individual's age and developmental stage will assist in guiding care. It is essential that pediatric individuals are not treated as little adults. Fear and emotional distress must be expected and continually assessed and appropriate comfort measures provided. The perioperative nurse gauges the needs of the parents/caregivers and considers their presence during each phase.

Nurses caring for children in the perioperative setting need to be knowledgeable in the varying vital sign parameters, developmental stages, and age-appropriate methods of assessment. For example, some children may be able to use faces on a pain scale to rate their pain as opposed to a Numeric Pain Intensity Scale (see Figure 11.1). Role playing, distraction and other comfort measures, and medications should all be considered to enhance the individual care experience.

Individuals 65 and Older

Physical changes in individuals 65 and older require special considerations that may put them at a higher risk for adverse outcomes. Alterations in the older population may include a decline in mobility or functional limitations, cognitive changes, cardiovascular alterations, respiratory changes, gastrointestinal alterations, genitourinary alterations including decreased kidney function, sensory changes, fragile or thin skin, presence of chronic disease(s), and considerations of other age-related disabilities.

Because of these alterations, age-appropriate assessment including knowledge of vital sign changes in older adults should be considered by the perioperative nurse. Individuals in later stages of life may need to consider the advantages and challenges related to their health status and the need for a procedure/surgery. Assessment and related care of the individual's nutritional status, fall risk, communication needs, support system, and learning needs contribute to the older individual's safe care.

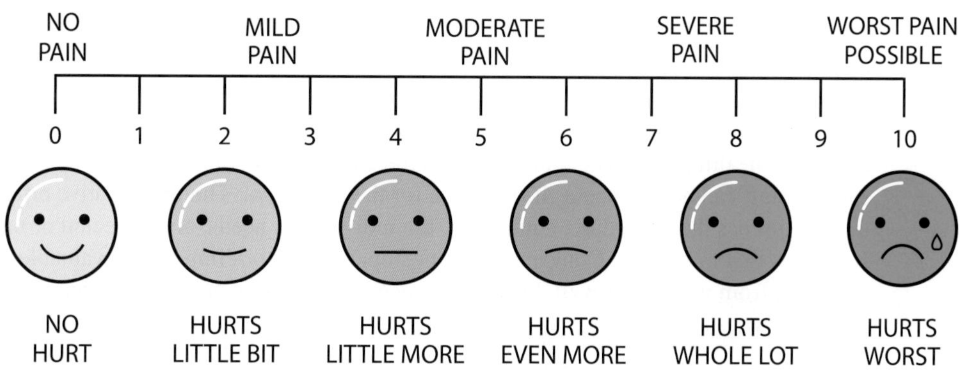

FIGURE 11.1 Horizontal pain measurement scale or pain assessment tool, vector.

Individuals With Health Issues

Chronic disease represents a unique challenge depending on the disease state and health of the individual at the time of the procedure. Specifically, obesity, cardiovascular disease, and diabetes mellitus present challenges to prepare for and include in the plan of care.

Obesity rates continue to increase, and "its associated comorbidities can have significant implications in perioperative ambulatory surgical care" (Prabhakar et al., 2017, p. 48). Obesity is defined as a body mass index of 30 kg/m² and greater. Respiratory and cardiovascular complications, in particular, may have an increased potential of occurrence (Prabhakar et al., 2017). An important screening preoperatively for this population is for obstructive sleep apnea (OSA) because it is more prevalent in the obese individual.

"OSA is a syndrome characterized by periodic, partial, or complete obstruction in the upper airway during sleep" (ASA, 2014, p. 268). Validated questionnaires provide a brief but validated way to screen individuals, because many may be undiagnosed. Individuals with OSA may require different methods of anesthetic delivery, should have pain management focused on nonopioid modalities when possible, and should have close monitoring during their postanesthetic encounter.

Cardiovascular diseases, respiratory conditions, and diabetes mellitus require preparation for complications that may occur as a result of the disease state or management-related issues.

Additionally, the individual's level of self-care and knowledge of their health can contribute to risks in ambulatory surgery. Hypertension, hyperlipidemia, presence of pacemakers or defibrillators, and history of myocardial injury require extra steps of preoperative assessment and monitoring perioperatively. Ventricular assist devices are found more commonly than in the past, but considerations for surgeries/procedures for this population should be closely examined for the level of care that can be provided in an ambulatory surgery setting.

Respiratory conditions, including asthma and COPD, may require additional preoperative assessments and therapy, as well as altered management during the perioperative period. Diabetes management in ambulatory settings may follow specific protocols, including time frames for monitoring of blood sugars, preoperative management of the individual's diabetes-related medications, including oral or insulin agents, and alterations in the medication regimen during the perioperative period.

Complications in Ambulatory Surgery

Additional complications related or unrelated to the individual's health status can occur in the ambulatory surgical setting. These complications include but are not limited to

- thermoregulation issues such as hypothermia, hyperthermia, and malignant hyperthermia
- oversedation
- cardiovascular complications, including dysrhythmias (sinus bradycardia, atrial fibrillation and flutter, supraventricular tachycardia), hypotension, and hypertension
- respiratory complications like airway obstruction, hypoxia, laryngospasm, and bronchospasm

Preparation of personnel and equipment that may be needed is critical in responding to the preceding list of complications, particularly for those individuals with the added complexity of additional health issues. The more prepared the environment, nurse, periprocedural team, and support staff can be, the better the outcome for the individual. The preoperative briefing is the time to discuss the procedure, equipment, the individual's needs, and expected or unexpected situations that may arise. Conversely, the postoperative debriefing is also valuable to discuss and learn from what went well during the procedure and what could have been improved.

Individual Safety: Ambulatory Surgery

"In healthcare, a culture of safety can be defined as sharing and implementing knowledge and beliefs which promote safe practice settings and safe care" (ASPAN, 2017–18, p. 14). It is the responsibility of all individuals within the bounds of the individual's periprocedural care to have a questioning and receptive attitude, which includes speaking up and listening when a member of the team or individual has a question or concern.

Closed loop communication is used in many settings to enhance individual safety and to ensure the message being relayed is being received as intended. Effective communication using safety tools for an individual, such as situation, background, assessment, recommendation (SBAR) or concerned, uncomfortable, and a method of raising concerns that require attention, in a safe and appropriate format. More information on both types of communication can be found at the Institute for Healthcare Improvement (IHI.org).

Overview and Characteristics: Infusion Centers

Infusion therapy, once used for the most critically ill, continues to grow and evolve as advances in techniques, technologies, and complex care plans progress. "Infusion therapy is a highly specialized form of treatment" delivered in hospitals and alternative care settings, including infusion centers (Alexander et al., 2010, p. 1). Infusion center settings include physician offices, hospital clinics, emergency departments, or freestanding infusion centers. "These centers allow for coordination of resources and efficient delivery of services" (Gorski et al., 2010, p. 116).

Individuals in infusion centers may receive one or more infusions including, but not limited to, parenteral nutrition, chemotherapy, antimicrobial therapy, pain relief therapies, fluids, and blood and blood components. These solutions, medications, nutritional products, and blood products are delivered via vascular access devices (VADs) inserted in veins, arteries, and bone marrow. Such devices may be temporary or provide longer term access for planned, repeated use. They may include an implanted port inserted subcutaneously into the vascular system or peripheral or central venous catheters (CVCs) inserted through the arm, neck, or chest into a large vein.

Standards: Infusion Centers

Infusion Nursing Standards of Practice define evidence-based practice, scope of practice, and educational requirements and provide criteria for safe infusion delivery. The Infusion Nurses Society (INS) standards are written for clinicians of multiple disciplines and are applicable to any patient care setting (Gorski et al., 2016). The standards address all aspects of infusion nursing specific to the specialty, with emphasis on individual and clinician safety, infection prevention and control, equipment, VAD selection and placement, VAD management, VAD complications, other infusion devices, and infusion therapies.

INS maintains a certification program for the formal recognition of infusion nurse specialists. Professional role certification designates the additional knowledge, education, and commitment for the specialty. Other professional organizations that provide input to infusion nursing include the National Home Infusion Associations, Association for Professionals in Infection Control and Epidemiology, and the American Society of Health-Systems Pharmacists.

Assessment and Care: Infusion Centers

Knowledge of anatomy and organ systems is essential for the safe administration of infusions. Vascular anatomy is of primary importance when locating and cannulating vessels (Alexander et al., 2010). Assessment of VAD site placement and ongoing management of the access site are skills essential for an individual's safety, proper infusion administration, and prevention of complications. Fluid and electrolyte balance require ongoing attention throughout the individual's care episode as well, because this is critical to care. Review of the individual's history and laboratory data when applicable will give an indication of the individual's risk for fluid or electrolyte imbalance. In addition, measurement of height, weight, vital signs, and pain assessment provides essential information into the individual's status during their infusion care.

Depending on the individual's history and current presentation, the nurse should be prepared to support the individual in their experience as the infusion encounter may be a single episode or repeated episodes. The infusion the individual receives will also require specific assessment, because the response, for example, to a chemotherapy medication can be very different from that to an antiviral medication. Intravenous administration guidelines describe specific assessments and/or an individual's responses to be alert in response to the infusion. Pre- and postinfusion assessment is based on the therapy administered.

Safety considerations and infection prevention interventions are standard and essential in infusion therapy. The risk of complications will be discussed later in this section, but the risk of an individual's adverse events varies depending on the type of vascular access (eg, peripheral intravenous catheter vs. CVC) and other individual-specific factors.

Collaboration and Support Services: Infusion Centers

Infusion centers have medical personnel on site to administer treatment plans and care for the individual during their therapy. Nurses, physicians, pharmacists, social workers, dietitians, administrative staff, and unlicensed healthcare personnel collaborate to efficiently and effectively provide client care (Alexander et al., 2010). Unlicensed healthcare personnel may include medical assistants, clinical assistants, or others who are not licensed but carry out delegated tasks within the nurse's supervision and according to standards. In many settings, nurses may work closely with laboratory technicians who are trained and certified.

The nature of the equipment needs and changes in infusion therapy also require support service coordinators to maintain adequate supplies, pumps and equipment, intravenous supplies, and other patient care supplies, including safety equipment such as gloves and masks.

Population Considerations: Infusion Centers

Consideration for special populations such as pediatrics, pregnant women, and older adults should take into account and is not limited to anatomic and physiologic differences, safety needs, and infusion administration. The following are some examples of these considerations:

- Pediatric patients need special consideration for their emotional needs, developmental stage, and the interactions of the family/caregivers, in addition to the physical differences. In particular, thermoregulation and warming should be considered.
- Securement of the access device also requires special attention with the pediatric or developmentally delayed individual.
- Pregnant patient considerations include additional assessment needs. Specific considerations of the infusion and safety are of utmost importance, as is collaboration with providers and pharmacists.
- Successful infusions in the older adult also require considerations for chronic conditions; physical changes, including veins that can be more difficult to access, thin or thickened skin; and drug considerations related to hepatic and renal changes (Coulter, 2016).

Complications and Emergencies: Infusion Centers

Complications that occur during infusion therapy encounters relate to the access device, solution being administered, and other factors. Common complications with peripheral intravenous access include phlebitis, infiltration, extravasation, and infection and are summarized as follows:

- Phlebitis is an inflammation of the wall of a vein, causing pain, erythema, swelling, and, possibly, thrombosis of the vein (Dychter et al., 2012).

- "Infiltration is defined as the inadvertent leakage of nonvesicant solution into surrounding tissue, and extravasation is the inadvertent leakage of a vesicant solution into surrounding tissue" (Dychter et al., 2012, p. 87).
- Infection can range from a minor, localized infection to a bloodstream infection resulting in septicemia.

The risk of infection is higher in individuals with VADs, because the integrity of the skin is disrupted and the risk of bacterial or fungal infection is increased (Alexander et al., 2010).

Central-line-associated bloodstream infections (CLABSIs) occur commonly in individuals with CVCs, are costly, and can be deadly (Centers for Disease Control and Prevention, 2011). CLABSI-related systemic inflammatory response syndrome, sepsis, or resulting septic shock are life threatening. The risk of any of these complications increases for individuals with susceptible immune systems.

Clinical signs of sepsis include fever, hypotension, hypothermia, apnea, bradycardia, and blood culture data (Alexander et al., 2010). There are national and local strategies to address CLABSI, which is the focus of hospital-acquired infection prevention efforts, including care bundles that group best practices when performed together, resulting in better outcomes. Infusion therapy center nurses are trained in basic life support and are knowledgeable in emergent care strategies that are performed while awaiting individual transfer to a higher level of care as indicated.

Individual Safety: Infusion Centers

Interventions for the individual, as well as clinician safety, should be at the forefront in infusion center environments. Medication-related safety applies to identification and administration, as well as storage and handling, particularly for hazardous medications. New comprehensive guidelines for hazardous drug handling in healthcare settings, called USP-800, are being updated to provide standards to minimize the risk of exposure to healthcare personnel, individuals, and the environment.

Standardizing staff education and products and evidence-based care delivery ensure that staff are familiar with equipment and that best practices are being followed. Nurse education should include individual monitoring requirements based on the specific infusion being administered. Needlesticks can be a risk to both individuals and clinicians, and prevention and tracking efforts are included in the standards from OSHA. Infection prevention efforts include aseptic technique for catheter insertion, care, and dressing changes, as well as hand hygiene.

Overview and Characteristics: Diagnostic and Therapeutic Centers

Diagnostic and therapeutic centers can include a wide range of services. They allow for outpatient procedures to determine/evaluate health conditions and, when appropriate, provide related treatment. Imaging and radiologic services, procedures for pain relief, gastrointestinal and cardiovascular procedures, and dermatology are just a few of the services provided. Imaging and diagnostic tools available at these centers provide valuable diagnosis of disease and altered health states.

Centers that perform gastroenterology services, such as colonoscopy or endoscopy, are prime examples of this type of episodic care. Colonoscopy procedures allow for screening and diagnosis by looking for abnormalities as well as taking biopsies and therapeutic care by removing polyps that are or have the potential to become cancerous growths.

Standards: Diagnostic and Therapeutic Centers

Standards guiding nursing practice in diagnostic and therapeutic centers are specific to the specialty practice. Like other standards, these set forth professional practice expectations, care, safety, and ethical expectations. In particular, the Association for Radiologic & Imaging

Nursing guides nurses in this specialty to provide safe quality individual care and offers specialty standards to address nursing care before, during, and after procedures. Nurses working in these environments can be highly specialized and develop specific skills within their scope and standards of practice.

Assessment and Care: Diagnostic and Therapeutic Centers

Nursing care and assessment of individuals in this type of episodic care will center on the individual's diagnosis, test, or need. In some cases, individuals may be given sedating medications for their diagnostic procedure, which requires additional monitoring to ensure individual safety. Sedation scales and capnography are used by trained nurses in moderate sedation in collaboration with anesthesia providers. Additionally, VADs are placed for some procedures in order to administer radiographic media or other medications. Nursing care includes managing the access device and the delivery of the medication, assessing the individual response, and watching for adverse events.

Collaboration and Support Services: Diagnostic and Therapeutic Centers

Radiologists, proceduralists, technicians, and support staff communicate and coordinate care for the individual during their diagnostic or therapeutic procedure. Individuals undergoing imaging services interact with x-ray technicians, have their images read by radiologists, and meet with a specialist to determine a plan of care. In centers that provide services for gastroenterologic needs, individuals may need sedation or anesthesia for their procedure, which includes care, as described earlier, by nursing, anesthesia, and the procedural team. An example of this would be a patient scheduled for a colonoscopy as illustrated in Box 11.4.

Complications and Emergencies: Diagnostic and Therapeutic Centers

Complications and emergencies can vary by the type of care the individual receives. Reactions to contrast material administered during imaging procedures are not uncommon. Reactions can range from rash and erythema to urticaria and angioedema. The emergency response depends on the individual presentation. Diagnostic and therapeutic centers that provide sedation require that staff have advanced cardiac life support training. As discussed in the infusion therapy section, many individuals with VADs are at risk for phlebitis, infiltration, and extravasation. Anaphylactic reactions may occur in diagnostic and procedural settings, which require a quick response by nursing and healthcare staff.

BOX 11.4 Collaboration in a Diagnostic Center

A 50-year-old woman reports for her first colonoscopy as recommended per national screening guidelines and after discussing it with her primary care provider. Her care team instructed her on her bowel preparation and discussed the procedure. She elected to have sedation for her procedure.

Upon check-in at her scheduled time, the desk attendant verifies she has had nothing by mouth today. The intake nurse then prepares her for her procedure, verifying that she fully completed her bowel preparation and discusses her health history, asking, in particular, about diabetes and blood-thinning medications. After completing the assessment, the nurse allows her to change into a gown and then starts a peripheral intravenous catheter infusion.

The nurse transports her to the procedure room, which has already been prepared by the procedural nurse, with equipment and medications in place, and the nurse anesthetist has prepared for her sedation. The proceduralist greets the individual and reviews the procedure, and then she is comfortably sedated while he performs the colonoscopy, assisted by the nurse. Biopsy samples are prepared and sent to the laboratory.

After the procedure, another nurse performs monitoring while the sedation wears off. When the individual is fully awake, the nurse reviews the postprocedure instructions and ensures she has a ride home. The procedural assistant takes the scope and equipment from the procedure to be disinfected and sterilized, following guidelines.

Individual Safety: Diagnostic and Therapeutic Centers

Individual and clinician safety include radiology safety in imaging areas. Dosimeter tracking is used for personnel, whereas shields and other protections are put in place for individuals. Safety also depends on the cleaning and sterilization of equipment, which is important in all care areas, but particular guidelines must be followed for scopes.

Overview and Characteristics: Urgent Care Centers

The Urgent Care Association of America (UCOA) defines an urgent care center "as a medical clinic with expanded hours that is specially equipped to diagnose and treat a broad spectrum of non-life or limb-threatening illnesses and injuries" (Stoimenoff & Newman, 2017).

Urgent care centers (UCC) have arisen out of the need for convenient care outside of "usual hours" in primary care clinics and the desire to avoid crowded emergency departments. These clinics encompass a range of customer-oriented innovations targeted toward swift, easily accessible, and more affordable care (Mehrotra, 2013).

Urgent care centers offer services such as imaging, which may not be found in other retail clinics, and the cost charged is often much less than emergency care according to the American Academy of Urgent Care Medicine. "Unscheduled care accounts for a substantial portion of outpatient visits" (Chang et al., 2018, p. 136) and contributes to the risk of fragmented care and reduced continuity and coordination of care. The increasing utilization of electronic health records to exchange individual health information helps to address these issues and assist in appropriate referrals.

Nurses in UCCs provide care for individuals in a wide range of ages and for a variety of acute symptoms, such as asthma, skin alterations/injuries, lacerations, and sprains, in addition to complications of chronic disease. A variety of interventions such as specimen collection, focused assessments, patient education, and other cares are routinely performed by nurses and others in UCC. Interprofessional practice, including delegation to unlicensed team members, is an important aspect of care in UCCs. It is also important for nursing staff to consider continuing care needs.

Standards: Urgent Care Centers

Scope and standards of practice for professional ambulatory care nursing promote the diverse care provided by ambulatory nursing, including nursing in UCCs (AAACN, 2017). The standards address the nursing process in ambulatory care as well as professional performance. Professional skills in evolving ambulatory settings require utilization of clinical skills, advanced reasoning, and working to a high scope of practice within teams.

These standards applied to clinical practice relate to individuals and populations, with population health becoming an ever-increasing focus of efforts and innovations in healthcare. Nurses in UCCs, like other ambulatory care settings, are responsible for identifying outcomes, planning needed services and interventions, implementing coordination of care, promoting health, and evaluating individual status. Additionally, professional practice standards set forth behaviors that can be applied to this setting, including performance improvement, leadership, and collaboration.

Assessment and Care: Urgent Care Centers

Nursing judgment and critical thinking based on thorough assessment alert the nurse in urgent care centers to individual status and identification of needs. Assessment of signs and symptoms may occur rapidly at times, as individuals move through this setting quickly, but are nonetheless as thorough as possible. Triage of individuals based on their presenting status and symptoms, not unlike in emergency room settings, may be a part of the nurse's role. Individuals with life-threatening presentations are stabilized and directed or transported to emergency services.

The nurse's skills in assessment are of utmost importance because the delegation of tasks to unlicensed personnel occurs frequently, in addition to the collaboration with providers based on the assessment findings. The common conditions treated in UCCs may allow the nurse to hone their skills of assessment, while becoming familiar with care, therapy, and medications indicated for the condition. Some of the most common conditions treated in UCCs include fevers, sprains, upper respiratory infections, lacerations, contusions, and back pain (Stoimenoff & Newman, 2017).

Collaboration and Support Services: Urgent Care Centers

Collaboration in UCCs can vary by the services provided but may include radiology, physical therapy, pharmacy, lab facilities, occupational health services, and health promotion services. The nurse must have skills for leading teams and communicating with departments and professionals providing care. As stated previously, delegation to unlicensed assistive personnel is an important aspect of care, and the nurse retains accountability for the duties and tasks carried out (Ashton, 2017).

"Nurses are increasingly called on to adapt to wider clinical teams" and foster working relationships in order to provide safe, quality patient care (Ashton, 2017, p. 52). Collaboration with providers facilitates a smooth flow for individuals through the UCC. Support staff in the clinic also contributes to efficiency, patient satisfaction, and a positive care experience.

Population Considerations: Urgent Care Centers

In a 2009 study, results indicated that populations at UCCs more closely mirrored those of primary care practices than emergency departments (Weinick et al., 2009). A subsequent national study, completed in 2016 by Le and Hsia, described geographic locations of the majority of UCCs as urban. Urban, suburban, and rural populations have varying needs and should be considered in these care locations.

Many centers are now designed specifically for pediatrics; however, an individual-friendly environment should be cultivated, whether it is pediatric only or not. In addition to assessment and care-related needs of pediatric individuals, adolescents seeking diagnosis, treatment, or care for concerns they wish to keep confidential such as sexually transmitted infections or contraceptive services may present to UCCs.

Complications and Emergencies: Urgent Care Centers

Owing to the services offered by urgent care centers and patient misunderstanding, individuals may present for urgent care but may actually be in need of emergent services. Life-threatening situations requiring emergency services include stroke, acute myocardial infarction, drug-related emergencies, and limb-threatening injuries. UCCs must be prepared to triage, stabilize, and provide supportive care and arrange transport to the nearest emergency facility.

Complications for individuals utilizing urgent care include the risk of fragmented care, which can result in poor outcomes or reduced quality of care. The need to plan for continuity of care should be considered for all consumers of healthcare in this setting.

Individual Safety: Urgent Care Centers

Regulations by groups, including OSHA and Clinical Laboratory Improvement Amendments, provide standards for the environment of care and establish quality for testing, treatment, and assessment of health. Additionally, infection prevention and competency training and education assist in developing safe practices for urgent care centers.

Episodic Home-Based Services

The need for a "health visitor" was first promoted by Florence Nightingale in 1893 at the International Congress of Charities, Correction, and Philanthropy (Buhler-Wilderson, 1985).

Public health nursing was the first to answer that call, arising in the early 1900s through the support and efforts of philanthropists who identified a need to bring health services to the home. These services, provided by nurses through visiting nurses' associations, were primarily provided to individuals who did not have the means to afford other treatment. The specialty of public health has expanded considerably and continues today with the provision of a wide variety of prevention programs and services.

Like public health services, home healthcare also provides in-home services. This service was originally developed to facilitate early hospital discharge, providing a bridge toward self-care (Welch et al., 1996). Care provided by certified home health agencies is reimbursable by the Centers for Medicare and Medicaid Services (CMS) and other third-party payers, in which qualification for services is regulated. Home health agencies continue to be a growing segment of the healthcare market, providing skilled nursing care; home health aides; physical, occupational, and speech therapy; and medical social services for individuals needing home-based services. These agencies must receive reimbursement or private payment in order to continue to offer services to individuals.

Population Strategies for Home-Based Services

Over time, additional home-based services have evolved. Hospitals, medical practices, and health systems are increasingly taking a population approach for service provision, seeking ways to improve quality and service and reduce cost. This is particularly true as organizations begin to move from traditional reimbursement models toward quality and cost control incentives. A variety of services have been introduced in response to adult and pediatric populations that are living longer with more severe chronic conditions. Although examples are numerous, this section will focus on home-based palliative and **transitional care services**.

Palliative and transitional care services target both frail adults and children with multiple comorbid conditions at vulnerable times in their lives. These individuals may have cognitive and/or functional limitations and may not qualify for reimbursable home health or hospice services. However, population-based services are often provided as an extension of the health system, rather than through external agencies.

Regardless of the source, services may also be provided through telehealth delivery modes, which may include telephone, web-based services, and/or remote monitoring. Many sources have the ability to perform home-based point-of-care laboratory testing or home lab draw services for more complex tests and select radiologic exams. These services are closely connected to primary care and specialty teams overseeing care in conjunction with RN care coordinators or other roles providing direct services.

Caring for individuals in their homes can be challenging. In the past, most health systems did not engage in the management of individuals beyond their institutional walls, leaving individuals to find their own solutions. However, as more systems move toward capitated payment, incentives to control cost, improve quality, and avoid unnecessary utilization justify implementation of expanded home-based services under a larger umbrella of acute and ambulatory care.

Palliative Home Care

Palliative home-based services have evolved to address gaps in care identified for adults and children with advanced medical illness. These gaps include lack of timely access for symptom management, inadequate preparation of individuals and caregivers, lack of comprehensive services without self-navigation and substantial effort, and inadequate caregiver support (Marshall et al., 2008). Individuals in home-based palliative care may need aggressive symptom management to prevent exacerbations that, if not controlled, may result in emergency department visits and hospitalization. If symptoms are not immediately addressed, and hospitalization is necessary, these services are high cost for the system and high risk for the individual.

Studies demonstrate that palliative home-based services improved quality of life scores, reduced total symptom burden, increased self-efficacy, and demonstrated a marked reduction in hospitalization (Brannstrom & Boman, 2014). RNs practicing in ambulatory care may provide home-based palliative care services as an extension of a hospital or medical practice or through an independent service. These nurses provide a valuable service utilizing all aspects of the nursing process and clinical reasoning skills to support individuals in their home settings.

Palliative care is a specialty for nursing and many other disciplines, and practice competencies have been developed by specialty organizations such as the Center to Advance Palliative Care. Certifications for nurses, physicians, social workers, and advanced practice providers (nurse practitioners/physician assistants) are available from professional organizations for hospital and community practice. TJC also offers an advanced certification for inpatient programs wishing to be recognized for excellence.

Transitional Care Services

Transitional care is defined as a broad array of short-term services designed to improve health continuity for individuals experiencing a transition between care settings and care providers (Naylor et al., 2011). During transitions of care, handoffs occur that put individuals at higher risk for errors, adverse clinical events, and unmet needs. Transitional care services are designed to improve health outcomes and reduce readmissions and other unnecessary utilization for at-risk populations (Naylor et al., 2011). A recent study conducted by the Patient-Centered Outcomes Research Institute identified transitional care as a critical component of a comprehensive care management system for at-risk individual populations (Naylor et al., 2017).

Transitional care models may be deployed through primary care, specialty care, hospital practice, or as an intermediary step between hospital and community care. Target populations commonly include at-risk children, adults with multiple comorbidities, individuals with severe or end-stage primary diagnoses (eg, COPD or heart failure), and frail elders.

Nurses have demonstrated great success in leading transitional care models, notably through nurse practitioner models (Grant et al., 2017), clinical nurse specialist models (Bryant-Lukosius et al., 2015), and RNs acting as transition managers. Some hospitals employ RN transition managers who not only help to arrange a smooth transition from hospital to home but also continue to follow the individual and address needs for 30 to 60 days postdischarge.

Many transitional care programs actively recruit individuals in a target population to participate in a postdischarge home visitation program, often led by advanced practice nurses and RNs with the support of an interdisciplinary team. In addition to home visits, a variety of telehealth-facilitated interventions such as remote monitoring, video visits, and regular telephone contact are utilized. RNs that work in transition management often have hospital and home health or community care experience and development specific to the role. Specialty certification is provided by professional organizations such as AAACN and case management organizations.

Summary

Ambulatory care settings are diverse and dynamic. Breakthroughs in pharmaceuticals and diagnostic, therapeutic, surgical, and home-based services have and will continue to revolutionize healthcare. As service settings continue to evolve, the role of the ambulatory care RN increases in importance in all areas of healthcare delivery. Utilizing steps of the nursing process, along with cognitive, psychomotor, and affective knowledge and skills, the RN provides expert clinical care throughout the care episode, while keeping the individual and family at the center of all decisions.

In the episodic care setting, RNs face unique challenges that often mirror those of the acute care setting but also require incorporating care coordination and transition principles from ambulatory care. Episodic ambulatory care nursing is a fast-paced, exciting, ever-changing career that offers nurses a unique opportunity to be at the forefront of the design and delivery of the healthcare system of the future.

Case Study

Part 1

Ms. Garcia is a 54-year-old woman who presents to the ASC for a carpal tunnel repair requiring conscious sedation. As Amy, the RN, is beginning the initial assessment, she notes that Ms. Garcia is having shortness of breath and appears very anxious. Amy elects to use a pulse oximeter to obtain oxygen saturation, which is 90%. Ms. Garcia has a history of COPD and appears to be having COPD-related symptoms. Ms. Garcia has used a rescue inhaler in the past but did not bring any of her medications. The nurse is concerned that Ms. Garcia may not be able to tolerate the procedure unless she intervenes.

1. Whom should Amy contact about this situation?
2. Using the SBAR format, describe how Amy would present the information.

Part 2

Amy obtains an order for a short-acting medication to try to bring Ms. Garcia's oxygen baseline back to her normal. She administers the medication, monitors Ms. Garcia's status, and within 1 hour the individual's acute symptoms have returned to baseline. The individual has the procedure, tolerates it well, and outcomes are met, except for the delay in start time.

After the procedure is over and during recovery, Ms. Garcia mentions that she is out of her COPD medications and is not refilling because of cost. Amy notes this in the chart but takes no further action.

1. How might Amy have assisted Mrs. Garcia with her medication issue? What referrals would have been appropriate?
2. Why is it important, even in an episodic setting, to address transitional care needs such as adherence to chronic care medications?

Key Points for Review

- Although episodic ambulatory care settings are diverse, the role of the RN is built on implementation of the nursing process along with the cognitive, psychomotor, and affective skills required in the specialty.
- Episodic ambulatory care settings are becoming increasingly complex and individual needs more acute and diverse.
- The ambulatory care RN role is becoming increasingly important in episodic care environments to provide expert clinical care and to coordinate care and services across the continuum.
- Ambulatory care RNs working in specialty practices implement standards of professional clinical care as well as standards of the specialty practice.
- Ambulatory surgery, diagnostic and therapeutic centers, urgent care, and home-based services are a few of the settings in which ambulatory care RNs practice.
- As payment models evolve, settings and services will also continue to evolve to meet quality, safety, service, and cost requirements.

REFERENCES

Alexander, M., Corrigan, A., Gorski, L., Hankins, J., & Perucca, R. (2010). *Infusion nursing: An evidence-based approach. Infusion nurses society* (3rd ed.). Saunders Elsevier.

Alfaro-LeFevre, R. (2009). *Applying nursing process. A tool for critical thinking* (7th ed.). Lippincott Williams & Wilkins.

American Academy of Ambulatory Care Nursing. (2017). In C. Murray (Ed.), *Scope and standards of practice for professional ambulatory care nursing* (9th ed.). Author.

American Nurses Association, Inc. (2015). *Nursing: Scope and standards of practice* (3rd ed.). Author.

American Society of Anesthesiologists. (2013). Practice advisory for preanesthesia/NAN. Evaluation: An updated report for the American Society of Anesthesiologists Task Force on preanesthesia evaluation. *Anesthesiology, 116*(3), 522–538. http://anesthesiology.pubs.asahq.org/article.aspx?articleid=2443414

American Society of Anesthesiologists. (2014). Practice guidelines for the perioperative management of patients with obstructive sleep apnea. *Anesthesiology, 120*(2):268–286. https://doi.org/10.1097/ALN.0000000000000053

American Society of Perianesthesia Nurses. (2017–18). *Perianesthesia nursing standard practice recommendations and interpretive statements*. Author.

Ashton, L. (2017). Urgent care: A growing healthcare landscape. *Nursing Management, Wolters Kluwer Health, 48*(9),49–54. https://doi.org/10.1097/01.NUMA.0000522176.46134.f2

Brannstrom, M., & Boman, K. (2014). Effects of a person-centered and integrated chronic heart failure and palliative home care. PREFER: A randomized control study. *European Journal of Heart Failure, 16*, 1142–1151. https://doi.org/10:1002/ejhf.151

Bryant-Lukosius, D., Carter, N., Reid, K., Donald, F., Martin-Misener, R., Kilpatrick, K., Harbman, P., Kaasalainen, S., Marshall, D., Charbonneau-Smith, R., & DiCenso, A. (2015). The clinical effectiveness and cost-effectiveness of clinical nurse specialist-led hospital to home transitional care: A systematic review. *Journal of Evaluation in Clinical Practice, 21*(5), 763–781. https://doi.org/10.1111/jep.12401

Buhler-Wilkerson, K. (1985). Public health nursing: In sickness or in health? *American Journal of Public Health, 75*(10), 1155–1161. https://doi.org/10.2105/ajph.75.10.1155

Center for Disease Control and Prevention. (2011). Vital signs: Central line-associated blood stream infections-United States, 2001, 2008, and 2009. *Morbidity and Mortality Weekly Report, 60*(8), 243–248.

Chang, J., Chokshi, D., & Ladapo, J. (2018). Coordination across ambulatory care: A comparison of referrals and health information exchange across convenient and traditional settings. *Journal of Ambulatory Care Management, 41*(2), 128–137. https://doi.org/10.1097/JAC.0000000000000227

Coulter, K. (2016). Successful infusion therapy in older adults. *Journal of Infusion Nursing, 39*(6), 352–358. https://doi.org/10.1097NAN.0000000000000196

Cronenwett, L., Sherwood, G., Barnsteiner, J., Disch, J., Johnson, J., Mitchell, P., Sullivan, D. T. & Warren, J. (2007). Quality and safety education for nurses. *Nursing Outlook, 55*(3), 122–131. https://doi.org/10.1016/j.outlook.2007.02.006

Dychter, S., Gold, D., Carson, D., & Haller, M. (2012). Intravenous therapy: A review of complications and economic considerations of peripheral access. *Journal of Infusion Nursing, 34*(2), 84–91. https://doi.org/10.1097/NAN.0b013e31824237ce

Goodman, T., & Spry, C. (2014). *Essentials of perioperative nursing* (5th ed.). Jones & Bartlett Learning.

Gorski, L., Miller, C., & Mortlock, N. (2010). Infusion therapy across the continuum. In M. Alexander, A. Corrigan, L. Gorski, et al. (Eds.), *Infusion nursing: An evidence-based approach* (3rd ed., pp. 102–126). Saunders Elsevier.

Grant, J., Lines, L., Darbyshire, P., & Perry, V. (2017). How do nurse practitioners work in primary health care settings? A scoping review. *International Journal of Nursing Studies, 75*, 51–57. https://doi.org/10.1016/j.ijnurstu.2017.06.011

Hall, M., Schwartzman, A., Zhang, J., & Xiang, L. (2017). Ambulatory surgery data from hospitals and ambulatory surgery centers: United States, 2010. U.S. Department of Health and Human Services, Centers for Disease and Control Prevention. *National Health Statistics Reports, 102*, 1–15.

Hoeve, Y. T., Jansen, G., & Roodbol, P. (2013). The nursing profession: Public image, selfconcept and professional identity. A discussion paper. *Journal of Advanced Nursing, 70*(2), 295–309. https://doi.org/10.1111/jan.12177

Hughes, R. G. (2011). Overview and summary: Patient-centered care: challenges and rewards. *OJIN: The Online Journal of Issues in Nursing, 16*(2). https://doi.org/10.3912/OJIN.Vol16No02ManOS

Laughlin, C., & Witwer, S. G. (2019). *Core curriculum for ambulatory care nursing* (4th ed.). American Academy of Ambulatory Care Nursing.

Le, S., & Hsia, R. (2016) Community characteristics associated with where urgent care centers are located: A cross-sectional analysis. *BMJ Open 2016, 6*, e010663. https://doi.org/10.1136/bmjopen-2015-010663

Levett-Jones, T., Hoffman, K., Dempsey, J., Jeong, S. Y., Noble, D., Norton, C. A., Roche, J., & Hickey, N. (2010). The "five rights" of clinical reasoning: An educational model to enhance nursing students' ability to identify and manage clinically "at risk" patients. *Nurse Education Today, 30*(6), 515–520. https://doi.org/10.1016/j.nedt.2009.10.020

Marshall, D., Howell, D., Brazil, K., Howard, M., & Taniguchi, A. (2008). Enhancing family medicine physician capacity to deliver quality palliative home care. *Canadian Family Physician, 54*(12), 1703–1703.e7.

Mastal, M. F., & Paschke, S. M. (2019). Overview: Specialty of ambulatory care nursing. In C. B. Baker & S. G. Witwer (Eds.), *Core curriculum for ambulatory care nursing* (4th ed.). AAACN.

Mehrotra, A. (2013). The convenience revolution for treatment of low-acuity conditions. *Journal of the American Medical Association, 310*(1), 35–36. https://doi.org/10.1001/jama.2013.6825

Munnich, E., & Parente, S. (2018). Returns to specialization: Evidence from the outpatient surgery market. *Journal of Health Economics, 57*, 147–167. https://www.sciencedirect.com/science/article/pii/S0167629617310743#bib0015

Naylor, M. D., Aiken, L. H., Kurtzman, E. T., Olds, D. M., & Hirschman, K. B. (2011). The care span: The importance of transitional care in achieving health reform. *Health Affairs (Millwood), 30*(4), 746–754. https://doi.org/10.1377/hlthaff.2011.0041

Naylor, M. D., Shaid, E. C., Carpenter, D., Gass, B., Levine, C., Li, J., Malley, A., Malley, A., McCauley, K., Nguyen, H. Q., Watson, H., Brock, J., Mittman, B., Jack, B., Mitchell, S., Callicoatte, B., Schall, J., & Williams, M. V. (2017). Components of comprehensive and effective transitional care. *Journal of the American Geriatric Society, 65*(6), 1119–1125. https://doi.org/10.1111/jgs.14782

Patient and Family-Centered Care. (2018). *From website: Institute for patient-and family-centered care.* http://www.ipfcc.org/about/pfcc.html

Prabhakar, A., Helander, E., Chopra, N., Kaye, A. J., Urman, R., & Kaye A. D. (2017). Preoperative assessment for ambulatory surgery. *Current Pain Headache Rep, 21*, 43–48. https://doi.org/10.1007/s11916-017-0643-7

Smith, S. (2013). Telehealth nursing. In C. B. Baker (Ed.), *Core curriculum for ambulatory care nursing* (3rd ed.). AAACN.

Stoimenoff, L., & Newman, N. (2017). Urgent care industry white paper 2018: The essential role of the urgent care center in population health. *Urgent Care Association of America (UCOA)*. www.ucaoa.org

Tanner, C. A. (2006). Thinking like a nurse: A research-based model of clinical judgment in nursing. *Journal of Nursing Education, 45*(6), 204–211. https://doi.org/10.3928/01484834-20060601-04

Weinick, R., Bristol, S., & DesRochest, C. (2009). Urgent care centers in the US: Findings from a national survey. *BMC Health Services Research, 9*, 79. https://doi.org/10.1186/1472-6963-9-79

Welch, H. G., Wennberg, D. E., & Welch, W. P. (1996). The use of Medicare home health care services. *The New England Journal of Medicine, 335*, 324–329. https://doi.org/10.1056/NEJM199608013350506

12

Medical Specialty Clinics

Rocquel Crawley and Mary Coffey

PERSPECTIVES

"Specialty clinic registered nurses are effective practitioners, care coordinators, health coaches, and advocates for individuals with acute and chronic conditions that cause serious and sometimes debilitating illness or premature death. They understand the nuance of clinical conditions, as well as the effects of the associated management and treatment. These nurses help individuals and families mitigate social determinants of health that diminish one's ability to manage their health and are the lynchpin to other healthcare providers and essential services. As team-based ambulatory care matures, the value of registered nurses in specialty clinics is evident."

Pamela F. Cipriano, PhD, RN, NEA-BC, FAAN, Dean and Sadie Heath Cabaniss Professor of Nursing, University of Virginia School of Nursing, 1st Vice President, International Council of Nurses

LEARNING OBJECTIVES

Upon completion of this chapter, the reader will be able to:

1. Understand the role of specialty clinics in the landscape of ambulatory care.
2. Describe the role of nursing in helping individuals navigate between specialty clinics and their primary care providers.
3. Describe the difference between clinics that address noncommunicable chronic disease and those that address infectious chronic diseases.
4. Understand the role of specialty clinics in serving as the primary healthcare source for some individuals.
5. Explain the role of telehealth and interprofessional communication between specialty and primary care clinics.

KEY TERMS

Care continuum
Chronic infectious diseases
Interprofessional teams
Mental health
Noncommunicable chronic diseases
Specialty practice
Substance misuse

Overview and Context

Many of the concepts, skills, and competencies overlap to all ambulatory settings; thus, to some extent, it is an artificial distinction to discuss different settings as though they were completely separate from other parts of ambulatory nursing. However, for the purposes of organization, this chapter focuses on the ambulatory settings that address a specific ongoing disease process or health challenge. Additional areas that might be considered specialties, such as infusion centers, ambulatory surgery, or diagnostics and procedures, were previously addressed in Chapter 11. Specialty populations (in contrast to **specialty practices**), such as pediatric and younger individuals, veteran care, and care of those experiencing homelessness, are discussed in Chapters 13 and 14. Certainly, any of these individuals might be in any of these clinics; however, the concepts and skills in this chapter relate to nursing care while the individual is in a specific clinic for a specific issue: clinics such as cardiology, oncology, or nephrology as well as newer health specialties such as pain management, **substance misuse**, or bariatrics.

It is not within the scope of this chapter to cover every possible specialty clinic. Rather, the objective is to provide principles related to specialty care, discuss ways that nursing in specialty care may be different and similar to that in primary or family care, and provide a few examples of these competencies and skills. Similarly, the topics of **mental health** and substance misuse are far broader than can be covered in this one chapter. The intent of this discussion is to provide some examples of ways that these areas may be addressed in ambulatory care and to touch briefly on some of the associated nursing interventions.

The role of the professional registered nurse (RN) in ambulatory care is evolving day by day and, in some cases, minute by minute. Common transitions of care include, but are not limited to, outpatient to higher level of care, inpatient to higher level of care (ie, transfer from general floor to an intensive care unit), inpatient to a skilled nursing facility or residential facility, and inpatient to an outpatient setting. Specialty care clinic nurses provide assistance with referrals to primary care, other specialties, and community resources. Care coordination and management between specialty care nurses is essential, because many patients treat their specialty provider as their primary care provider (PCP). Communication must be timely, accurate, and complete, in order for members of the patient's care team to develop well-thought-out plans of care. Ambulatory nurses are at the forefront of these transitions and have the ability to influence and improve patient outcomes each and every day.

Figure 12.1 illustrates a conceptual framework developed by the American Academy of Ambulatory Care Nursing to highlight the work completed by RNs in an office setting and providing the context of specialty care within that framework (Figure 12.1).

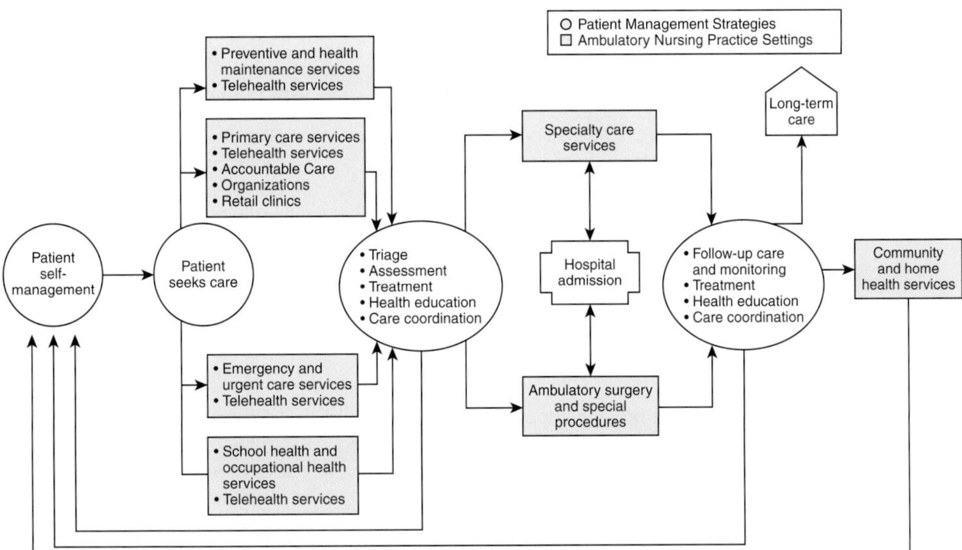

FIGURE 12.1 Context for ambulatory care nursing practice. (American Academy of Ambulatory Care Nursing. [2017]. In C. Murray [Ed.], *Scope and standards of practice for professional ambulatory care nursing* [9th ed.]. Author. Used with permission of American Academy of Ambulatory Care Nursing [AAACN], aaacn.org)

As noted earlier, although some specialty clinics may primarily address a specific medical issue, others may be the primary source of healthcare for its individuals. For example, a renal or orthopedic specialist may have a shorter individual involvement, whereas the human immunodeficiency virus (HIV) or congenital heart disease specialist may provide both specialty and primary care for the individual from diagnosis until the individual's health issue is resolved.

Individuals with these issues may see their specialist more often and may have an established and trusting relationship. The individual spends a great deal of time at the specialist care team to manage their disease, and the individual, individual's family, specialist, and specialty interprofessional care team have a greater opportunity to develop an interpersonal relationship and communicate frequently with each other. In this context, the specialist may address issues that are not directly related to their specialty concern, such as renewing medications that the PCP would normally renew.

Nursing Role in Specialty Practice

As noted earlier, the overarching principles of ambulatory care nursing apply in all settings. Some competencies of ambulatory care that will be discussed in the context of specialty care include education, empowerment of the individual, care coordination and transition management, and interprofessional collaboration. However, there are many ways in which the RN roles in specialty and primary care are different. Table 12.1 compares ambulatory nurses in a primary care setting with those in a specialty care setting.

The ambulatory care RN in specialty care practice has a key role empowering, encouraging, motivating, educating, and partnering with individuals to be engaged in all aspects of their care to achieve their healthcare goals. The Institute of Medicine (2001) identified that increased patient satisfaction improved health outcomes, and quality of decisions was linked to patient engagement through shared decision-making. Funnell (2016) stated, "Empowerment is based largely on the work of the educator Paulo Freire and first applied to healthcare in the 1980s. Empowerment is essentially based on the theory of self-determination, a general theory of

TABLE 12.1 PRIMARY CARE VERSUS SPECIALTY CARE

	Primary Care	Specialty Care
Coordination of care	• RNs provide a consistent point of contact for patients and families • Educate patients and families on chronic disease processes • Assess overall patient health needs • Request and review any and all past medical/surgical history from specialty or prior healthcare providers • Referrals to specialists as needed	• RNs provide a consistent point of contact for patients and families • Educate patients and families on episodic disease processes or acute injury • Assess focused health needs related to specialty • Request and review any and all past medical/surgical history from primary care • Coordinate referrals from primary care
Navigation of care	• RNs provide support (psychosocial and emotional) for chronic illness/disease • Develop and maintain a nurturing relationship with patient and family members • Coordinate provider appointments, diagnostic testing, and procedures related to chronic or new disease diagnosis • Identify missing medical and/or surgical history information and works to obtain	• RNs provide support (psychosocial and emotional) for episodic or acute illness/disease • Develop and maintain a nurturing relationship with patient and family members • Coordinate provider appointments, diagnostic testing, and procedures related to specialty care • Identify missing medical and/or surgical history information and works to obtain

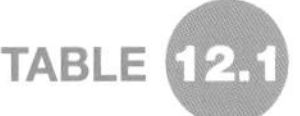

TABLE 12.1 PRIMARY CARE VERSUS SPECIALTY CARE (CONTINUED)

	Primary Care	Specialty Care
Management of care	• Monitors chronic patient conditions and updates specialty team on progress to goals • Determines follow-up related to primary care—frequency, urgency, and setting needed • Assess and assist patient with DME needs • Educate patient on the need for routine and well visits • Evaluate family support and identify community resources needed to manage care in the home setting • Refer patients to specialty care as needed	• Monitors acute patient conditions and updates primary care team on progress to goals • Determines follow-up related to specialty care—frequency, urgency, and setting needed • Assess and assist patient with DME needs • Educate patient on the need for acute visit and routine visits • Refer patients to primary care to establish care for chronic disease and wellness management

Note. DME = durable medical equipment; RN = registered nurse.

motivation" (p. 1921). The specialty care practice RN supports the individual's autonomy in prioritizing needs, preferences, and values while assisting individuals to examine the cognitive, emotional, and social aspects of their lives and the impact of their decisions (Haas et al., 2014). The RN provides psychosocial and emotional support for the individual and their family for episodic or acute illnesses.

Care Coordination and Transition Management

The RN in specialty care practice is central to coordinating the care of the individual across the continuum of care and transition management. An example of care coordination and transition management for specialty practice may be seen in the case study in Box 12.1.

The specialty care practice RN's aptitude regarding social determinants of health and the impact on the individuals' health outcomes is essential in order to establish goals and connect the individuals to internal and community resources needed to effectively manage the individual's care in the home.

BOX 12.1 Care Coordination and Transition Management in a Specialty Clinic

Mr. J., an individual with COPD, has a follow-up visit in the pulmonary specialty practice. The RN along with the interprofessional team (provider, social worker, pharmacy) engages the individual and family regarding the care plan, review of goals, goals achieved, barriers to achieving goals, and compliance with treatment. The role of the specialty care practice RN is to counsel the individual and family regarding COPD symptom management and lifestyle choices to improve prognosis because the individual continues to smoke 10 cigarettes a week.

The RN educates the individual and family regarding COPD disease process while utilizing appropriate individual engagement and activation skills such as motivational interviewing. In addition, the specialty care RN is the point of contact for the individual and family throughout the individual's treatment or disease management. The RN coordinates specialty provider appointments, referrals from primary care, diagnostic testing, and procedures related to the specialty care. The RN triages the individual for acute illnesses and determines urgency for an appointment if needed or provide the appropriate disposition for care.

Note. COPD = chronic obstructive pulmonary disease; RN = registered nurse.

Interprofessional Care Teams

The Institute of Medicine (2001) report, *Crossing the Quality Chasm*, identified five core competencies that provide patient-centered care: "Work in interdisciplinary teams, employ evidence-based practice, apply quality improvements, and utilize informatics." These competencies are essential for all healthcare team members to effectively address the 21st-century healthcare needs (Yellowitz, 2016, p. 61). Individuals are living longer with more complex and chronic healthcare needs that benefit from a holistic approach best addressed by **interprofessional teams**. The goal of interprofessional care teams in a specialty care practice is to bring together competent and skilled experts in their specialty to establish a partnership between the healthcare team members and the individuals to provide a coordinated approach to shared decision-making regarding health and social determinants of health issues (Kent et al., 2016).

Interprofessional collaboration is an essential aspect of providing care in specialty care settings. Additionally, it is critical for the interprofessional team, specialists, and primary care to communicate and stay abreast of the individual's plan of care and progress. Utilizing a shared electronic health record (EHR) is key in order for all healthcare team members to update and review the individual's plan of care; diagnostic, imaging, and lab results; and medications across the **care continuum**.

Oncology care provides an excellent example of interprofessional collaboration. In this specialty, dietary, medicine, nursing, social services, and other specialties regularly collaborate to optimize the treatment regimen for their individuals. The specialty care RN requests and reviews all of the individual's past specialty and/or primary care records from external providers so that the healthcare information can be scanned into the EHR and is accessible by the entire healthcare team.

Specialty Clinics for Noncommunicable Chronic Diseases: Four Examples

The number of Americans living with noncommunicable diseases (NCDs) continues to rise. Heart disease, cancer, and diabetes are considered some of the costliest NCDs, often preventable and commonly manageable through early screening and lifestyle changes. These and other NCDs may require management in specialty clinics, which often become the individual's primary care source. In these settings, RNs play a significant role in transforming the current delivery of chronic care management and care coordination.

In this discussion of specialty care, four common NCDs will be used as exemplars of the nursing role in ambulatory specialty settings. Heart disease (particularly heart failure [HF]), diabetes, cancer, and chronic obstructive pulmonary disease (COPD) are specialties whose individuals rely on them to manage or have significant input on all aspects of their care. These examples do not cover all clinics that may fall into this category, and clinics addressing ongoing health challenges such as sickle cell disease, degenerative neurologic disorders, and hematologic issues, only to name a few, also may provide holistic care for their individuals. However, many of the concepts discussed here would apply to those settings as well.

Heart Disease

Heart disease refers to various types of heart conditions and is the leading cause of death in the United States (Centers for Disease Control and Prevention [CDC, 2017]). Individuals with coronary heart disease are living longer and have an improved quality of life because of the advancement of medications, procedures, and treatments. Individuals under the care of cardiology may be there for a variety of reasons: an individual with a congenital heart defect may have been under this care since infancy, one with a recent myocardial infarction may need care for a limited time, an elderly individual with HF may need ongoing follow-up and coordination with all aspects of healthcare.

The RN in cardiology may educate the individual and family about a variety of issues regarding heart disease such as the individual's treatment plan, treatable risk factors, or early warning signs of cardiac complications. As an example, if the individual is transferred to the care of the HF clinic, the RN engages and empowers the individual to make necessary lifestyle changes to improve their quality of life and to reduce the incidence of hospital readmissions.

As an example of RN intervention for HF management, the specialty practice RN collaborates with the interprofessional team to identify the individuals admitted in the hospital who are at the highest risk for readmission in order to allow the maximum resources to be directed at keeping the individual well and out of the hospital. Remote telemonitoring strategies may be initiated before discharge by identifying the individuals at greater risk. After discharge, telemonitoring devices allow for transmission of the individual's vital signs, weight, oximetry, and symptoms (Dunbar-Yaffe et al., 2015). The specialty care RN contacts the individual on a regular basis to assess the individual and self-care compliance. The RN keeps the specialist and primary care abreast of the individual's status and coordinates the individual's appointments between the specialist, PCP, and other interprofessional team members.

The RN interested in cardiology needs to be knowledgeable of cardiac problems and the disease process, procedures, and treatment methods. In addition, the RN should be familiar with various medical equipment for diagnostics and monitoring (ie, electrocardiogram [ECG/EKG] equipment, continuous dysrhythmia monitors, stress testing equipment, automated external defibrillator [AED], pacemakers). Some of this equipment involves remote monitoring with RN oversight, discussed later in the section on telemedicine.

The cardiology practice RN can obtain the following certifications: Basic ECG Board Certification, 12-Lead ECG Board Certification, and Cardiovascular Nursing Board Certification (CVRN-BC).

Cancer

According to the National Cancer Institute (2017) and the Centers for Disease Control and Prevention (CDC, 2017), cancer is the second leading cause of death in the United States. The role of the RN in oncology practices has expanded over the last decade because of advances in treatment and research. The oncology specialty practice RN educates and validates that the individual and their family are able to describe the state of the disease, therapy goals, treatment schedules, and side effects of treatment; provide psychological and physical preparation for treatment; offer psychological and physical comfort measures and community resources; and identify emergencies related to disease and/or therapy (Oncology Nursing Society, 2017). The RN partners with the individual and their family to collaborate with the PCP, pharmacy, social worker, medical oncology, surgical oncology, radiation oncology, and other interdisciplinary team members in response to the individual's individualized needs to coordinate the individual's plan of care.

In addition, the RN performs prescreening and individual assessment prior to chemotherapy administration, provides care in the management of side effects, and coordinates long-term follow-up care for the individual (Oncology Nursing Society, 2017). The Oncology Nursing Society (ONS, 2017) offers a chemotherapy training course for nurses who administer chemotherapy and biotherapy, which includes administration of antineoplastic drugs (all routes), handling and disposal of antineoplastic, and management of allergic reactions and documentation.

Depending upon the RN's area of specialty in oncology, the following certifications are available for the nurse to obtain: Oncology Certified Nurse (OCN), Certified Pediatric Hematology Oncology Nurse (CPHON), Certified Breast Care Nurse (CBCN), Advanced Oncology Certified Nurse (AOCN), Advanced Oncology Certified Clinical Nurse Specialist (AOCNS), and Blood & Marrow Transplant Certified Nurse (BMTCN).

Diabetes

Diabetes is a chronic metabolic disorder in which high levels of blood glucose result from defects in insulin production and/or insulin action and was the seventh leading cause of death in 2016 (Xu et al., 2018). Diabetes can lead to serious health complications and premature death if not managed appropriately through diet, physical activity, and the appropriate use of insulin and other medications to control blood sugar levels.

The RN working in a diabetes or endocrinology clinic addresses the individual's current knowledge regarding their disease, health beliefs, cultural needs, emotional and psychosocial concerns, family support, financial status, health literacy, numeracy, and other factors that influence the individual's ability to achieve the challenges of self-management (Powers et al., 2016). The RN assesses the individual's ability for self-management and educates the individual living with diabetes about the need to make a multitude of self-management decisions daily. The RN in an endocrinology specialty care practice is knowledgeable about diabetes disease process, treatable risk factors, complications, diabetes self-management education and support (DSME/S), medication treatment options, carbohydrate counting, and management of hypoglycemia and hyperglycemia. The ambulatory care RN in endocrinology educates the individual and family how to use a glucometer and, if appropriate for the individual, to administer insulin and/or glucagon injections, insulin pumps, and continuous glucose monitoring devices.

The RN completes a comprehensive foot examination on the individual during the clinic visit to evaluate for foot ulcers and any neuropathic symptoms. The RN educates the individual and family about proper foot care; the importance of the individual checking their feet daily for sores, skin tears or openings, numbness, and pain; and the need to notify the nurse immediately. In addition, the RN coordinates a variety of specialist appointments (eg, ophthalmology, podiatry, nutritionist), PCP appointments, diagnostic and lab testing, and community resources related to specialty care. The RN monitors the individual for acute and episodic illnesses; educates the individual and family regarding the need for acute visits, appropriate use of the emergency department (ED) versus routine follow-up visits, importance of medication and dietary compliance; and assesses and assists the individual with durable medical equipment (DME) needs. The specialty care practice RN reevaluates the individual's diabetes care goals and self-management needs throughout the individual's life span and critical transition periods into adulthood, hospitalizations, skilled nursing facility, correctional facility, or rehabilitation center (Powers et al., 2016).

The RN in specialty care practice for endocrinology can earn a certification as a certified diabetes educator (CDE) if they possess comprehensive knowledge and experience in prediabetes, diabetes management, and diabetes prevention. A CDE promotes self-management and supports the individual to achieve individualized behavioral and treatment goals. Another certification is Board Certified-Advanced Diabetes Management (BC-ADM). The individual who is BC-ADM manages complex individual needs that are within their scope of practice.

Respiratory Disorders

Various respiratory conditions impact the overall quality of health for many individuals. Two of the most common respiratory conditions are asthma and COPD. Several risk factors contribute to asthma and COPD such as smoking, air pollution, dust, and chemicals.

Asthma is a common pulmonary condition characterized by periods of reversible airflow obstruction and is one of the most common noncommunicable chronic childhood diseases (CDC, 2017). According to the CDC (2017), asthma impacts an estimated 23 million people, including over 6 million children. Asthma symptoms occur or worsen with changes in weather, stress, exercise, infections, exposure to allergens and irritants, or other factors.

The RN in a pulmonary specialty practice has in-depth knowledge about respiratory disorders and the disease process, respiratory treatment options, interventions, diagnostic testing, medications, and pulmonary rehabilitation. The specialty practice RN responsibilities include educating the individual about self-management and how to manage their asthma, self-monitoring to recognize either symptoms or peak flow monitoring for asthma worsening, compliance with long-term control and quick relief medications, appropriate inhaler and peak flow technique, and reducing the risk of exacerbations. The RN provides emotional support and encouragement to the individual to achieve targeted goals in the plan of care; collaborates and communicates closely with the interprofessional team, specialist, and PCP to keep everyone updated regarding the individual's status; and coordinates individual visits and referrals.

COPD is a group of progressive, debilitating respiratory conditions that include emphysema, chronic bronchitis, and small airways diseases, which cause airflow blockage and breathing-related problems (Cunningham et al., 2014, p. 1033). In 2016, chronic lower respiratory disease, which includes COPD as well as chronic bronchitis and asthma, was the fourth leading cause of death in the United States (Xu et al., 2018).

The specialty practice RN engages and empowers the individual living with COPD to make the necessary lifestyle changes to improve their quality of life. The most significant lifestyle change is to quit smoking and avoid secondhand smoke. The RN may refer the individual to a smoking cessation program in order to help slow or halt the progression of COPD. The RN connects the individual to support groups to help manage coping strategies and appropriate internal and external resources, as well as educating and supporting the individual regarding self-management of COPD to keep the individual out of the ED and hospital.

Another chronic pulmonary disease is cystic fibrosis (CF), a chronic, progressive, and frequently fatal genetic lung disease characterized by early colonization and infection of the airways (Cantin et al., 2015). According to the Cystic Fibrosis Foundation (2017), more than 70,000 people worldwide are living with CF. Because of research and medical advances in CF there have been dramatic improvements in the treatment, and today the predicted survival age is close to 40 years. For this reason, individuals who previously would only have been treated by pediatric pulmonary specialists are transitioning to adult care.

Asthma and CF are both noncommunicable childhood diseases for which the specialty practice RN will address adolescent to adult care transition. As part of this care, the RN may administer the validated Transition Readiness Assessment Questionnaire (TRAQ) to assess performance of chronic disease self-management skills and measure readiness for transition. A TRAQ summary score >4 is equivalent to respondents reporting that they are beginning to perform necessary disease self-management skills. Another tool is the Patient Activation Measure, which gauges individuals' self-efficacy and confidence to manage one's own disease and healthcare on a scale of 0 to 100, with 100 representing functioning independently as an adult with chronic disease (Huang et al., 2014).

Safe and effective healthcare transition for adolescents with a chronic disease from child-centered to adult-oriented healthcare systems is critical to achieving positive health outcomes (Huang et al., 2014). The specialty care RN plays a key role engaging, supporting, and preparing the adolescent individual and family for the care transition. This includes educating and preparing adolescents to independently self-manage their disease and to communicate effectively with their specialist, PCP, and interprofessional team regarding their disease.

Chronic Infectious Diseases

Chronic infectious diseases such as HIV and hepatitis B and C are spread directly or indirectly from one person to another, which distinguishes them from noninfectious chronic diseases that are not spread from individual to individual. This distinction can have an impact on individual education that may need to include difficult topics such as sexual or lifestyle implications related to transmission. Because of the holistic nature of this care, individuals also may feel that these clinics provide a safe setting for them to receive all of their primary care requirements.

The discussion of chronic infectious diseases is specific to HIV. However, the general principles related to the RN role in HIV care also apply to individuals with hepatitis or other diseases transmitted through intimate contact.

Human Immunodeficiency Virus

The RN in the HIV practice assesses the individual's understanding regarding their disease, antiretroviral regimen, potentially harmful behaviors, risk reduction interventions, and readiness for change. The RN performs a detailed assessment of sexual and substance use behaviors per visit, an HIV transmission risk assessment, including the individual's sexual practices with each partner, and needle use practices, if applicable. In this setting, it is important that the RN provide nonjudgmental and emotional support for the individual and family, also facilitating partner notification, counseling, and testing and coordinating appropriate referrals. These may include social work, psychosocial and behavioral services, community resources, and obstetrician for prenatal care, if applicable.

HIV specialty care practices serve an important role in primary care, including assessing at each appointment the individual's need for preventive care, because the specialty clinic may be the only primary care source for these individuals. The RN educates the individual regarding prevention interventions with emphasis on the individual's health and the health of their partner(s). Engagement and collaboration with the interprofessional team are key as the individual is empowered to set goals and target behavior change if needed. To further support prevention, as needed, the HIV specialty practice may furnish the individual with supplies to provide increased protection against infection of others.

The RN specializing in HIV/acquired immunodeficiency syndrome (AIDS) nursing practice can achieve formal recognition of HIV/AIDS nursing knowledge by becoming certified in Advanced HIV/AIDS Certified Registered Nurse (AACRN) or AIDS Certified Registered Nurse (ACRN) certifications.

Registered Nurse Roles in Chronic Infectious Disease Care

Regardless of the chronic infectious disease, the specialty care RN addresses a variety of needs. These may include:

- develop and maintain a nurturing relationship with the individual and their family
- serve as the point of contact for communication and emotional support to the individual and family
- complete focused assessments of risks and health needs
- educate and ensure the individual and family have a clear understanding of the disease, treatment, and risk reduction interventions
- coordinate specialist and interprofessional team appointments, diagnostic testing, and procedures
- keep the specialist, PCP, and interprofessional team members abreast of the individual's plan of care and challenges with achieving goals.

Mental Health and Substance Misuse in Specialty Care

Mental health nursing may be considered a separate specialty as well as a component of nursing care in all situations. In particular however, living with chronic health conditions presents many challenges and stressors for individuals and their families. Some of the stressors consist of managing their complex chronic health conditions and multiple medications, making highly complex medical decisions, covering costs related to frequent and multiple provider visits, and enduring hospitalizations that are often exacerbated by depression (Roper et al., 2017). It is essential for both primary care and mental health specialty practices to communicate and provide effective coordination of care to ensure the well-being of the individual.

Mental health services are often not available or not easily accessed by all those in need. Individuals with mental health disorders may require frequent visits to mental healthcare professionals and various support services, or individuals in immediate crisis or harm may seek help in the ED. Specialty sites for mental health services are available in local health departments, psychiatry clinics, and behavioral health facilities. However, in recognition of the ongoing need, some primary care practices have tackled mental health access issues by embedding behavioral health specialists. This aspect of mental healthcare is discussed in Chapter 10. However, some of the principles that apply to mental health and substance misuse in both primary and specialty care also will be addressed here.

Substance Misuse

Opioid abuse has escalated in the United States. According to Brady et al. (2016), "Prescription opioids are now the most commonly initiated drugs, second only to marijuana, with approximately 1.9 million new initiates per year" (p. 18). In addition to opioid issues, misuse of alcohol, tobacco, marijuana, and addictive drugs remains an ongoing challenge for healthcare providers. This includes providers in the primary as well as the specialty care clinics, particularly specialty care providers who also serve as the primary care source for their individuals.

As all providers become more aware of the challenges related to substance misuse, RNs in both specialty and primary care are in a position to provide screening for these issues. For individuals who require follow-up or further evaluation, the RN may work with the provider to coordinate referral and care. A few of the screening tools used for substance misuse are summarized by the U.S. Substance Abuse and Mental Health Services Administration and are listed in Box 12.2.

BOX 12.2 Selected Screening Tools for Substance Misuse

Instrument	Population(s)	Description	Access/More Information
ASSIST	Adults, Adolescents	An 8-item screening tool developed for the WHO by an international group of substance abuse researchers to detect and manage substance use and related problems in primary and general medical care settings. Includes a patient feedback report card. Available in several languages.	http://www.who.int/substance_abuse/activities/assist/en *The Alcohol, Smoking and Substance Involvement Screening Test (ASSIST): Manual for Use in Primary Care* (Humeniuk et al., 2010)
AUDIT	Adults, Adolescents	A 10-item screening tool developed by the WHO to identify persons whose alcohol consumption has become hazardous or harmful to their health. Available in English-, Spanish-, and Slovenian-language versions.	http://www.who.int/substance_abuse/activities/sbi/en/index.html *AUDIT: The Alcohol Use Disorders Identification Test Guidelines for Use in Primary Care, Second Edition* http://whqlibdoc.who.int/hq/2001/WHO_MSD_MSB_01.6a.pdf
AUDIT-C	Adults	The first three questions of AUDIT (those that focus on alcohol consumption).	http://www.hepatitis.va.gov/provider/tools/audit-c.asp#S1X
CAGE (**C**ut down, **A**nnoyed, **G**uilty, **E**yeopener)	Adults (people older than age 16)	A 4-item, nonconfrontational questionnaire for detecting alcohol problems. Questions are usually phrased as "have you ever" but may also focus on present alcohol problems.	https://www.hopkinsmedicine.org/johns_hopkins_healthcare/downloads/all_plans/CAGE%20Substance%20Screening%20Tool.pdf

(continued)

BOX 12.2 Selected Screening Tools for Substance Misuse (continued)

Instrument	Population(s)	Description	Access/More Information
CRAFFT (**C**ar, **R**elax, **A**lone, **F**orget, **F**amily or Friends, **T**rouble)	Adolescents	A 6-item screening instrument. Test covers alcohol and drugs and situations that are relevant to adolescents.	https://docs.clinicaltools.com/pdf/sbirt/CTI_CRAFFT.pdf
DAST (**D**rug **A**buse **S**creening **T**est)	Adults	A 20- and 28-item adaptation of the MAST to detect consequences related to drug abuse without being specific about the drug, thus alleviating the necessity of using different instruments specific to each drug.	20-item instrument: https://adai.uw.edu/instruments/pdf/Drug_Abuse_Screening_Test_105.pdf
DAST-A	Adolescents	A 28-item DAST for adolescents	https://www.smartcjs.org.uk/wp-content/uploads/2015/07/DAST-A.pdf
Fagerstrom Test for Nicotine Dependence	Adults	A 6-item test evaluating cigarette consumption, the compulsion to use, and dependence. Screens for nicotine dependence. Severity rating can be used for treatment planning.	https://cde.drugabuse.gov/instrument/d7c0b0f5-b865-e4de-e040-bb89ad43202b
MAST (Michigan Alcohol Screening Test)	Adults, Adolescents, Seniors	A 24-item instrument providing a general measure of lifetime alcohol problem severity that can be used for choosing treatment intensity and guiding inquiry into alcohol-related problems. A 13-item version (Short MAST) and geriatric version (MAST-G) are available.	Updated MAST: https://www.anitamcleodcounseling.com/userfiles/4702580/file/MAST%20updated.pdf Short MAST: https://hopequestgroup.org/wp-content/uploads/2011/09/SMAST-Short-Michigan-Alcohol-Screening-Test.pdf Short MAST-Geriatric Version http://vtspc.org/wp-content/uploads/2016/12/SMAST-G.pdf
NIDA Drug Use Screening Tool	Adults	A 1- to 7-question screening tool adapted by the National Institute on Drug Abuse from the WHO's ASSIST.	Summary chart of screening and assessment tools: https://www.drugabuse.gov/nidamed-medical-health-professionals/screening-tools-resources/chart-screening-tools
TWEAK (**T**olerance, **W**orried, **E**ye-openers, **A**mnesia, [**K**] Cut down)	Adults, Pregnant women	A 5-item scale to screen for risky drinking.	Instruments for pregnant women: https://pubs.niaaa.nih.gov/publications/arh25-3/204-209.htm

Note. ASSIST = Alcohol, Smoking, and Substance Involvement Screening Test; AUDIT = Alcohol Use Disorders Identification Test; WHO = World Health Organization. Substance Abuse and Mental Health Services Administration. (2013). *Systems-level implementation of screening, brief intervention, and referral to treatment*. Technical Assistance Publication (TAP). Series 33. HHS Publication No. (SMA) 13-4741. Author.

Anxiety and Depression

Mental health conditions affect individuals of all ages, and mental health conditions are the leading cause of disability. Depression is the most common mental health disorder, with more than 300 million people suffering from depression worldwide (Goodrich et al., 2013, p. 2). The World Health Organization (WHO, 2017) reported that there is an interrelationship between depression and other health conditions. The symptoms of depression and anxiety are multifactorial and result from complex interactions of psychological, social, and biologic factors. If depression and anxiety are not adequately treated, they can become disabling and predispose the individual to suicidal ideations (Yohannes & Alexopoulos, 2014, p. 346). Bhattacharya et al. (2014) found depression and anxiety to be associated with chronic physical conditions such as diabetes, asthma, heart disease, cancer, HIV/AIDS, and COPD.

Depression and anxiety are frequently treated by PCPs. The role of the RN in primary care is central to screening and assessing the individual for depression and follow-up and is discussed in Chapter 10. Similarly, though, the role of the specialty practice RN is crucial because the specialist clinic sometimes serves as the individual's PCP. The Patient Health Questionnaires with two and nine questions (PHQ-2 or PHQ-9) are the most common tools utilized to screen the individual for signs and symptoms of depression (Haas et al., 2014, p. 47). The PHQ-2 score can range from 0 to 6. A score of 3 or more requires the individual to be further evaluated with the PHQ-9 or other diagnostic tools. A screening tool used for anxiety is the Generalized Anxiety Disorder (GAD-7), which is a seven-question tool that identifies whether a comprehensive assessment for anxiety is needed.

A screening tool to identify individuals with probable posttraumatic stress disorder is the Primary Care (PC)—PTSD-5, a five-item tool designed to use in the primary care setting. Similarly, the traumatic events screening inventory for children (TESI-C) is a 16-item tool that assesses a child's experience of various potential traumatic events such as domestic violence, disasters, physical and sexual abuse, and many other events. The interpretation of the results should be done by clinicians.

The role of the RN is to assess the individual and identify stressors, such as financial problems, difficulties at work, or physical or mental abuse, and sources of support, such as family members and friends. From this assessment, the RN can identify the appropriate internal and community resources to alleviate stressors and ensure the maintenance or reactivation of social networks and social activities. By effectively screening and assessing individuals, the healthcare team can coordinate the needed resources to ensure the safety and well-being of the individual. As noted in previous sections, the RN team member coordinates provider appointments and referrals, keeps the specialist abreast of the individual's plan of care and overall health status, and educates the individual and family regarding the importance of the individual keeping scheduled appointments and compliance with plan of care.

Virtual Care in Specialty Clinics

As telemedicine becomes more accessible, more specialty care providers are turning to this format to improve their reach and offer care to patients regardless of their geographic location. This may be especially important for specialty services that may not be easily available to individuals in remote or underserved settings.

As mentioned in the section on cardiac diseases, specialty clinics may have specific remote monitoring equipment such as cardiac dysrhythmia monitors or HF monitoring. Likewise, neurology clinics may monitor individuals with movement disorders or seizures. RNs in these and other specialty areas review the data from these devices and have ongoing contact with the individuals for any related challenges or changes in condition.

The topics of telehealth and virtual care are covered in more detail in Chapter 9; however, specialty care nurses may have specific responsibilities that include but are not limited to:

- assisting the patient to obtain needed DME
- educating and supporting the individual in the use and care of monitoring equipment, as well as any potential associated complications
- monitoring and intervening as needed based on telemedicine data
- from a remote location, supporting telemedicine conferencing by coordinating with the specialty provider and, as needed, providing on-site assessment
- from a specialty office, maintaining ongoing communication with remote individuals and coordinating care with the specialist as needed

Referrals to Primary Care

High-level primary care and the patient-centered medical home (PCMH) are team-based care delivery models that target improving the patient experience, access, population health, care coordination, and cost. Care coordination between specialty clinics and these primary care settings is especially important to avoid adverse events.

Inadequate coordination of care transition results in fragmented care, medication errors, adverse outcomes, decreased individual satisfaction, delays in treatment, increased ED utilization, and inpatient readmissions.

Collaboration and communication between the high-level primary care or PCMH, specialty practices, and other key services such as social work and community health workers are important to stay abreast of the individuals' plan of care and well-being. To ensure appropriate referrals and safe transitions of care across many specialists, the specialty care RN collaborates with the interprofessional team and serves as the primary contact to coordinate the transitions and communicates with the primary care setting when the individual experiences a care transition.

Specialty Registered Nurses and Accountable Care Organizations

The Centers for Medicare and Medicaid Services considers accountable care organizations (ACOs) as groups of doctors, hospitals, and other healthcare providers, who come together voluntarily to give coordinated high-quality care to their Medicare patients. The goal of coordinated care is to ensure that patients, especially the chronically ill, get the right care at the right time, while avoiding unnecessary duplication of services and preventing medical errors. Quality is measured in four domains: patient/caregiver experience, care coordination/patient safety, preventive health, and clinical care for at-risk populations (ie, diabetes, ischemic vascular disease, hypertension, HF, coronary artery disease, and depression). Ambulatory specialty care RNs have the ability to positively impact all four of the quality domains and ultimately improve patient outcomes.

Specialty care RNs can serve in the following roles within established ACOs: care coordinator, communicators, advance practice nurses, quality improvement managers, and expert health education coaches. The specialty RN works collaboratively within the ACO, many times supporting a preferred provider. The specialty support encompasses case management, disease management, community resource coordination, information and data analyst, process management, discharge/transition planner, and health coach (Jones, 2011). As organizations integrate these roles, the skill set and knowledge brought to the table by specialty RNs will enhance and enrich the lives of the patients and providers they serve.

Diagnostic Testing

The role of a professional RN in a specialty care setting related to diagnostic testing takes on many forms. First, the RN is a content expert who helps the care team approach and holistically care for the patient. Next, the RN is responsible for understanding the provider's needs and the workflow and processes associated with the diagnostic test. They then communicate the patient's needs, ensuring that all members of the team are working as one fluid unit. Third, the RN plays the dynamic role of an educator. This includes education about the test; expectations related to pretest, intratest, and posttest; follow-up care and monitoring; and any medications or treatments dictated by the provider's plan of care. Finally, the specialty RN is responsible for communicating test results to patients and family members, other providers, and ancillary services as needed. Clear and concise communication regarding the outcomes of the diagnostic tests is the responsibility of the RN, thus creating an accurate account of the care provided.

Summary

Individuals are living longer with complex chronic health conditions and are challenged with navigating a fragmented healthcare system. These healthcare complexities often entail the individual visiting multiple specialty clinics, some of which may be short term and others that may include care to the end of life. In the specialty clinic setting, this requires an RN who is competent in a specific medical specialty as well as in longitudinal care across the care continuum. The longitudinal care plan allows the interprofessional team to communicate regarding the individual's healthcare needs, healthcare goals, and care plan across all settings.

Individuals often get lost in the system and fail to receive the appropriate follow-up, treatment, and management of their healthcare needs. The RN is a key partner to transforming how healthcare is delivered in the United States. By engaging individuals to partner with the interprofessional team and to be empowered to make decisions regarding their healthcare, the RN supports individuals to achieve their healthcare goals.

Case Study

Ms. Wise is a 58-year-old woman who presents to the orthopedic clinic after being seen in the ED for a fractured ankle 2 days prior, for which she is wearing a "boot." She is alone, sitting in a chair, appears pale, and has a dry cough. Vital signs are: blood pressure 160/90, heart rate 102, respiratory rate 22, pulse oximetry 95% on room air, and temp 97.8°F.

Ms. Wise reports no complications from her fracture, and her pain relief is adequate. She is able to mobilize as needed for daily activities. However, during her health history, she reports dyspnea when walking even before the injury, especially long distances, and has noticed that she wheezes. She has not been able to go upstairs to her bedroom because of her ankle and dyspnea. She feels fine at rest. Both her ankles are swollen, but she dismissed it because of fracture. She has been coughing a lot and feels tired. She is having nocturia, getting up two to three times during the night, and loss of appetite the last 2 days. She denies any previous heart problems or chest pain.

Her only medications are pain medications provided to her for ankle pain. Her physical examination reveals crackles in the bilateral upper lung fields and 3+ edema to her bilateral ankles.

(continued)

Case Study (*continued*)

She does not have a PCP since moving 2 years ago from another state and losing her insurance coverage. The provider orders x-ray of lungs, EKG, and labs, in addition to treatment for her ankle, and will determine disposition after results. The RN meets with Ms. Wise to discuss the care plan.

1. Because Ms. Wise has not been seen by a PCP for 2 years, what medical issues might be of concern given her age, vital signs, and symptoms? What potential diagnoses and referrals would the RN expect?
2. What follow-up questions might the RN ask related to the cause of the injury? These might include home safety issues or other causes for ankle injury.
3. What are the next steps in care coordination for the RN if Ms. Wise is discharged home? What questions would the RN ask regarding support systems? What other resources and referrals would be appropriate for her socioeconomic situation?

Key Points for Review

- The specialty care RN plays a key role empowering, encouraging, motivating, educating, and partnering with the individual to be engaged in all aspects of their care to achieve their healthcare goals.
- Specialty clinics may provide short-term care or specialty plus primary care for their individuals.
- RNs in specialty clinics need to have specific knowledge of their specialty, as well as the competencies to coordinate care and support care transition as needed.
- The RN is well positioned to coordinate the care for individuals living with multiple chronic health conditions as well as short-term specialty needs.

REFERENCES

Bhattacharya, R., Shen, C., & Sambamoorthi, U. (2014). Excess risk of chronic physical conditions associated with depression and anxiety. *BMC Psychiatry, 14*(10). http://www.biomedcentral.com/1471-244X/14/10

Brady, K. T., McCauley, J. L., & Back, S. E. (2016). Prescription opioid misuse, abuse, and treatment in the US: An update. *American Journal of Psychiatry, 173*(1):18–26. http://doi.org/10.1176/appi.ajp.2015.15020262

Cantin, A. M., Hart, D., Konstan, M. W., & Chmiel, J. F. (2015). Inflammation in cystic fibrosis lung disease: Pathogenesis and therapy. *Journal of Cystic Fibrosis, 14*(4), 419–430. http://doi.org/10.1016/j.jcf.2015.03.003

Centers for Disease Control and Prevention. (2017). *Chronic disease prevention and health promotion*. https://www.cdc.gov/chronicdisease/stats/index.htm

Cunningham, T. J., Ford, E. S., Croft, J. B., Merrick, M. T., Rolle, I. V., & Giles, W. H. (2014). Sex-specific relationships between adverse childhood experiences and chronic obstructive pulmonary disease in five states. *International Journal of Chronic Obstructive Pulmonary Disease, 9*, 1033–1043. http://doi.org/10.2147/COPD.S68226

Cystic Fibrosis Foundation. (2017). *About cystic fibrosis*. https://www.cff.org/What-is-CF/About-Cystic-Fibrosis/

Dunbar-Yaffe, R., Stitt, A., Lee, J. J., Mohamed, S., & Lee, D. S. (2015). Assessing risk and preventing 30-day readmissions in decompensated heart failure: Opportunity to intervene? *Current Heart Failure Reports, 12*, 309–317. http://doi.org/10.1007/s11897-015-0266-4

Funnell, M. M. (2016). Patient empowerment: What does it really mean? *Patient Education and Counseling, 99*(12), 1921–1922. http://doi.org/10.1016/j.pec.2016.10.010

Goodrich, D. E., Kilbourne, A. M., Nord, K. M., & Bauer, M. S. (2013). Mental health collaborative care and its role in primary care settings. *Current Psychiatry Reports, 15*(8), 2–17. http://doi.org/10.1007/s11920-013-0383-2

Haas, S. A., Swan, B. A., & Haynes, T. S. (2013). *Developing Ambulatory Care Registered Nurse Competencies for Care Coordination and Transition Management*. College of Nursing Faculty Papers & Presentations. Paper 61. https://jdc.jefferson.edu/nursfp/61

Haas, S. A., Swan, B. A., & Haynes, T. S. (2014). *Care coordination and transition management core curriculum*. American Academy of Ambulatory Care Nursing.

Huang, J. S., Terrones, L., Tompane, T., Dillon, L., Pian, M., Gottschalk, M., Norman, G. J., & Bartholomew, L. K. (2014). Preparing adolescents with chronic disease for transition to adult care: A technology program. *Pediatrics, 133*(6), e1639–e1646. http://doi.org/10.1542/peds.2013-2830

Humeniuk, R. E., Henry-Edwards, S., Ali, R. L., Poznyak, V., and Monteiro, M. (2010). The Alcohol, Smoking and Substance Involvement Screening Test (ASSIST): manual for use in primary care. Geneva, World Health Organization. https://www.who.int/management-of-substance-use/assist/

Institute of Medicine. (2001). *Crossing the quality chasm: A new health system for the 21st century*. National Academies Press.

Jones, P. (2011, April). *The nurse's role in accountable care [Briefing Paper]*. Milliman Healthcare Reform. https://us.milliman.com/-/media/milliman/importedfiles/uploadedfiles/insight/healthreform/nurses-role-accountable-care.ashx

Kent, F., Francis-Cracknell, A., McDonald, R., Newton, J. M., Keating, J. L., & Dodic, M. (2016). How do interprofessional student teams interact in a primary care clinic? A qualitative analysis using activity theory. *Advances in Health Sciences Education: Theory and Practice, 21*(4), 749–760. http://doi.org/10.1007/s10459-015-9663-4

National Cancer Institute. (2017). *What is cancer?* https://www.cancer.gov/about-cancer/understanding/what-is-cancer

Oncology Nursing Society. (2017). *Role of the oncology nurse navigator throughout the cancer trajectory*. https://www.ons.org/make-difference/advocacy-and-policy/position-statements/ONN

Powers, M. A., Bardsley, J., Cypress, M., Duker, P., Funnell, M. M., Fischl, A. H., Maryniuk, M. D., Siminerio, L., & Vivian, E. (2016). Diabetes self-management education and support in type 2 diabetes: A joint position statement of the American Diabetes Association, the American Association of Diabetes Educators, and the Academy of Nutrition and Dietetics. *Clinical Diabetes: A Publication of the American Diabetes Association, 34*(2), 70–80. http://doi.org/10.2337/diaclin.34.2.70

Roper, K. L., Ballard, J., Rankin, W., & Cardarelli, R. (2017). Systematic review of ambulatory transitional care management (TCM) visits on hospital 30-day readmission rates. *American Journal of Medical Quality, 32*(1), 19–26. http://doi.org/10.1177/1062860615615426

Selzer, M. L. (1971). The Michigan Alcoholism Screening Test: The quest for a new diagnostic instrument. *The American Journal of Psychiatry, 127*(12), 1653–1658. https://doi.org/10.1176/ajp.127.12.1653

World Health Organization. (2017). Depression. https://www.who.int/en/news-room/fact-sheets/detail/depression

Xu, J. Q., Murphy, S. L., Kochanek, K. D., Bastian, B., & Arias, E. (2018). Deaths: Final data for 2016. *National Vital Statistics Reports, 67*(5):1–76.

Yellowitz, J. A. (2016). Building the ideal interdisciplinary team to address oral health. *Generations, 40*(3), 60–65.

Yohannes, A. M., & Alexopoulos, G. S. (2014). Depression and anxiety in patients with COPD. *European Respiratory Review: An Official Journal of the European Respiratory Society, 23*(133), 345–349. http://doi.org/10.1183/09059180.00007813

13

Population Health: Ambulatory Care Focus

Cynthia L. Murray and Aleesa M. Mobley

PERSPECTIVES

"The ambulatory care nurse ensures optimally coordinated healthcare for individuals, families, communities and populations that improve holistic well-being."

Margaret F. Mastal, PhD, MSN, RN, founding member and past president, American Academy of Ambulatory Care Nursing.

LEARNING OBJECTIVES

Upon completion of this chapter, the reader will be able to:

1. Understand the principles of population-focused nursing practice.
2. Explain the social, economic, and policy influences leading to and having an impact on population-focused specialty practice nursing.
3. Understand the following roles as they relate to population-focused nursing: coordination/transition management, health promotion/disease prevention, risk stratification, chronic disease management, and telehealth.
4. In selected settings, describe the roles and functions of the registered nurse in clinics caring for those populations.

KEY TERMS

Correctional health
Occupational health
Population health
School-based healthcare
Veterans' health
Women's health

Overview

This chapter begins with an overview of population-focused practice and external influences on the field, including the impact of policy on ambulatory care populations in general. This is followed by a description of the general principles related to **population health** and the roles of the registered nurse (RN) that are common to all areas of these populations. The final section will address specific population practice settings.

In healthcare, the word "population" can have different meanings in different settings; an ambulatory care practice may consider all individuals to be that practice's population.

Alternately, a public health perspective may consider a population as being defined by a geographic area, or by a health challenge such as diabetes or hypertension. In health stratification terms, a population defined as "at risk" may have specific medical criteria, but vary widely in classifications such as age, socioeconomic status, or cultural background.

The populations in this chapter are classified by a common setting or background rather than by a medical condition. With the exception of **women's health**, the individuals in these populations are not defined by gender, age, or a specific medical history. However, their environment of school, work, or prison influences their healthcare delivery. Likewise, individuals classified under women's health or veterans care changes the lens through which nurses see their health needs.

This chapter focuses on the characteristics that give these care delivery sites a particular identity and how those characteristics affect healthcare for their individuals. This chapter is not meant to be a comprehensive list of populations that might fall into this category; rather, it is meant to provide some of the more common examples of populations that transcend categorization by age, sex, or disease classification, but instead are made up of individuals who share a common setting or history.

Population-Focused Practice in Ambulatory Care

Population health nursing focuses on the assessment needs and care management of all physical, biologic, social, psychological, and environmental influences on the health of a defined population. The RN in this field must stay current with new legislation, developing healthcare policy, payment and reimbursement models, as well as emerging trends in the provision of healthcare design and delivery in the populations managed. Compliance with governmental and accrediting bodies is essential for the RN functioning within any of these population-focused clinics.

A record of purposeful population-focused nursing practice in the United States dates back to the late 1800s with Clara Barton's care of Civil War soldiers and the formation of the American Red Cross; Lillian Wald's founding of the Henry Street Settlement for the sick and indigent of New York City; and the early 1900s when Margaret Sanger opened the nation's first birth control clinics. Public health nurses from the late 1800s to the early 1900s traveled at times by horseback to remote rural areas, such as the American Appalachia and the American Western frontier, providing nursing health clinics to those underserved populations where medical providers were nonexistent.

Population-focused nursing practice is characterized by defined settings where care is centralized to a distinct subset of the general population based on the patient's physical location, gender, eligibility for service, work setting, or connection with an education plan. Population-focused nursing practice has historically served and continues to serve both local and national public health initiatives. Within the provision of infectious disease surveillance and monitoring, nursing practice includes administering mass immunizations in various settings, thereby decreasing the risk of pandemics and improving the overall health of the nation. RNs interact with these populations through formal clinic facilities and mobile health units for face-to-face encounters or through telehealth and virtual technologies to interface with patients at a distance and as members of the interprofessional healthcare team.

The Patient Protection and Affordable Care Act (PPACA) enacted into law in 2010 aimed to reform healthcare by focusing on health promotion, disease prevention, and increased access through insurance reform. Healthcare received through specialized population-focused health clinics is essential to ensuring the expansion of access to primary care. The use of RNs in the coordination of healthcare services and evidence-based practice improves outcomes based on healthcare quality indicators and by ultimately decreasing the cost to the consumer (Melnyk et al., 2014).

Emerging Policies and Healthcare Agencies

Health policy addresses questions concerning how effectively healthcare is being delivered, how we want it to be delivered in the future, and available alternatives. The importance of health policy in the context of specific populations is related to the effect it has both on healthcare as a whole and on individual populations as indicated further. RNs have the potential to significantly impact health policy in their care of and advocacy for the individuals in their population group. A more detailed discussion about political influences on healthcare may be found in Chapter 3; however, a few points may be brought out as they relate to population health.

The policy process involves problem identification, process definition, analysis, assessment, evaluation and choice, implementation, planning, and finally feedback. "An unusual aspect of healthcare in the United States is the low level of influence that health professionals have on policy formation" (McLaughlin & McLaughlin, 2019, p. 74). It is, therefore, extremely important for RNs to remain vigilant in their advocacy for and adoption of new and emerging healthcare policies and practices. The RN is often the initial advocate or voice for a practice change that the nursing profession can then contribute to the policy process.

As an example of policy changes for population health, supported by nurse-led initiatives, Gurol-Urganci et al. (2013) demonstrated how the use of mobile technology could provide an inexpensive delivery method for healthcare appointment reminders. This type of research outcome was used to promote policies aimed at changes in practice as well as changes in technology encryption standards. The role of the RN in practice-oriented policy development and ambulatory care management is important for regulatory compliance and health promotion adherence, as private physician practices continue to shift from individual ownership to Accountable Care Organizations (ACOs) and larger health systems. The following are some of the many agencies involved in healthcare policy.

Agency for Healthcare Research and Quality

The Agency for Healthcare Research and Quality (AHRQ) houses the National Quality Measures Clearinghouse (NQMC), an agency that provides population-based structured, standardized summaries for use by practitioners, providers, health plans, and other health professionals (NQMC, 2013). The mission of the AHRQ is to produce evidence that can be used to make healthcare safer, higher quality, more accessible, equitable, and affordable. AHRQ also works with other Health and Human Services agencies to ensure that evidence is easily understood and disseminated.

Healthcare Effectiveness Data and Information Set

Healthcare Effectiveness Data and Information Set (HEDIS) is a healthcare quality tool made up of 94 performance measures across seven domains of care developed and maintained by the National Committee for Quality Assurance (NCQA, 2018). The tool is used by more than 90% of America's health plans.

Centers for Medicare and Medicaid Services

The Centers for Medicare and Medicaid Services (CMS, 2018) provides the minimum health and safety and Clinical Laboratory Improvement Amendments (CLIA) standards for provider and suppliers who desire reimbursement for their participation in CMS. As a federal insurance program, CMS providers and suppliers are subject to federal healthcare quality standards and certified by State Survey Agencies who have an agreement with the secretary of the Department of Health and Human Services.

Occupational Safety and Health Administration

The Occupational Safety and Health Administration (OSHA) is a branch of the U.S. Department of Labor. The mission of OSHA is based on the General Duty Clause of the OSH Act of 1970. The Act requires employers to provide a safe workplace, that is, an environment free of any known hazards that cause or have the potential to cause death or severe injury. The OSHA standards have particular importance for RNs working in **occupational health**.

The Joint Commission

The mission of The Joint Commission (TJC) is to evaluate healthcare organization and inspire those agencies to excel in the provision of high quality and value with the aim to continuously improve healthcare for the public. TJC is an independent, not-for-profit, nationally recognized organization that certifies nearly 21,000 healthcare organizations and programs within the United States, including primary care providers and nonsurgical settings such as medical group practices and community health centers (TJC, 2018).

Specialty Populations

Population health refers to assessing the healthcare needs of a specific group of people and making healthcare decisions based on the needs of that group. The term *population* encompasses "all persons within a defined subgroup with specific common characteristics, such as diagnosis, age group, or claims history" (American Academy of Ambulatory Care Nursing [AAACN], 2016, p. 34). Five population-focused healthcare clinics will be discussed in this chapter, including **veterans' health**, women's health, school-based health, corporate and occupational health, and **correctional health**. An individual's membership in the population served by these specialized clinics is based upon their eligibility for the healthcare service, that is, veteran's discharge status, female gender, primary education enrollment, work or disability status, and incarceration, respectively.

Roles of the Registered Nurse in Population-Focused Clinics

The needs, beliefs, and attitudes of a certain community or group of people are typically the focus of population health. Population-focused healthcare is driven by a need to control a specific condition or avoid a potential problem within a specific population. The RN practicing in a population-focused clinic functions in a variety of roles with the aim to develop evidence-based healthcare plans and health promotions for the intended population. In the ambulatory care setting, the RN acts as a key member of the interprofessional healthcare team and is actively involved in one or more of the following roles:

1. care coordination and transition management
2. health promotion
3. disease prevention
4. risk stratification
5. chronic disease management
6. telehealth or virtual care

Care Coordination and Transition Management

As the first-line communicator between external service providers, unlicensed clinic staff, certified medical assistants, and healthcare providers, in addition to patient educator, the RN has a principal role in care coordination. Care coordination is defined as: "The deliberate organization of patient care activities between two or more participants (including the patient) involved in a patient's care to facilitate the appropriate delivery of healthcare services. Organizing care involves the marshalling of personnel and other resources needed to carry out all required patient care activities and is often managed by the exchange of information among participants responsible for different aspects of care" (Haas et al., 2014, p. 189).

Transition management involves assisting in the provision of coordinated services between healthcare settings. The RN acts as an essential patient advocate during transition management. "Transition Management in the Context of Ambulatory Care RNs—the ongoing support of patients and their families over time as they navigate care and relationships among more than one provider and/or more than one health care setting and/or more than one health care service. The need for transition management is not determined by age, time, place, or health care condition, but rather by patients' and/or families' needs for support for ongoing, longitudinal individualized plans of care and follow up plans of care within the context of health care delivery" (Haas et al., 2014, p. 196).

Care coordination and transition management are discussed more fully in Chapter 7; however, it may be noted that the common principles of care coordination cross all boundaries of diverse populations.

Health Promotion

The purpose of health promotion is to engage and activate individuals and populations in health practices through appropriate education that reduces identified health risks with the goal to prevent disease (Kemppainen et al., 2013). The RN role as health educator is based on the fundamental concepts of health promotion and illness prevention, that is, "lifestyle coaching designed to promote optimal health, quality of life and wellbeing" (Saylor, 2004, p. 97).

In the context of population management, health promotion is especially fundamental to school and occupational health. In both areas, it is well recognized that success in education and work is dependent upon the health of the participant.

Disease Prevention

Disease prevention is characterized by those principles applied to treatment plans for individuals and populations with or without current risk factors for disease development. Disease prevention activities aim to protect patients and other members of the public from actual or potential health threats and their harmful consequences.

In all settings, healthy lifestyle coaching, health education, promotion of optimal dietary intake, daily physical activity, and appropriate medication management are utilized by population health-focused RNs to prevent disease from occurring. However, in occupational nursing, disease prevention activities may encompass addressing risks directly related to the workplace, such as exposure to cancer-producing chemicals or respiratory irritants.

Risk Stratification

Risk stratification, represented by a risk score (a standardized metric), demonstrates the likelihood of experiencing a particular outcome. Risk estimates may be made on individuals or populations. When risk calculation is performed on the number of individuals exposed, it is considered a population risk, expressed in units of expected increased cases per a specified time. When the total number of individuals exposed is not taken into consideration, it is a calculation of individual risk, expressed in units of incidence rate per a specified time.

Risk stratification is used to proactively identify and institute outreach to at-risk patients to initiate patient-centered care planning (Haas et al., 2014). A platform to stratify patients according to risk is "key" to the successful management of population health initiatives (Haller et al., 2015). The platform for care planning and risk calculation by the RN occurs through the utilization of health informatics within the electronic health record.

Chronic Disease Management

"Chronic disease management consists of an organized, proactive, patient centered approach to health care delivery that involves all members of a defined population who have a specific medical condition or a population with specific risk factors" (Norris et al., 2003, p. 477). Management of chronic disease may best be achieved with a designated team member with whom a patient can receive continuity of care through successive routine appointments.

Chronic disease care is essential in all areas of population health. The RNs caring for the veteran with heart disease, or the student with asthma, or supporting healthy choices for employees of a large company are all addressing the burden of chronic disease on the healthcare system.

Telehealth/Virtual Care

Telehealth and virtual care are forms of healthcare delivery that include health management and the coordination of care and services across distances. These services integrate electronic information and telecommunication technologies to increase access, improve outcomes, and contain or reduce costs associated with healthcare (Rutenberg & Greenberg, 2012).

Telehealth and virtual services allow the RN to use telephonic connections, secure messaging, e-mails, texts, and virtually interfaced encounters to interact remotely with patients. Information from these interactions and encounters can be obtained, stored, and forwarded using the virtual assessment platforms that provide high-quality digital images and video for interpretation and diagnosis at a later time by a remote provider or specialist. A more complete discussion on telehealth and virtual care is found in Chapter 9.

Population-Specific Settings

The scope and emphasis of population health is influenced by changing demographics. Population-specific growth affects the long-range planning of community health and medical facilities. Alterations in age-range composition, residential migration, the composition and size of racial/ethnic groups, industrial work environments, local environmental exposures, and changes in population densities require meaningful surveillance and local adaptations by healthcare facilities and providers.

The following sections address some of the most common population-based types of care in ambulatory nursing. Each section will include an overview of the population-specific care, purpose of the clinics, and the roles of the RN. As appropriate, additional areas such as virtual care or risk stratification will also be discussed.

Veterans' Health

Veterans' benefits and healthcare assistance can be traced to the war between the Pilgrims and the Pequot Indians in 1636. During that time, a law was passed stating that the colony would support disabled soldiers. Throughout its history, the mission of the Veterans Health Administration (VHA) has reflected the words of Abraham Lincoln, "to care for him who has borne the battle, his widow and orphan," that is, providing care for service-connected injuries caused by their military service. It was not until 1994 that the primary focus of that care became the prevention of disease and the promotion of health through the Veterans Administration's Primary Care Directive requiring all veteran healthcare facilities to provide primary care (Weber & Clark, 2016). To be eligible for healthcare at a VHA facility, a veteran must meet certain eligibility requirements including time in active service requirement and discharge status (Szymendera, 2016).

The VHA expanded primary care from the medical centers into the community by leasing or building Community-Based Outpatient Clinics (CBOCs) across the country to provide primary care, mental health services, women's health, specialist services, diagnostics, and treatment closer to the veteran population being served. The VHA is America's largest integrated healthcare system.

In 2010, the VHA launched the patient-aligned care team (PACT) model to transform the delivery of primary care by requiring the presence of an RN on each team to function in the role of a care manager (Veterans Administration, n.d.). The PACT consists of a medical provider; RN; clinical assistant in the form of a licensed practical nurse (LPN), licensed vocational nurse (LVN), or health technician (HT); and an administrative associate all managing the healthcare needs of a defined panel of patients as a team. Currently, nursing is the largest professional presence within the VHA. As such, the future of VHA nursing is poised to transform the delivery of healthcare from a medical model to a patient-centered model across the care continuum (Jabbarpour et al., 2017).

Purpose

The purpose of the Veterans Affairs (VA) healthcare system is to promote well-being and optimal health for eligible veterans at all stages of the life cycle. Veterans' clinics provide primary care, comprehensive women's healthcare, mental healthcare, specialty care services, health surveillance, immunizations, diagnostic testing for routine health screening, health education, disease prevention, health and wellness planning, minor injury care, illness care, and acute care referral.

Role of the Registered Nurse

Nurses are key members of the veterans' health PACT, providing acute, chronic, and ongoing care. The complexity of care that veterans require demands that nurses have specialized knowledge with strong assessment and clinical decision-making skills. The RN working in the VHA is a federal employee who, although licensed by a specific state, has the ability to move seamlessly between any of veteran's clinics within the United States and its territories.

Care Coordination

The care coordination role encompasses all existing health needs for the optimization of well-being including specialized care referrals. The transition management role follows the individual during the specialized care referral to a higher level care within the VHA or within the civilian community and ends with transitioning the individual back to the clinic. Because the VHA has a seamless electronic health record that follows the veteran across the United States and its territories, the RN has nearly immediate medical record access to care coordination and transition of care information.

Risk Stratification

The risk stratification role requires the RN to facilitate the interprofessional healthcare team's plan of care for individuals based on their assessed medical risks, potential for disease onset, or progression of disease within this specialized population. Veteran health risk assessments include military service exposure registries that identify potentials for the development of multiple disease conditions secondary to exposures, such as Agent Orange that may lead to chronic disease conditions including diabetes mellitus, prostate disease, thyroid disorders, integumentary diseases, cancers, and other sequelae.

Chronic Disease Management

In the chronic disease management role, the RN coordinates and aligns various activities of the interprofessional healthcare team in the complex management of chronic diseases that are of greater prevalence and specificity to active military action compared to the general civilian population, including blast injuries, traumatic brain injury, Agent Orange exposure, tobacco use, anxiety, depression, and posttraumatic stress disorder (PTSD). Chronic conditions are high among the veteran population, with the most common conditions being cardiovascular disease, diabetes, arthritis, and pain management. The goal of the RN in this role is to support optimal health, decrease exacerbation episodes, and increase optimal well-being.

Telehealth/Virtual Care

In most locations, telehealth in the VA system is a robust component of care. Providers have the ability to virtually connect with their individuals, sometimes with the collaboration of the RN who provides information and physical assessment through remote access. Other virtual care is provided through RN-led monitoring of chronic issues such as hypertension, diabetes, mental health, and cardiac rehabilitation.

Women's Health

The focus of women's health has evolved in the past century from one based primarily on reproductive healthcare to one encompassing the totality of healthcare concerns for women as a distinct population. Historically, the medical model was based on a presumption that men and women's health needs were the same, not focusing on the intrinsic biologic and physiologic differences in men and women's health (Hart, 2015). Women's health facilities provide comprehensive primary care services with a focus on women throughout their life span, across a continuum of care, and are no longer solely focused on reproductive needs. The RN has been an advocate of health promotion from puberty to end of life that is provided in the context of coordinated services for women (Association of Women's Health, Obstetric and Neonatal Nurses, 2014).

Purpose

The purpose of women's healthcare is to promote well-being and optimal health for women at all stages of the life cycle beginning with puberty. Women's health includes a range of focus areas (MedlinePlus, 2018), including:

1. Birth control, sexually transmitted infections (STIs), and gynecology
2. Breast cancer, ovarian cancer, and other female cancers
3. Mammography
4. Menopause and hormone therapy
5. Osteoporosis
6. Pregnancy and childbirth
7. Sexual health
8. Women and heart disease
9. Benign conditions affecting the function of the female reproductive organs

Women's health provides primary care, health surveillance, immunization, diagnostic testing for routine health screening, health education, disease prevention, health wellness planning, reproductive healthcare, and minor to acute urgent care needs as well as specialty referrals all based upon the physiologic and biologic needs of women (Office of Disease Prevention and Health Promotion, 2016).

Role of the Registered Nurse

The RN practicing in women's health provides acute, chronic, and ongoing nursing care. Nurses must possess strong assessment skills and a broad knowledge base of the complex medical conditions and health states that present and impact women differently than men. The RN who practices in this setting must be well versed in care coordination and care transitions as women's health may be the only source of primary care a patient has. In addition, RNs in this setting should be familiar with family planning options and be aware of their own beliefs and how they may have an impact on individual education and advisement.

Care Coordination

The care coordination role encompasses the comprehensive health needs of women with the goal to optimize their health status and the coordination of specialized care referrals. For specialty care, the RN transition management role in women's health may be concerned with engaging the patient with a primary care provider, who can then make any needed specialized care referral.

Health Promotion and Disease Prevention

The health promotion and disease prevention role in women's health necessitates that the RN possess the knowledge and skills for education and activities pertaining to general primary care health concerns as well as the specialized health concerns of women. Women's health is specifically concerned with issues such as breast care in the developing female; menstruation education; female sexual development; reproductive issues; pregnancy and pregnancy prevention; lactation and breast care for new mothers; breast, cervical, and ovarian cancer screenings; and perimenopausal health needs. The goal of health promotion in women's health is to optimize patient engagement in self-care activities and those health practices that prevent the disease development.

Chronic Disease Management

In the chronic disease management role, the RN aligns the activities of the interprofessional healthcare team in the complex management of chronic disease specific to women's health. Chronic disease management in women's health includes conditions such as polycystic ovarian disease, uterine fibroids, endometriosis, dysmenorrhea, infertility, and pelvic floor dysfunction. The goal of chronic disease management and focus is to minimize acute care needs throughout the life span and provide for optimum quality of life outcomes similar to all other populations.

School-Based Healthcare

Student health services provided during secondary education (vocational schools, colleges, and universities) are more similar to services obtained through a general primary care practice, whereas **school-based healthcare** provided within elementary school systems varies widely in the composition and complexity of the services provided. School-based healthcare may be provided in the form of a traveling school nurse with only an intermittent on-site presence to that of a fully operational health clinic staffed with providers, nurses, and ancillary support personnel.

There is no standard (local, state, or national) requirement to provide on-site healthcare outside of the current realm of an elementary school nurse for disease prevention, health surveillance, or acute care referral. The goal of increasing access to basic healthcare services for children, adolescents, and young adults in school settings is to focus on health promotion, illness and injury prevention, and mitigate the long-term effects of chronic disease following the completion of elementary education (Leroy et al., 2017).

Purpose

The purpose of the school-based clinic is to promote well-being and optimal health status throughout a student's formal primary education. Elementary school-based clinics involved in primary education span a variety of healthcare services including primary care, health surveillance, immunizations; diagnostic testing for routine health screening; medication management; health education, reproductive education and care, disease prevention; health and wellness planning; chronic disease management; minor injury and illness care; acute assessments; and referrals for health emergencies (Galemore et al., 2016).

Role of the Registered Nurse

The RN is the primary healthcare provider in many elementary educational settings and may be the sole clinician for multiple locations within a school district (National Association of School Nurses, 2016). The school-based RN is often the first-line provider of care for elementary students with chronic disease such as diabetes mellitus, asthma, anaphylaxis, and mental health conditions that require coordinated care to support their participation in the teaching and learning process and other school activities. The RN who practices in an elementary school-based setting must possess strong assessment skills and a broad knowledge base of complex medical conditions and health states that may impact student learning (American Academy of Pediatrics, 2016).

As the complexity of care increases in school systems overall, the role of the school nurse becomes increasingly important and challenging. Students with potentially severe issues with allergies, asthma, diabetes, and congenital complications may strain a system that depends on local funding. In many schools, this strain is exacerbated by location in a less-affluent district that cannot afford the needed level of RN support.

Care Coordination

The care coordination role of the RN in school-based health encompasses all existing health needs for the optimization of health and includes specialized care referrals. The RN may have access to on-site medical management for minor episodic exacerbations of chronic conditions or may be required to coordinate the health plan with a private pediatrician, primary care provider, or specialist depending on the comprehensive nature of the settings. The role of care coordination in elementary education settings includes responsibilities to:

1. communicate with families;
2. share information about observations regarding student behaviors;
3. obtain blood sugar test results;
4. promote student successes in self-management.

The RN is also involved in correlating recommendations for treatment and community resources (Centers for Disease Control and Prevention, 2018; McClanahan & Weismuller, 2015) that include:

1. Engaging families in the development and evaluation of the school and health and medical management plans
2. Facilitating referrals within the school and community
3. Relaying emotional support and parental education

The RN in the transitions management role follows the individual during the specialized care referral to a higher level care and ends with transitioning the individual back to the school-based health clinic.

Health Promotion and Disease Prevention

The health promotion and disease prevention role encompass all aspects of nursing care delivery to students in elementary education settings. According to research compiled for analysis by Maughan (2003), the role of the school nurse has a positive influence on the rate of absenteeism. The school nurse is in a position to promptly identify and address health needs in the management of episodic and chronic disease conditions.

The overarching goal is to use available resources in health education for the student, family, and caregiver to engage in self-care, health promotion for overall well-being, improved quality of life, and health practices that prevent the formation or spread of disease. All of these activities optimize the student's ability to participate in the teaching and learning environment and support academic success. In some settings, specific activities may include actual delivery of vaccinations and immunizations, or the school RN may implement and encourage healthy choices to slow the increase in obesity and type 2 diabetes mellitus in younger children.

Chronic Disease Management

In the role of chronic disease management, the RN aligns the activities of the interprofessional healthcare team's efforts in the complex management of chronic disease within the student health population. The RN also assesses the impact of the chronic disease on the student's educational environment and manages the health plan accordingly to optimize the student participation in teaching and learning activities. The RN must remain knowledgeable of common chronic conditions (asthma, seizure disorder, immobility, behaviors related to autism spectrum disorders), as well as common episodic illnesses of school-aged children including chicken pox, common cold, influenza (flu), impetigo, pink eye (conjunctivitis), head and body lice, ringworm (tinea corporis), scabies, strep throat, and pinworm.

Corporate and Occupational Health

Healthcare clinics have been a part of industrial America since the 1800s, focusing mainly on the care of injury and exposure to industrial hazards. In the early 1900s, rudimentary healthcare clinics were operated by local civilian hospitals and schools of medicine in industrial cities, and labor unions were beginning to negotiate health insurance plans. In the mid-1900s, the agricultural industry began to provide health services to migrant farm workers and their families in the form of traveling clinics composed of doctors and nurses for the treatment of communicable diseases.

On April 28, 1971, the OSHA (U.S. Department of Labor, 2016) was enacted by President Richard Nixon to standardize and mandate the reporting of occupational exposure, illness, injury, and death, as well as for the prevention of illness, injury, death, and disease in the workplace. According to the World Health Organization (2018), occupational health "deals with all aspects of health and safety in the workplace and has a strong focus on primary prevention of hazards. The health of the workers has several determinants, including risk factors at the workplace leading to cancers, accidents, musculoskeletal diseases, respiratory diseases, hearing loss, circulatory diseases, stress related disorders and communicable diseases and others" (para 1).

Corporate health and wellness programs offer discounts and incentives through health enhancement opportunities such as access to exercise equipment, fitness classes, and health and fitness consultations. Many large corporations offer on-site-managed or contracted health clinics that provide cost-effective comprehensive primary care services, management of chronic diseases, and preventive healthcare services (O'Keefe & Anderson, 2017). These clinics may also be under contract to manage the occupational health needs of the employee population. As the industrial work setting has changed in the 21st century, health surveillance, risk stratification, health promotion, disease prevention, chronic disease management, care coordination, and transition management have become major focuses of occupational and corporate health. The goal is to improve access to affordable healthcare and decrease overall health costs to both the employee and employer, and ideally increase the productivity by reducing lost work days because of illness, injury, and time off to access primary healthcare at distant locations (Bolnick et al., 2013; Caloyeras et al., 2014).

Purpose

The purpose of occupational health is to promote overall well-being and optimal health status of employees and disabled workers. According to McCauley and Peterman (2017), clinics provide primary care and occupational health management. These services may include:

1. certified driver's license (CDL)
2. disability exams
3. functional capacity exams
4. health surveillance
5. immunizations
6. diagnostic testing for routine health screening
7. health education
8. disease prevention
9. health and wellness planning
10. minor injury and illness care and acute assessment
11. urgent specialist referral

Role of the Registered Nurse

Nurses are primary healthcare providers in most corporate and occupational health facilities for acute, chronic, and ongoing care needs. The complexity and level of care that the workplace population requires demand specialized knowledge with strong assessment and clinical decision-making skills (Moore & Moore, 2014). The RN must have current and ongoing knowledge of occupational health and safety standards and the ability to promptly identify potential environmental health risks. It is part of the RN's responsibility to mitigate potential health hazards in the workplace.

Care Coordination

The care coordination role in the occupational health clinic is utilized in the treatment plan for employee work-related injuries, exposures, and illness needs for specialized care referrals. The RN in this type of setting may be more commonly involved with emergency medical service (EMS) interventions and life-saving first aid practices depending on the industrial nature of the workplace and injury potentials. The same coordination role is utilized in the corporate health clinic setting for the provision of industrial and primary care needs.

The transitions management role occurs throughout a treatment event for specialized care needs or higher level of care referral and ends with transitioning the individual back to the clinic for resumption of health oversight for occupational health clinics and primary care needs within the corporate health clinics.

Health Promotion and Disease Prevention

The goal of health promotion and disease prevention in occupational and corporate health is to optimize patient activation in self-care, health promotion, and health practices that prevent injury, the formation of disease, and spread of disease within the confines of the work environment. The RN utilizes available educational resources to improve the health literacy of the employees promoting safe work practices as well as healthy lifestyles.

In addition to general healthcare, the RN in occupational health is also required to develop and track health and safety education programs consistent with the industry needs and federal regulations. The RN ensures workers are compliant with personal protective equipment and other specialized gear used to prevent injuries in the workplace and reduce workers' compensation claims.

Risk Stratification

The risk stratification role requires the nurse to identify workplace hazards and surveillance of real or potential exposures to health hazards in the work environment. The RN facilitates the interprofessional healthcare team's plan of care for individuals based on their risk for medical events, potential for disease or progression of disease at the work site for occupational health clinics as well as general primary care health concerns for corporate health clinics.

Chronic Disease Management

In the chronic disease management role, the nurse facilitates the development of alternative work plans to assist employees affected by chronic illness. These illnesses may or may not be related to the workplace environment, but in either case they would have an impact on worker productivity. The RN coordinates the interprofessional healthcare team's activities in the complex management of chronic diseases within the work setting with the goal of optimal health and productivity of each individual.

Chronic diseases that are managed by the RN in the occupational clinic setting include repetitive motion ailments, pulmonary, cardiac, endocrine, dermatologic, cancers, and bloodborne pathogens. In corporate clinics where there may be less risk potential for occupational injury, the RN is even more likely to be focused on health promotion and wellness activities including weight loss and smoking cessation. As the focus in occupational health moves from one of avoiding injury to one of optimizing health, the role of RNs will also shift to that of an advocate for healthy lifestyles.

Correctional Health

The Prison-Industries Act of 1979 provided for the employment of inmate labor in state correctional institutions. Inmates could be involved in the private manufacturing of certain products under specific conditions. The Act set forth the requirements and responsibilities of the state commission of corrections, the governor, other officers and agencies regarding inmate employment and the distribution of products and proceeds from inmate employment.

The complexity of correctional health clinics falls in a range that encompasses both occupational health and primary care. Correctional health also resides within various settings (city and county jails, adult and juvenile detention centers, state and federal prisons) that have differing internal acute and chronic healthcare support systems.

To describe the primary distinctions between these facilities, jails are places of confinement under the jurisdiction of a local government (such as a county) for the confinement of persons awaiting trial or those convicted of minor crimes. Detention centers are allegedly short-term holding institutions for the housing of illegal immigrants, refugees, persons awaiting trial or sentencing, or youthful offenders. Prisons (also referred to as penitentiaries) are under state or federal jurisdiction for the confinement of persons convicted of serious crimes.

Correctional health clinics may be managed by a private contractor agreement with local civilian health centers or by independent contracted health services. They may have self-sustained health clinics managed internally that are linked together by state or federal jurisdictions to local law enforcement centers across the country. The clinics can be standalone units within a correctional facility without access to specialists or internal acute care treatment facilities, or they may be part of an ambulatory care service line within a correctional medical center. The populations (typically divided by gender) range in age from school-aged children to older individuals with acute and chronic health needs (Almost et al., 2013).

The RN working within the Federal Bureau of Prisons is duly appointed as a federal law enforcement officer. That is, the RN must pass an annual competence for requirements in legal activities, correctional functions, theory, and firearms proficiency in addition to a physical test that may include a variety of challenging activities.

Purpose

In 1976, the Supreme Court codified the "evolving standard of decency" for the provision of healthcare in correctional institutions (Macmadu & Rich, 2015). The purpose of the correctional health clinic is to prevent injury and promote well-being and the optimal health of incarcerated individuals. The clinic(s) may provide primary care, women's health, health surveillance, immunizations, diagnostic testing for routine health screening, health education, disease prevention, health wellness planning, pharmaceutical management, minor injury and illness care, and acute care assessment with referral.

In a federal corrections setting, healthcare is considered a constitutional right. This is based on the understanding that withholding care is considered cruel and unusual punishment, which is prohibited by the eighth amendment of the Constitution (Williams & Hevey, 2014).

Role of the Registered Nurse

The RN is the primary healthcare provider in most correctional settings for acute, chronic, and ongoing care needs (Schoenly, 2013). The complexity of care that the incarcerated population requires demands nurses to have specialized knowledge with strong assessment and clinical decision-making skills (American Nurses Association, 2013). The RN remains responsible and accountable to patient advocacy even when practicing in what may be a highly biased environment.

Care Coordination

The care coordination and transition management roles begin with the medical intake process for the newly incarcerated individual, devising the plan of care and coordination of all existing health needs. Transitions management will occur throughout the incarcerated event for specialized care needs and ending with transitioning the individual to a different level of correctional healthcare authority or transfer of the individual to a civilian healthcare provider upon release. "Over 95% of incarcerated individuals will eventually return to their communities, and their health problems and needs will often follow" (Macmuda & Rich, 2015, p. 1).

Health Promotion and Disease Prevention

The goal of health promotion and disease prevention is to optimize patient activation in self-care and health practices that prevent the formation of disease or spread of disease within the confines of the correctional environment. Communicable diseases are of great concern because of the close proximity of prison inmates to each other, as well as the prison employees. "Over half of state prisoners and up to 90% of jail detainees suffer from drug dependence, compared with only 2% of the general population. Hepatitis C is nine to 10 times more prevalent in correctional facilities than in communities" (Macmuda & Rich, 2015, p. 1).

Mental health disorders are often exacerbated during incarceration either because of changes in medication formulary or the stress of confinement. Major depression typically does not result in overt behavioral expressions, resulting in delayed diagnosis or misdiagnosis. Patients with mood disorders may cycle between episodes of depression and mania resulting in behavioral outbursts. "Over half of all inmates in jails and prisons suffer from drug dependence, and have a substantial need for evidence-based drug treatment" (Macmadu & Rich, 2015, p. 5). The RN must be alert to patients who may be incarcerated without divulging their substance abuse history, resulting in the need to manage acute withdrawal.

Chronic Disease Management

In the chronic disease management role, the RN coordinates all aspects of care to limit the progression or exacerbation of disease and aligns the activities of the interprofessional healthcare team and referrals to specialists in the complex management of chronic disease within the confines of the correctional health environment. Akin to the general aging population, chronic health conditions, such as diabetes, hypertension, and asthma, comprise a growing proportion of correctional healthcare needs.

"Female inmates have a greater burden of disease than their male counterparts" and "post-traumatic stress disorder is particularly common among incarcerated women, about a third of whom experienced physical abuse and a third of whom experienced sexual abuse prior to incarceration" (Macmadu & Rich, 2015, p. 3). Additionally, providing optimal prenatal care and delivery for pregnant incarcerated women is a challenge for the mothers as well as the infants who will be transferred to care outside of the prison (Baker, 2019).

Summary

From Florence Nightingale's tender care of the sick and indigent in the wards of England and the Crimea to the battlefields of the modern era, nursing has provided and continues to provide patient-focused healthcare in the environment of the population served. Nurses are key health agents in identifying, assessing, and addressing healthcare risks, reduction of medical errors, inefficiencies in delivery systems, and implementing measures to improve overall health outcomes (AAACN, 2017).

Ambulatory care nurses are at the forefront of patient care in diverse settings. As healthcare reform continues to evolve, the depth, breadth, and scope of practice for the RN in the ambulatory care setting become essential to the health and wellness of specialty populations.

Population health nursing focuses the needs of defined populations. Hence, the RN must remain current with state legislation, healthcare policies, issues of third-party payment, and reimbursement models as well as emerging technology trends in healthcare design and delivery.

The unique domain of the RN practice focuses on healthcare for individuals, families, groups, communities, and populations. Increased utilization of ambulatory care services (office visits, telehealth, and virtual platforms) outside of traditional acute care facilities emphasizes the advantages of RN interventions. The RN brings basic skilled nursing to the interprofessional team as well as the essential skills of ambulatory care coordination, health promotion, disease prevention, and chronic disease management—professional skills that utilize various forms of technology, risk stratification, patient education, and advocacy to improve overall health outcomes.

Case Study

A 41-year-old woman, wife of a retired veteran who has posttraumatic stress disorder (PTSD), is covered by her husband's health insurance, TriCare for Life, and presents to your ambulatory care clinic with a complaint of nausea, without vomiting or fever. She has transient dizziness and unexplained weight gain. Her history is significant for mild hypertension, hypothyroidism, attention deficit hyperactivity disorder (ADHD), and hyperlipidemia. She is taking an extended release combination of amphetamine and dextroamphetamine 20 mg daily, levothyroxine 50 µg daily, simvastatin 20 mg daily, and amlodipine 5 mg daily. She is seen and examined by the eligible provider on duty who orders a point-of-care pregnancy test that comes back positive and a referral to obstetrics/gynecology (OB/GYN). The patient and her husband live about 40 minutes from the ambulatory care clinic, but almost 2 hours from the nearest OB/GYN specialist who takes her insurance. The patient is noticeably distraught.

Discussion Questions

1. When performing medication review, what potential issues should the RN address for a pregnant individual?
2. What health promotion measures should be implemented for this individual with a high-risk pregnancy?
3. What questions might the RN ask this individual in order to assess her possible resources, needs, and state of mental health?

Key Points for Review

- RNs in population health must be aware of external influences on the populations they care for, including influences of policy, legislation, and regulations.
- Nurses work in a variety of population-focused specialty clinics, including veterans' health, women's health, school-based health, corporate and occupational health, and correctional health.
- The roles of population-focused specialty practice nursing include care coordination/transition management, health promotion/disease prevention, risk stratification, chronic disease management, and telehealth.
- The challenge for population-focused nursing today is to embrace leadership role opportunities in all ambulatory care settings by promoting and engaging nurses at all levels of professional practice as providers of care.

REFERENCES

Almost, J., Gifford, W. A., Doran, D., Ogilvie, L., Miller, C., Rose, D. N., & Squires, M. (2013). Correctional nursing: A study protocol to develop an educational intervention to optimize nursing practice in a unique context. *Implementation Science*, *8*(1), 71. https://doi.org/10.1186/1748-5908-8-71

American Academy of Ambulatory Care Nursing. (2016). *Scope and standards of practice for registered nurses in care coordination and transition management*. Author.

American Academy of Ambulatory Care Nursing. (2017). American Academy of Ambulatory Care Nursing position statement: The role of the registered nurse in ambulatory care. *Nursing Economics, 35*(1), 39–47.

American Academy of Pediatrics. (2016). Role of the school nurse in providing school health services council on school health. *Pediatrics, 137*(6), e20160852. https://doi.org/10.1542/peds.2016-0852

American Nurses Association. (2013). *Correctional nursing scope and standards of practice*. Author.

Association of Women's Health, Obstetric and Neonatal Nurses. (2014). Nursing care quality measurement (position statement). *Journal of Obstetric, Gynecologic & Neonatal Nursing*, *43*(1), 132–133.

Baker, B. (2019). Perinatal outcomes of incarcerated pregnant women: An integrative review. *Journal of Correctional Health Care, 25*(2), 92–104. https://doi.org/10.1177/1078345819832366.

Bolnick, H., Millard, F., & Dugas, J. P. (2013). Medical care savings from workplace wellness programs. What is a realistic savings potential*? Journal of Occupational and Environmental Medicine, 55*(1), 4–9. https://doi.org/10.1097/JOM.0b013e31827db98f

Caloyeras, J. P., Liu, H., Exum, E., Broderick, M., & Mattke, S. (2014). Managing manifest diseases, but not health risks, saved PepsiCo money over seven years. *Health Affairs, 33*(1), 124–131. https://doi.org/10.1377/hlthaff.2013.0625

Centers for Disease Control and Prevention. (2018). *Healthy schools: Care coordination*. https://www.cdc.gov/healthyschools/shs/care_coordination.htm

Center for Medicare and Medicaid Services. (2018). *Quality, safety & oversight—certification & compliance*. https://www.cms.gov/Medicare/Provider-Enrollment-and-Certification/CertificationandComplianc/index.html

Galemore, C. A., Bowlen, B., Combe, L. G., Ondeck, L., & Porter, J. (2016). Whole school, whole community, whole child-Calling school nurses to action. *NASN School Nurse*, *31*(4), 217–223. https://doi.org/10.1177942602X16651131

Gurol-Urganci, I., deJongh, T., Vodopivec-Jamsek, V., Atun, R., & Car, J. (2013). Mobile phone messaging reminders for attendance at healthcare. *Cochrane Database of Systematic Reviews, 2013(12)*, CD007458. https://doi.org/10.1002/14651858.CD007458.pub3

Haas, S. A., Swan, B. A., & Haynes, T. S. (Eds.). (2014). *Care coordination and transition management core curriculum*. American Academy of Ambulatory Care Nursing.

Haller, I. V., Johnson, B. P., VanScoy, M., VonRueden, C., Hitz, P. J., & Bianco, J. (2015). Risk stratification and population management: Validation of the patient stratification model based on electronic health record. *Journal of Patient-Centered Research and Reviews, 2*, 124–125. https://doi.org/10.17294/2330-0698.1160

Hart, T. (2015). *Health in the city: Race, poverty, and the negotiation of women's heath in New York City, 1915–1930*. New York University Press.

Jabbarpour, Y., DeMarchis, E., Bazemore, A., & Grundy, P. (2017). *The impact of primary care practice transformation on cost, quality, and utilization*. Patient Centered Primary Care Collaborative and the Robert Graham Center. https://www.pcpcc.org

Kemppainen, V., Tossavainen, K., & Turunen, H. (2013). Nurses' roles in health promotion practice: An integrative review. *Health Promotion International, 28*(4), 490–501. https://doi.org/10.1093/heapro/das034

Leroy, Z. C., Wallin, R., & Lee, S. (2017). The role of school services in addressing the needs of students with chronic health conditions: A systematic review. *The Journal of School Nursing, 33*(1), 64–72. https://doi.org/10.1177/1059840516678909

Macmuda, A., & Rich, J. D. (2015). Correctional health is community health. *Issues in Science and Technology, XXXII*(1), 10 pp. http://issues.org/32-1/correctionalhealth-is-community-health/

Maughan, E. (2003). The impact of school nursing on school performance: A research synthesis. *The Journal of School Nursing, 19*(3), 163–171. https://doi.org/10.1177/10598405030190030701

McCauley, L., & Peterman, K. (2017). The future of occupational health nursing in a changing health care system. *Workplace Health & Safety*, *65*(4), 168–173. https://doi.org/10.1177/2165079917699641.

McClanahan, R., & Weismuller, P. C. (2015). School nurses and care coordination for children with complex needs: An integrative review. *The Journal of School Nursing, 31*(1), 34–43. https://doi.org/10.1177/1059840514550484

McLaughlin, C. P., & McLaughlin, C. D. (2019). *Health policy analysis: An interdisciplinary approach* (3rd ed.). Jones & Bartlett Learning.

MedlinePlus. (2018). *Women's health*. U.S. National Library of Medicine. https://medlineplus.gov/ency/article/007458.htm

Melnyk, B. M., Gallagher-Ford, L., Long, L. E., & Fineout-Overholt, E. (2014). The establishment of evidence-based practice competencies for practicing Registered Nurses and Advanced Practice Nurses in real-world clinical settings: Proficiencies to improve healthcare quality, reliability, patient outcomes, and costs. *Worldviews on Evidence-Based Nursing*, *11*(1), 5–15. https://doi.org/10.1111/wvn.12021

Moore, P., & Moore, R. (Eds.). (2014). *Fundamentals of occupational and environmental health nursing: AAOHN Core Curriculum*. American Association of Occupational Health Nurses.

National Association of School Nurses. (2016). Framework for 21st century school nursing practice. *NASN School Nurse*, *31*(1), 45–53. https://doi.org/101177/1942602x15618644

National Committee for Quality Assurance. (2018). *HEDIS and quality compass*. http://www.ncqa.org/hedis-quality-measurement/what-is-hedis

National Quality Measures Clearinghouse. (2013). *Mission*. Agency for Healthcare Research and Quality. http://www.ahrq.gov/cpi/about/otherwebsites/qualitymeasures.ahrq.gov/index.html

Norris, S. L., Glasgow, R. E., Engelgau, M. M., O'Connor, P. J., & McCulloch, D. (2003). Chronic disease management: A definition and systematic approach to component interventions. *Disease Management and Health Outcomes, 11*(8), 477–488. https://doi.org/10.2165/00115677-200311080-00001

Office of Disease Prevention and Health Promotion. (2016). *Access to health services*. https://www.healthypeople.gov/2020/topics-objectives/topic/Access-to-Health-Services

O'Keefe, L. C., & Anderson, F. (2017). Benefits of on-site clinics. *The Online Journal of Issues in Nursing, 22*(2). https://doi.org/10.3912/OJIN.Vol22No02PPT51

Rutenberg, C., & Greenberg, M. E. (2012). *The art and science of telephone triage: How to practice nursing over the phone*. Telephone Triage Consulting, Inc.

Saylor, C. (2004). The circle of health: A health definition model. *Journal of Holistic Nursing, 22*(2), 97–115. https://doi.org/10.1177/0898010104264775

Schoenly, L. (2013). Context of correctional nursing. In L. Schoenly & C. M. Knox (Eds.), *Essentials of Correctional Nursing* (pp. 1–18). Springer.

Szymendera, S. D. (2016). *Who is a "veteran"?—Basic eligibility for veterans' benefits*. Congressional Research Service report 7-5700. https://www.fas.org/sgp/crs/misc/R42324.pdf

The Joint Commission. (2018). *Ambulatory health care*. https://www.jointcommission.org/accreditation/ambulatory_healthcare.aspx

U.S. Department of Labor. (2016). *All about OSHA. Occupational Safety and Health Administration* 3302-11R 2016. www.osha.gov/Publications/all_about_OSHA.pdf

Veterans Administration. (n.d.). *Your VA primary care provider and PACT team*. https://www.va.gov/health-care/about-va-health-benefits/your-care-team/

Weber, J., & Clark, A. (2016). Legislative: Providing veteran-specific healthcare. *Online Journal of Issues in Nursing, 21*(2), 9. https://doi.org/10.3912/OJIN.Vol21No02LegCol01

Williams, T., & Heavey, E. (2014). How to meet the challenges of correctional nursing. *Nursing, 44*(1), 51–54. https://doi.org/10.1097/01.NURSE.0000438716.50840.04

World Health Organization. (2018). *Health topics: Occupational health*. http://www.who.int/topics/occupational_health/en/

14

Underserved Populations and Cultural Considerations

Helen Baker and Debra L. Cox

PERSPECTIVES

"You are not here to teach me how to fish. I already know how to fish. You just fish differently. Let us not waste time on who fishes better but learn from each other what we can, so that we might both grow in the best ways possible. Let's fish together."

Source unknown.

LEARNING OBJECTIVES

Upon completion of this chapter, the reader will be able to:

1. Identify the social, economic, research, and policy influences impacting disparities in healthcare.
2. Describe the challenges and opportunities of rural ambulatory care nursing practice and nursing care of those seeking refuge and immigrants.
3. Describe the health challenges specific to individuals experiencing homelessness.
4. Discuss the issues and nursing approach to care of Native American and Alaskan Native individuals.
5. Understand the concepts that prepare ambulatory nurses to demonstrate cultural humility when caring for populations of different cultures.
6. Apply culturally sensitive care to individuals from a variety of backgrounds.

KEY TERMS

Cultural humility
Health disparities
Health equity
Immigrants
Native American and Alaska Native
Refugees
Rural communities
Social determinants of health

History and Overview

The art of nursing care across cultures is ageless and the science of multicultural nursing is a foundational competency for all nurses across the continuum of care. Providing care to individuals from diverse backgrounds and cultures is complex and presents challenges to both novice and expert nurses. However, if healthcare is to be delivered well to a growing pluralistic society, learning **cultural humility** and recognizing and addressing healthcare disparities are critical. Political and social influences on health and healthcare have been discussed from a policy and economic perspective in Chapter 3; the focus of this chapter is on the nursing response to these challenges. Toward that goal, transcultural assessments and tools are discussed that can prepare nurses to provide culturally humble care in the ambulatory setting.

Multicultural health is a concept that has gained increasing focus across the country and the world, as cultural background is now recognized as a critical component influencing the health and well-being of individuals and populations. A summary of influences on health is provided in Box 14.1.

Healthcare professionals must consider individuals, families, and populations within a cultural context to ensure that effective services can be provided in a manner that respects the individual's lifestyle and approach to maintaining health. Healthcare professionals must also be aware of their own cultural context and biases when providing care to others. To begin to address multicultural health issues, assessments, and interventions, it is helpful to understand the history, policy, and regulatory environments that have an impact on the role that culture plays in health and wellness.

On the national level, legislation from as early as 1946 to the passage of the Affordable Care Act (ACA) has addressed issues of healthcare disparity and discrimination. In 1946, the Hill-Burton Act ensured that hospitals receiving federal construction funds could not discriminate based on race, color, national origin, or creed and must provide some amount of free or subsidized care for a portion of their indigent individuals. By the time hospital construction through Hill-Burton funds was coming to an end, the Civil Rights Act of 1964 was passed, which prohibited any federally funded programs from discriminating on the basis of race, color, or national origin. This was followed in 1965 by the passage of the bill leading to Medicare and Medicaid.

Healthcare laws such as the Patient Protection and ACA and the option of expanded Medicaid were designed to provide greater access to all populations; however, individual state laws and ongoing national debates have a significant impact on the implementation of national policy. It is important for ambulatory care registered nurses (RNs) to understand both state and national policies and political influences on healthcare access because these policies have a direct impact on the ability of ambulatory care individuals to adhere to treatment regimens.

In addition to addressing the needs of those who face healthcare disparities because of race or income, the U.S. health system also has come to recognize that those from different cultures also face challenges and obstacles. The Health and Human Services Office of Minority Health (OMH) has developed national standards for Culturally and Linguistically Appropriate Services in Health Care (CLAS). According to the U.S. Department of Health and Human Services (USDHHS), the CLAS standards are "intended to promote **health equity**, improve quality, and help eliminate healthcare disparities by providing a blueprint for individuals and health care organizations to implement culturally and linguistically appropriate services" (U.S. Department of Health and Human Services, Office of Minority Health, n.d.). The Joint Commission and Centers for Medicare and Medicaid Services (CMS) have standards requiring that providers of healthcare show respect for individuals' cultural and spiritual beliefs and

BOX 14.1 Influences on Health

"Culture affects people's perception of their health and illness, how they pursue and adhere to treatment, their health behaviors, beliefs about why people become ill, how symptoms and concerns about problems are expressed, what is considered to be a health problem and ways to maintain and restore health."

Note. Ritter, L. A., & Graham, D. H. (2017). *Multicultural health*. Jones and Bartlett.

preferences to ensure highest safety and quality care delivery. To assist in this effort, researchers have developed conceptual care models and tools for cultural assessment and interventions for diverse individual and population needs based on the science of transcultural nursing and supported by changes in societal mores, legislation, and policy. Some of these tools are described further, in discussions of specific populations.

Health Equity and Disparities

To address health equity, healthcare professionals must understand the contributing forces toward disparities in healthcare across the country. The identification of **health disparities** is a major assessment factor when addressing both short-term and long-term plans of care in the ambulatory care setting. Health disparities "are differences in health outcomes and their determinants between segments of the population, as defined by social, demographic, environmental and geographic attributes" (Centers for Disease Control and Prevention, Division of Community Health, 2013, p. 4). Social, economic, and policy factors, as well as access to and the delivery of healthcare all contribute to health disparities. Disparities are most often identified along racial and ethnic lines, but may also be based on characteristics such as sex, income, education, residence (rural vs. urban), sexual orientation, body habitus, and many others.

The Healthy People 2020 report launched by the USDHHS identifies the elimination of health disparities as critical for the achievement of maximum health across the nation. The four goals are:

1. Attain high-quality, longer lives free of preventable disease, disability, injury, and premature death.
2. Achieve health equity, eliminate disparities, and improve the health of all groups.
3. Create social and physical environments that promote good health for all.
4. Promote quality of life, healthy development, and healthy behaviors across all life stages (U.S. Department of Health and Human Services, 2014).

Social determinants of health (SDOH) are the conditions in which people are born, grow, live, work, and age (World Health Organization [WHO], 2016). These conditions—socioeconomic position, residential location, environmental living conditions, occupational risks and exposures, health risk and health-seeking behaviors, along with limited access to medical care—contribute to disparities in health status and health outcomes for certain individuals and groups (Braveman, 2014).

Differences in health outcomes are closely connected to the degrees of social disadvantage. Many living conditions can contribute to adverse health outcomes. For instance, individuals may lack the economic resources to purchase goods and services, or reside in neighborhoods with high concentrations of poverty and crime. Even limited green space and a lack of neighborhood grocery stores create risk for adverse health outcomes. The resources needed for health are not just limited to access to medical care but also include health-promoting physical and social conditions in homes, neighborhoods, and workplaces (Braveman, 2014).

Safe neighborhoods and schools, education and health literacy, ample access to healthy food, and various other social supports underpin population health. Without making progress in addressing the SDOH, it is difficult to make real progress in addressing healthcare costs, which is now understood as a fundamental basis for achieving true parity in healthcare. These vulnerable or at-risk populations discussed in this chapter include individuals experiencing homelessness, **immigrants** or individuals from another country, those seeking refuge, and migrant workers, as well as underresourced populations in rural areas or Indian reservations.

The healthcare industry increasingly recognizes that improvements in health and health equity will only be possible after addressing SDOH, including socioeconomic status, education, neighborhood and physical environment, social support networks, and access to healthcare. For these reasons, healthcare organizations are becoming actively involved in community and public health partnerships to address gaps in social determinants, with positive results (Peeler, 2019).

In addition to direct care and education for individuals negatively affected by SDOH, RNs also may have an impact on gaps in care through their advocacy, both on an individual level and in the policy arena at the local and national levels. Nursing advocacy is discussed in more detail in Chapter 8.

Assessment of Health Risks

Assessment of SDOH and socioeconomic factors, such as access to transportation, health literacy, food access, and housing stability, can make the difference between an individual successfully avoiding or managing a chronic disease, or becoming a victim to it. Housing and transportation issues, language and literacy barriers, lack of social support, and other nonclinical challenges frequently confound high-risk individual care plans in the ambulatory care setting.

Standard screening tools for various identified SDOH have been available for many years; however, the use of these tools is still debated, for a variety of reasons (Andermann, 2018; Garg et al., 2016). These include provider reluctance because of time constraints, lack of knowledge or comfort in using the tools, and feeling uncertain as to what they could do with the information. Additionally, some believed that it was inappropriate to screen on an individual level for issues that are best addressed at a societal/political level or even that it was unethical to screen if the provider was unable to offer referral or help for identified problems.

Although arguments may exist against formal screening for the impact of SDOH, there is value for individual assessment of these risks even without use of a specific screening tool. Conducting in-depth psychosocial risk assessments for high-risk individuals enables the nurse and care team members to develop a better understanding of the individual's environment outside of the clinic, which in turn allows for proper customization of the care plan, as well as providing the level and type of support required. Housing security is a critical health issue for vulnerable populations; access to affordable housing is a key component to improve the health of communities and advance the economic, social, and environmental conditions for health. Food security and transportation also are key environmental impacts that must be included in risk assessments.

The informal screening of individuals, including a thorough assessment of the individual's current status in terms of housing, food, transportation, and safety, is the most important data to collect. This is especially true in a setting that cares primarily for individuals who are experiencing homelessness and/or have limited resources. SDOH information can provide a springboard for conversation with the RN and an opportunity for the RN to offer resources and referrals.

Mental Health and Addiction Considerations

In recent years, there has been a growing understanding that mental health issues are a significant challenge for all populations. Addictions, including chemicals, gambling, sexual behavior, and opioid use, are a growing societal problem and a leading cause of death. A full discussion of the mental health and addiction implications for both overall health and healthcare disparities is beyond the scope of this chapter. However, the following brief discussion will touch on screening and general ambulatory care considerations for these pervasive and important issues that have a significant impact on the SDOH of individuals suffering from mental health or addiction concerns.

There are a number of screening tools to assist in identification of mental health and addiction risk. The Patient Health Questionnaire with nine and two questions (PHQ9 or PHQ2) is a tool frequently used to screen for depression; this and other depression screening tools support early detection of potential mental health issues (Howe, 2020). A variety of tools are also available for substance abuse screening, including the Clinical Opiate Withdrawal Scale (COWS) (Wesson & Ling, 2003), and tools from the National Institute on Drug Abuse and the American Society of Addiction Medicine (AMSAM, n.d.; National Institute on Drug Abuse, n.d.). AMSAM also provides tools and criteria to assess for and help determine treatment type and location for substance use disorder. These tools may be used by other members of the healthcare team as well as RNs; for instance, mental health assessments for trauma and torture are administered by a licensed mental health professional utilizing standardized tools and processes.

Once risks have been identified, interventions may take a variety of forms and levels of intensity and will include all members of the healthcare team for pharmacologic, behavioral, and lifestyle changes. Principles of behavior change and individual education are covered in more detail in Chapter 7. However, some interventions that have demonstrated effectiveness for individuals who are underserved and/or experiencing homelessness include the Community Resiliency Model (Figure 14.1) for trauma-informed care (Trauma Resource Center, n.d.) and resources through the Substance Abuse and Mental Health Services Administration (SAMHSA, n.d.).

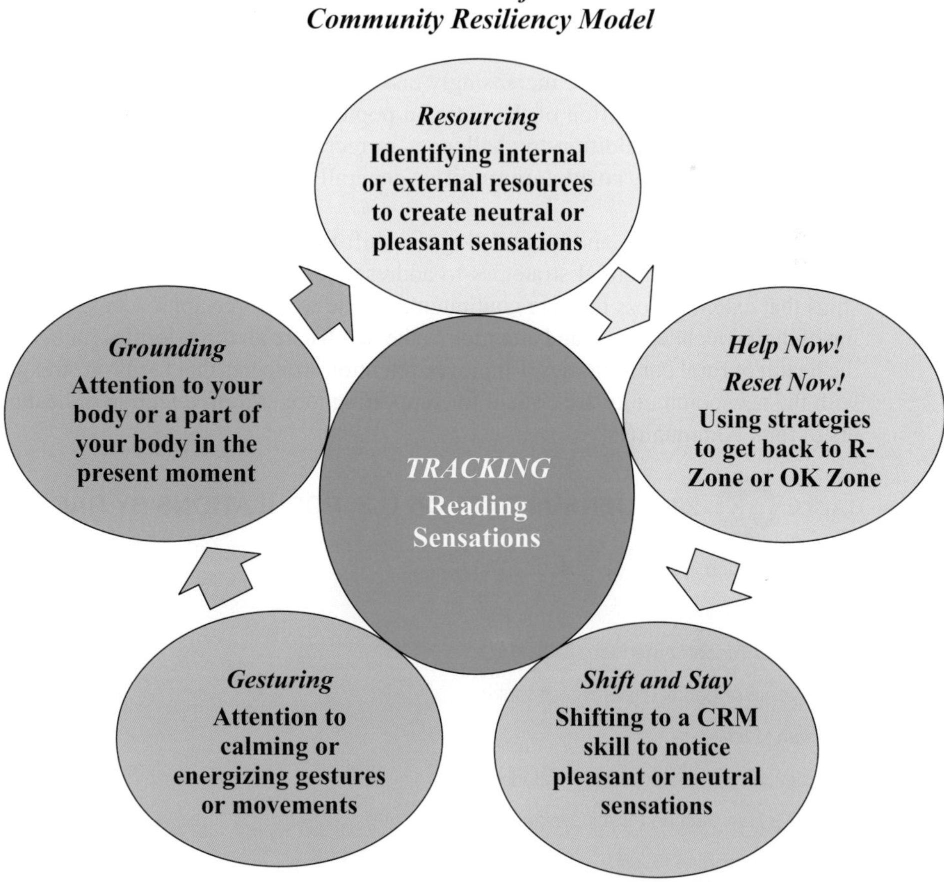
The Skills of the
Community Resiliency Model
Resourcing
Identifying internal or external resources to create neutral or pleasant sensations
Help Now!
Reset Now!
Using strategies to get back to R-Zone or OK Zone
Shift and Stay
Shifting to a CRM skill to notice pleasant or neutral sensations
Gesturing
Attention to calming or energizing gestures or movements
Grounding
Attention to your body or a part of your body in the present moment
TRACKING
Reading Sensations

FIGURE 14.1 Community resiliency model skills (Trauma Resource Institute).

Diversity in Research

For many individuals, clinical trials offer a chance to benefit from promising new treatments not yet available in their healthcare provider's office. However, not all people have the same access to these research study opportunities. Groups such as racial minorities, older individuals, and those with low income are less likely than others to participate in clinical trials, according to government agencies. For example, in 2016 racial and ethnic minority groups represented 25% of drug trial participants in the United States (U.S. Food and Drug Administration, n.d.). However, minority groups (excluding Hispanic) make up about 27% of the population and about 16% of any race identifying as Hispanic, according to the 2010 U.S. census (Humes et al., 2011). These data are summarized in Table 14.1.

Lack of diversity in drug trials means that research findings and subsequent treatment regimens may not apply to all members of the population. Health disparities research seeks to understand how disparities in treatment response arise and how they may occur at multiple levels, ranging from molecular mechanisms to population-level investigations. It may be argued that differences in treatment effectiveness may be more of a socioeconomic and societal problem than one of biologic response to medication. This argument can only be resolved through meticulous and ongoing research with the greatest possible diversity of individuals. Ultimately, the goal is to determine ways to address and resolve any discrepancies between populations and to tailor treatment appropriately.

Rural Communities

Rural healthcare leaders are increasingly tasked with the responsibility of providing health access to a large proportion of the national population with a small percentage of the provider workforce. In addition to challenges in recruitment and retention of individuals for community practices, **rural communities** generally also have limited individual access to specialty services.

Resource utilization and accelerating the shift to a more integrated and sustainable rural health system are potential strategies to address these problems. Additionally, new partnerships that extend across the care continuum, unique workforce approaches, effective leveraging of digital technologies, and attention to the SDOH are all top priorities for better managing the health of rural communities. Employee retention strategies that focus on strengthening ties with the new community are critical for supporting longer term retention of healthcare workers in rural communities.

TABLE 14.1 **2010 CENSUS DATA ON U.S. POPULATIONS BY RACE**

Total population in 2010 census: 308,745,538
White (72.4%)
Black or African American (12.6%)
Hispanic or Latinx (16% of all population)
Asian (4.8%)
American Indian and Alaska Native (0.9%)
Native Hawaiian and Pacific Islander (0.2%)
Some other race (6.2%)

Note. Data from Humes, K. R., Jones, N. A., & Ramirez, R. R. (2011). *Overview of race and Hispanic origin: 2010: 2010 census briefs.* www.census.gov/prod/cen2010/briefs/c2010br-02.pdf

Nursing Considerations

Professional nursing practice in rural settings has both challenges and rewards. Ambulatory care nurses identify a broad range of assessment and technical nursing skills that are applied across the individual's life span in small rural clinics and critical access hospitals; some nurses serve in both individual and ambulatory roles. Knight et al. (2016) identified the current conceptualized practice of ambulatory rural nurses as problematic in that it does not recognize the intangible complexities of this environment or the "mastery of ambiguity" that is necessary for success in this challenging clinical arena. A common challenge in rural or areas of small population is that ambulatory care nurses in these settings may be caring for known community members, friends, and families. Additionally, they are seeking to identify creative resources in shrinking rural communities with dwindling resources.

Rural nurses identify a number of strategies as being effective in sustaining them in their practice in an environment with competing stakeholder needs and limited resources and options for care. These include identification of rural policy that supports their practice, education opportunities for their growth, supportive recruitment and retention strategies, and clinical governance over practice (Knight et al., 2016).

Nurses and care teams are increasingly relying on connected care technologies to bridge the distance between individuals and other providers. Toward that goal, Medicare regulatory support is growing for enhancement of telemedicine or virtual healthcare reimbursements to address resource and distance challenges in the rural healthcare setting. Video conferencing is an effective support strategy for both individuals and professional staff. Individuals can connect with online communities, receive education and support in new forums, as well as receive specialty consultation while still located in a rural office setting. Nurses identify access to both education and support through online conferences and video as critical to their skill building and confidence in rural practices.

Innovative models of care are emerging to better support the current realities of rural healthcare including nurse-practitioner- and physician-assistant-led teams in rural locations that rely on physician support through video telemedicine services. Additionally, community paramedic programs are offering a new model of care capitalizing on their mobility and skill set. In these programs, sometimes known as mobile integrated healthcare or community paramedicine, emergency medical services personnel make follow-up visits to high-risk individuals in order to avoid hospitalizations and address health issues before they become major problems (Choi et al., 2016).

Care Coordination and Transition Management (CCTM) RNs in primary care also are participating in home visits as they develop longitudinal plans of care for diverse individual populations. The goal of the CCTM RN is to support individuals in the identification of their health needs, assist in preventing costly and unnecessary emergency room visits, decrease hospitalizations, and prevent hospital readmissions. In a rural setting, the CCTM RN incorporates an assessment of social determinants of care for complex individuals and partners with community resources to activate services for individuals striving to improve their health. Care coordinators in rural settings have unique opportunities to provide care throughout the life span.

Individuals Seeking Refuge and Immigrants

Foreign-born individuals make up 13.5% of the U.S. population, with most (76%) of the individuals living legally in the country. The majority of immigrants or individuals from another country in the United States arrive from Mexico, followed by China, India, the Philippines, and El Salvador. Just under half of the nation's immigrants live in three states: California, Texas, and New York. Educational level for individuals from another country varies by origin location. Individuals from Mexico and Central American have lower levels of education than the general U.S. population, whereas individuals from South and East Asia, Europe, Canada, the Middle East, and sub-Saharan Africa are more likely than U.S.-born residents to have a bachelor's or advanced degree (Lopez et al., 2018). Understanding key terms related to migration may help in the discussion of this topic (Box 14.2).

Migrants, those seeking refuge, and displaced persons can be some of the most vulnerable populations in the world. Individuals migrate for numerous reasons, including conflict, poverty, natural and man-made disasters, inequality, globalization, and lack of access to work. This population can be exposed to discrimination, violence, exploitation, detention, limited access to education, human trafficking, malnutrition, and limited access to preventative and/or essential healthcare services (International Council of Nurses, 2018). Children, pregnant individuals, the elderly, and individuals with physical and intellectual disabilities and victims of torture can be at additional risk for challenges during the migration journey.

BOX 14.2 Key Migration Terms

Asylum seeker: A person who seeks safety from persecution or serious harm in a country other than their own and awaits a decision on the application for refugee status under relevant international and national instruments. In case of a negative decision, the person must leave the country and may be expelled, as may any non-national in an irregular or unlawful situation, unless permission to stay is provided on humanitarian or other related grounds.

Emigration: The act of departing or exiting from one state with a view to settling in another.

Forced migration: A migratory movement in which an element of coercion exists, including threats to life and livelihood, whether arising from natural or man-made causes (eg, movements of those seeking safety from their country and internally displaced persons as well as people displaced by natural or environmental disasters, chemical or nuclear disasters, famine, or development projects).

Immigration: A process by which non-nationals move into a country for the purpose of settlement.

Internally Displaced Person: Persons or groups of persons who have been forced or obliged to flee or to leave their homes or places of habitual residence, in particular as a result of or in order to avoid the effects of armed conflict, situations of generalized violence, violations of human rights or natural or human-made disasters, and who have not crossed an internationally recognized State border (United Nations Guiding Principles on Internal Displacement, 2004).

Migrant: The International Organization for Migration (IOM) defines a migrant as any person who is moving or has moved across an international border or within a State away from their habitual place of residence, regardless of (1) the person's legal status, (2) whether the movement is voluntary or involuntary, (3) what the causes for the movement are, or (4) what the length of the stay is (IOM, n.d.). IOM concerns itself with migrants and migration-related issues and, in agreement with relevant States, with migrants who are in need of international migration services.

Refugee: An individual who, "owing to a well-founded fear of persecution for reasons of race, religion, nationality, membership of a particular social group or political opinions, is outside the country of his nationality and is unable or, owing to such fear, is unwilling to avail himself of the protection of that country" (UNHCR The UN Refugee Agency, n.d.) (the Convention relating to the Status of Refugees, Art. 1A(2), 1951 as modified by the 1967 Protocol). In addition to the refugee definition in the 1951 Refugee Convention, Art. 1(2), 1969, the Organization of African Unity (OAU) Convention defines a refugee as any person compelled to leave their country "owing to external aggression, occupation, foreign domination or events seriously disturbing public order in either part or the whole of his country or origin or nationality" (UNHCR The UN Refugee Agency, 1969). Similarly, the 1984 Cartagena Declaration states that refugees also include persons who flee their country "because their lives, security or freedom have been threatened by generalised violence, foreign aggression, internal conflicts, massive violations of human rights or other circumstances which have seriously disturbed public order" (UNHCR The UN Refugee Agency, 1984).

Nursing Considerations

The American Nurses Association House of Delegates in 2010 held the position that healthcare is a basic human right and that all individuals who reside in the United States should have access to healthcare, regardless of their immigration status (American Nurses Association, 2010). This position is shared by the International Council of Nurses, which outlines that the individual nurse should:

- develop and enhance their own cultural competence and ensure it is incorporated into care delivery for all individual groups.
- empower and support migrants, **refugees**, and displaced peoples to navigate the health system of their host country including being able to identify and access available healthcare services.
- provide ethical, respectful, culturally sensitive, and dignified care to migrants, those seeking refuge, and those who are experiencing displacement and their families, that acknowledges the interconnectedness of their physical, psychosocial, spiritual, cultural, and social needs and challenges.
- engage in research to contribute to evidence that expands understanding of issues that relate to the physical, psychosocial, spiritual, cultural, and social needs of migrants, refugees, and displaced peoples and that can improve healthcare service delivery and support the development of consistent and comparable measures to facilitate this research (International Council of Nurses, 2018).

Most individuals from another country coming to the United States have historically been healthy and young. Research studies show that the age of immigration has a great impact on health and mortality; for example, one study found that when individuals from another country enter the United States after the age of 24 years, they are more likely to keep their diet and health practices of their home countries, which can provide protection from obesity, hypertension, and cardiovascular disease seen in the U.S. population (Holmes et al., 2015). However, individuals from another country are less likely to have all of their immunizations and can be more likely to have infectious diseases such as hepatitis B, tuberculosis, and parasites (Cesario, 2017). Psychological issues, such as posttraumatic stress disorder and depression, also may be present because of psychological trauma (Bertelsen et al., 2018).

When individuals seeking refuge first arrive in the United States, community health nurses are often involved in their initial assessment, which includes preliminary health screening including screening for tuberculosis. They will then have a medical evaluation with a primary care physician who will assess their immunizations. When those seeking refuge are resettled in the United States, they receive short-term health insurance called Refugee Medial Assistance, which is available for up to 8 months. Some refugees may be eligible for Medicaid or Children's Health Insurance Programs for several years. When this temporary health assistance is over, the refugee is expected to receive health insurance through their employment or on the ACA marketplace insurance exchanges.

There are many issues that potentially arise when working with individuals from another country in the ambulatory care setting. The Centers for Disease Control and Prevention (CDC) has profiles for individual refugee groups to give key health and cultural information about specific refugee groups resettled in the United States (Centers for Disease Control and Prevention, 2018):

- Priority health conditions
- Background
- Population movements
- Healthcare and conditions before arrival
- Medical screening of those seeking refuge in the United States

- Postarrival medical screening
- Health information

This information can help nurses and other healthcare providers determine appropriate interventions and services needed for individuals of the specific refugee group. This will assist nurses with providing care for the specific refugee population to understand their background, circumstances of the displacement, living conditions while they were seeking asylum, and common health conditions of this group. One example of a clinic designed to assist individuals from other countries and those seeking refuge is found in Box 14.3.

Individuals Experiencing Homelessness

Any of the individuals described in this chapter, as well as those in other population categories may be experiencing homelessness. People who are homeless or who are facing housing insecurity bring a set of challenges that are additional to any health issues the individual may already have. The social and political issues around homelessness are discussed in Chapter 3; however, some health implications will be discussed here.

Mental health is a pervasive issue for those who are experiencing homelessness, both as a potential root cause and as an effect of homelessness. Individuals with untreated or undertreated mental health issues may have difficulty maintaining steady jobs or relationships, which in turn can result in homelessness and begin a spiral of inadequate access to care, poor control of mental health issues, and further deterioration of living conditions and overall

BOX 14.3 Global at Home: Clinic for Immigrants and Those Seeking Refuge

Clarkston, Georgia, is a major resettlement area for those seeking refuge located just outside of the city of Atlanta. Resettlement activity in this area has grown rapidly since the late 1980s because of its close location to a major city, access to public transportation, and an abundance of affordable housing. According to the 2000 census, the foreign-born population hails from more than 50 countries (spanning six continents) within this 1.1 square mile enclave, leading Clarkston to be described as the most diverse square mile in America. In 2009, the foreign-born population of this area was estimated to be 31.8% compared with the State of Georgia average of 7.1%.

Clarkston Community Health Center (CCHC), founded in May 2013, is a nonprofit 501c(3) clinic that provides an individual-centered medical home for low-income residents of the City of Clarkston and its surrounding communities. The clinic's primary populations are those seeking refuge and individuals from other countries, but it also accepts any individuals without insurance. In February 2015, CCHC began a once-weekly clinic to provide much-needed medical care that is culturally and linguistically sensitive for the diverse population of Clarkston. Subsequently, services were expanded to provide laboratory testing and to offer adult primary care clinics twice weekly, women's health once a week, and mental health and other specialty services on a periodic basis.

CCHC has evolved into an interprofessional facility with multiple clinic days per week, with nurse practitioner-led clinics, collaboration between nursing and medical schools, and an interprofessional clinic that includes students from nursing, public health, and medicine.

Challenges for this facility have included finding reliable methods to obtain interpreters for a variety of languages, translating health information handouts, and ensuring that there are protocols and updated standards of care for the variety of providers. Because the great majority of workers are volunteers, it can be difficult both to provide continuity in standards of practice and to ensure organizational efficiency. These challenges have in part been addressed by creating a salaried position of clinic director; however, as with any clinic that serves an indigent population, the persistent need is that of funding to support clinic services.

health. Similarly, the insecurity, stress, and trauma of homelessness can result in depression and stress-related illnesses in even the healthiest of individuals.

The physical challenges of homelessness also have a major impact on this population of individuals. These range from specific issues such as inadequate foot care to general health and medication-related obstacles. Even when individuals who are experiencing homelessness are able to receive adequate treatment, adherence may be complicated by barriers that are not common for individuals with a home but are significant for those without. A few examples of treatment and physical challenges specific to homelessness include:

- Lack of refrigeration for medications such as insulin and some antibiotics
- Challenges when dosing of medications requires specific timing with meals
- Theft of personal possessions, including medications
- Food considerations for specific issues such as diabetes, hypertension, or heart failure
- Skin breakdown from wet or inadequate footwear
- Physical trauma

Nursing Considerations

Nursing care of individuals experiencing homelessness takes many forms, from established free clinics and shelters to mobile outreach to faith-based or "pop-up" occasional interventions. These settings provide excellent opportunities for nursing care, screening, and care coordination. Issues such as foot and wound care can be addressed by nursing protocols and delegated orders. In other cases, the RN might refer to and collaborate with other health professionals for services such as mental health, diagnostic testing, and treatment options.

Individual education and care coordination are two of the strengths of nursing education and provide an invaluable service for individuals whose healthcare may be intermittent and fragmented. In addition to these skills, nurses who are able to work at their full scope of practice also may increase access to care for a population that frequently is overlooked and underserved.

Native Americans and Alaska Natives

According to the 2010 U.S. census, 5.9 million people reported being American Indian or Alaska Native along or in combination with one or more other race; 78% of these individuals lived outside of American Indian or Alaska Native areas (ie, Reservations, Villages) (Norris et al., 2012). It should be noted that the term "American Indian" is used by the US Census Bureau; however the term Native Americans is preferred in this textbook and will be used when not quoting Census Bureau statistics.

The states with the largest numbers of American Indian and Alaska Native in 2010 were California, Oklahoma, Arizona, Texas, New York, New Mexico, Washington, North Carolina, Florida, and Michigan (Norris et al., 2012). There are 567 tribal nations located in 35 states; each of these nations has its own sovereignty over the land and its own legally defined tribal government recognized by the federal government of the United States (National Congress of American Indians, n.d.).

When working with individuals who self-identify as Native Americans or Alaska Natives, it is critical to acknowledge that each individual's personal and family history will shape their cultural identity and practices and that this identity may change throughout their life (SAMHSA, CDC, IHS, & CMS, 2009). **Native American and Alaska Native** identities may fall on a continuum from living traditional culture every day, to identifying as "Indian" or "Native" with a small amount of knowledge and/or interest in traditional cultural practices, or everything in between. Historical trauma, including forced boarding school attendance and adoption to non-Native Americans or non-Alaska Natives, influences the attitudes, identity, and trust of individuals in this population (SAMHSA et al., 2009).

Nursing Considerations

Native Americans and Alaska Natives often view concepts of health and wellness as living in harmony and balance of spirit, mind, body, and the environment; this view can be different from the way individuals involved in providing "Western medicine" may view health and wellness (SAMHSA et al., 2009). Individuals who identify as Native Americans and Alaska Native may use a combination of traditional and Western medicine in their daily lives in different proportions. It is important when working with this population to understand that there is not a strict dichotomy between traditional practices and Western medicine, and it is not necessary for the individual to choose one or the other approach. Both can be used in a complementary approach to benefit the individual.

Native American and Alaska Native people have experienced health outcome disparities and lower life expectancy in comparison to other groups in the United States. This may be related to unequal access to education, higher levels of poverty, and discrimination within the healthcare system (Indian Health Service, 2018). Chronic conditions such as heart diseases, cancer, unintentional injuries, and diabetes are the leading causes of death in this population; the life expectancy for Native Americans and Alaska Natives born today is 5.5 years less than that of the U.S. population as a whole (averaged). Additionally, mortality rates calculated from 2009 to 2011 from accidents, diabetes, alcohol, chronic liver disease and cirrhosis, and assault are all at least two times higher than in the U.S. population as a whole (Indian Health Service, 2018).

Although the native population may experience health inequalities, it is also critical to keep in mind the strengths of the community. This includes extended family and kinship ties, shared sense of collective community responsibility, indigenous generational knowledge and wisdom, historical perspective, and strong connection to the past. Other strengths may include survival skills and resiliency when dealing with challenges, retention and reclamation of the traditional language and cultural practices, the ability to move between different cultures, and community pride (SAMHSA et al., 2009).

RNs working in this community need to know about Native American- and Alaska Native-specific healthcare resources. Nurses also should give individuals different options and levels of care and ensure that they are addressing the individual's cultural and spiritual needs, if relevant. Preventative health is critical in this population and must include supporting the strengths of the community as well as individuals and families. RNs should take into consideration the cultural differences in health and symptoms prior to drawing conclusions about the presenting health problem and make every effort to collaborate with local cultural advisors when they have questions about symptoms or treatment options for this population (SAMHSA et al., 2009).

It is important to stress that individuals may not have to choose between modern and traditional ways, nor do they have to commit to a single program of care. The nurse can take a plan of care one step at a time. Specific strategies for care in this community may include the following:

- Refer to culturally appropriate places, such as native recovery partners or online resources.
- Be aware of intergenerational aspects; consider the entire family when one member is being treated.
- Be mindful of traumas that individuals may have experienced, such as boarding schools or other intergenerational trauma.
- Start support groups of native people in the clinic.

The role of the nurse in this setting is summarized in this description by IHS:

> "Ambulatory Nursing provides comprehensive health care and education to the individual and family in the ambulatory setting, through provision of nursing care and/or services utilizing the nursing process, and in coordination with the medical plan of care and other health care providers. Continuity of care is accomplished through coordination of services with individual and community health programs and utilization of community resources in the promotion/maintenance of health. Ambulatory Nursing services are directed towards meeting the needs of individuals, families, and the community during times of health and illness." (Indian Health Service, n.d.)

Cultural Humility

The 2010 census indicates that minority and ethnic populations have increased in the last 10 years by 9.7% (Humes et al., 2011). This growth, which is likely to continue, makes it imperative for healthcare professionals to understand the various populations with which they interact. Table 14.1 summarizes the 2010 census information on U.S. populations.

There has been some discussion about the term used to describe this field, including options such as: cultural awareness, cultural humility, cultural sensitivity, cultural competence, and structural competency. Although recognizing that there are arguments for and against each term, for the purposes of consistency the term "cultural humility" will be used here. Cultural humility occurs when an individual or organization has the ability to function effectively within the cultural context of beliefs, behaviors, and needs of the individuals or community it serves. Chambers and Laughlin (2013) provide the following guidance for the RN working in CCTM for this population:

- Cultural disparities in health and healthcare: racial and ethnic minorities experience a lower quality of health services and are less likely to receive even routine medical procedures than Caucasians. Perceptions of illness, disease, and their causes vary by culture.
- Cultural competency: "An ongoing process in which the health care professional continually strives to work within the cultural context of the individual, individual, family and community" (p. 221).
- Cultural safety: "Providing culturally safe care requires the nurse to be respectful of nationality, culture, age, sex, and political and religious beliefs" (p. 222).

Haas et al. (2014) suggest additional guidelines for the RN in CCTM:

- "Strategies to improve cultural knowledge and skills: the RN in CCTM learns basic information about the predominant culture groups served within the care setting of responsibility and influence; learns and understands culturally influenced health behaviors; and develops culture-specific assessment skills.
- Cultural differences in disease incidence and management: the RN in CCTM needs to identify disease prevalence that commonly occurs within given ethnic populations and design screening and care interventions that meet the needs and unique characteristics of the populations served." (Haas et al., 2014, pp. 118–119)

Nursing Considerations

What may be considered cultural considerations also applies to groups not previously identified in this chapter, such as those with impaired vision or hearing or with mobility issues, or considerations related to religion or gender identity. Many online resources are available to nurses and healthcare teams initiating a cultural assessment for a new individual or population that may fall in any of these categories. Institutional-based diversity and inclusion programs are responding to regulatory requirements to ensure that healthcare teams have access to readily available resources to support inclusive healthcare no matter the time or setting. These web-based tools provide immediate access to information about various cultures and are designed to enhance general knowledge on topics such as language and communication, spirituality, pharmacology, family decision-making, health and wellness, death and dying, and views on mental illness.

For example, as was noted in the overview of this chapter, the USDHHS OMH offers online resources for healthcare workers to become more culturally humble and competent. The Culturally and Linguistically Appropriate Services in Health and Health Care (the CLAS Standards) supply a framework for healthcare workers to use in providing care to a diverse population, as is offered in their website: https://thinkculturalhealth.hhs.gov/. Additional resources also may be found through population-specific websites for individuals with physical or mental health challenges, gender identification, or other cultural considerations. These websites may offer healthcare workers a broader understanding of their individuals' perspective.

In addition to the need for cultural humility among care providers, simply achieving common communication may be one of the greatest challenges when providing care to individuals for whom English is not their first language. Best practices require that care teams must use a certified interpreter when communicating with individuals who have a second language need. However, this is difficult if no certified interpreter is available. Too often, healthcare workers are forced to rely on family members for communication, especially children who may have been introduced to English at an earlier age than their parents. If the information needed is intimate or inappropriate for the child or even a spouse, the RN may have to defer this part of assessment until an interpreter can be obtained by phone or other means. This is only one of many obstacles faced by individuals from non-English-speaking cultures, but arguably is one of the most significant. Ineffective communication has an impact on full assessment of the individual's health issues, adherence to care, understanding of potential complications, and success of treatment.

To provide context as ambulatory care nurses initiate their journey toward gaining cultural sensitivity, the following quotes and statistics offer information about a few of the challenges underserved individuals may experience:

- About 8 million adults identify as lesbian, gay, bisexual, or transgender, comprising 3.5% of the U.S. population. These individuals face health disparities linked to social stigma and discrimination. Recent electronic health record changes now recognize individual choice for gender identification—male, female, or other (Ritter &Graham, 2017, p. 269).
- Farmworkers and migrants tend to be regionally isolated; their mobility makes access to healthcare difficult. Unsanitary work and housing conditions, chemicals, and heavy work raise the risk for many healthcare problems (Ritter & Graham, 2017, p. 281).
- Individuals from another country may have poor health because of escape from locations with long-standing conflict. The CDC recommends three aims: promote and improve the health of those seeking refuge, prevent disease, and familiarize those individuals with the U.S. healthcare system (Ritter & Graham, 2017, p. 285).
- Native Americans and Alaska Natives are affected by the negative consequences of poverty, limited access to health services, and cultural dislocation. Inadequate education, high rates of unemployment, discrimination, and cultural differences all contribute to unhealthy lifestyles and disparities in access to healthcare (Ritter & Graham, 2017, p. 175).

This chapter has provided only a small overview of this complex and important topic. RNs in ambulatory care have the opportunity to make a long-lasting impact on individuals from a diversity of backgrounds, cultures, countries or who are underserved or in a minority in terms of race, physical ability, or gender identification. Cultural humility toward all individuals in the healthcare system reduces barriers to optimal healthcare delivery and supports the best possible outcomes in care.

Diversity Within the Nursing Workforce

Overall, foreign-born nurses in the United States make up about 15% of all RNs. The majority of foreign-born RNs were concentrated in just five states: California, New York, Florida, Texas, and New Jersey. In 2012, the top five countries of origin for foreign-born RNs were the Philippines, India, Jamaica, Canada, and Nigeria (Hohn et al., 2016).

Why does workplace diversity matter in nursing? Diversity among employees allows for a wide array of different perspectives and sensitivities. The same diversities occur in nurses as those that occur in nurses' clients and patients: age, gender, race, religion, culture, ability, national origin, socioeconomic class, sexual orientation, work experience, and career goals. When supported, these diversities can be a valuable asset in the healthcare setting.

Past programs and research have focused on assimilating individuals of different genders, races, ethnicities, religions, and sexual orientations into organizations. Progress has been made with this approach; however, diversity may have a broader definition. Organizations have also come to realize the value of identifying and appreciating the cultural, generational, and geographic differences of their employees. These varied perspectives offer the potential for a richer work environment that, in turn, helps healthcare workers to provide fully individual-focused care.

Summary

Care for the members of any society is a challenging endeavor, made more difficult in settings of limited resources or commitment to these populations. A few of the groups and populations that may be considered as underserved are included in this chapter, although it is not in any way a comprehensive list. Among those addressed here, however, two common themes are identified: barriers to access and continuity of care.

Barriers to access to care may be the most pervasive, persistent, and challenging issue. For individuals from another country, this may be reflected in communication barriers. For those in rural areas, the biggest hurdle may be distance. For some cultures, it may be difficult even to trust medical practitioners grounded in a U.S. perspective of healthcare. For those experiencing homelessness and are underresourced, financial barriers are steep. These barriers represent only a few examples.

An additional theme that cuts across most populations identified here is that of continuity of care. Because many underserved populations in the U.S. society use urgent care clinics, emergency departments, or safety-net clinics for care, it is often difficult or impossible to provide true care coordination and continuity. This lack of continuity occurs on both sides of the stethoscope; individuals may seek care from a variety of sources that are unable to share information, but provider turnover or inconsistency may be high even within the context of established care in a single clinic.

The problems mentioned here are beyond the ability for any single person to solve; however, the RN in ambulatory care can be aware of the political and societal elements that have an impact on these health issues. On an individual level, RNs can increase their comfort and competence in providing care to individuals from different backgrounds. Given the growth in our diverse society, it is impossible for nurses to understand all elements of cultural health for their individuals; however, it is possible for nurses to develop strong skills in cultural assessment and interventions so they are able to deliver culturally sensitive care to all individual populations.

Equally important, ambulatory care RNs are in a prime position to assess for healthcare disparities based on gaps in social determinants of healthcare. Nurses can incorporate assessments and interventions into the longitudinal plan of care to assist the interprofessional team in delivering respectful, quality care, incorporating beliefs and values of the individual, family, and community. RNs also can advocate for healthcare equity through advancing understanding of diversity, cultural awareness, importance of inclusive research, as well as demonstrating leadership and partnership with communities and local and federal government agencies to address gaps in healthcare for underserved members of society.

Case Study

Elizabeth is an RN volunteer at a free clinic in a large urban area. She is assessing Mr. James, a man seeking assistance with multiple health issues, including previous diagnoses of hypertension, diabetes, and alcohol misuse. He currently is experiencing homelessness and is living in a shelter, but is in danger of losing his place because he broke the shelter rule about not having alcohol on the premises. They have given him one more chance, and he is anxious about being put back on the streets.

Mr. James recently lost his job as a restaurant worker because it required him to be there at 7 in the morning. He had to take two buses to the restaurant, and the earliest time he could catch the first bus was 6 am. He was fired for being frequently late when the first bus would be delayed, causing him to miss his connection for the second.

His blood pressure this morning is elevated, and his hemoglobin A_{1c} indicates poor control of his diabetes. Neither issue is critical, although they are of concern to the RN.

Mr. James' family lives in the metropolitan area, but they have told him that they cannot provide him any financial or housing assistance. He used to be a member of a Protestant church that offers programs for people who are homeless, but lost touch with the members there.

Discussion Questions:

1. What assessment tools might Elizabeth use to evaluate Mr. James?
2. List the possible challenges related to his current living environment, especially in terms of security or nutrition.
3. List two primary issues and achievable goals for this individual.
4. What support systems in the family and community could the RN draw upon to help Mr. James address the challenges and achieve his goals?

Key Points for Review

- Over time, the United States has implemented legislation to address social, racial, and financial disparities; however, much work remains to be done on a national level.
- It is important for RNs to understand the terms SDOH, health disparities, health equity, and cultural humility and ways these issues have an impact on nursing care.
- Cultural humility in an RN allows for acceptance and understanding of an individual's specific cultural influences and the impact it may have on care delivery.
- There are specific challenges for optimal health and nursing care of those experiencing homelessness, those in rural settings, native Americans, individuals from another country, those seeking refuge, and those who face other physical, cultural, or societal barriers.
- Minority and diverse populations often have been underrepresented in medical research. As a result, there is less information about differences in response to treatment, which impedes the ability of healthcare professionals to determine appropriate interventions.
- Diversity in the nursing workforce provides additional perspectives to nursing care that can be a valuable part of healthcare delivery.

REFERENCES

American Nurses Association. (2010). *Healthcare for undocumented immigrants (Resolution from 2010 House of Delegates).* https://www.nursingworld.org/~4af0ba/globalassets/docs/ana/ethics/nursing-without-borders_-access-to-care-for-immigrants.pdf

American Society of Addiction Medicine. (n.d.). *Screening and assessment tools.* https://elearning.asam.org/screening-assessment

Andermann, A. (2018). Screening for social determinants of health in clinical care: Moving from the margins to the mainstream. *Public Health Reviews, 39*, 19. https://doi.org/10.1186/s40985-018-0094-7

Bertelsen, N. S., Selden, E., Krass, P., Keatley, E. S., & Keller, A. (2018). Primary care screening methods and outcomes for asylum seekers in New York City. *Journal of Immigrant And Minority Health, 20*(1), 171–177. https://doi.org/10.1007/s10903-016-0507-y

Braveman, P. (2014). What are health disparities and health equity? We need to be clear. Nursing in 3D: Workforce diversity, health disparities, and social determinants of health. *Public Health Reports, 129*(1) [Supplement 2], 5–8. https://doi.org/10.1177/00333549141291S203

Centers for Disease Control and Prevention. (2018). *Refugee health profiles.* https://www.cdc.gov/immigrantrefugeehealth/profiles/index.html

Centers for Disease Control and Prevention, Division of Community Health. (2013). *A practitioners guide for advancing health equity: Community strategies for preventing chronic disease.* U.S. Department of Health and Human Services.

Cesario, S. K. (2017). Immigration basics for nurses. *Nursing for Women's Health, 21*(6), 499–505. https://doi.org/10.1016/j.nwh.2017.10.004

Chambers, P., & Laughlin, C. (2013). Transcultural nursing care. In C. B. Laughlin (Ed.), *Core curriculum for ambulatory care nursing* (3rd ed., pp. 217–231). American Academy of Ambulatory Care Nursing.

Choi, B., Blumberg, C., & Williams, K. (2016). Mobile integrated health care and community paramedicine: An emerging emergency medical services concept. *Annals of Emergency Medicine, 67*(3), 361–366. https://doi.org/10.1016/j.annemergmed.2015.06.005

Garg, A., Boynton-Jarrett, R., & Dworkin, P. (2016). Avoiding the unintended consequences of screening for social determinants of health. *Journal of the American Medical Association, 316*(8), 813–814. https://doi.org/10.1001/jama.2016.9282

Haas, S. A., Swan, B. A., & Haynes, T. S. (Eds.) (2014). *Care coordination and transition management core curriculum.* American Academy of Ambulatory Care Nursing.

Hohn, M. D., Witte, J. C., Lowry, J. P., & Fernández-Peña, J. R. (2016). *Immigrants in health care: Keeping Americans healthy through care and innovation.* https://iir.gmu.edu/archive-2017/iir-projects/healthcare

Holmes, J. S., Driscoll, A. K., & Heron, M. (2015). Mortality among US-born and immigrant Hispanics in the US: effects of nativity, duration of residence, and age at immigration. *International Journal of Public Health, 60*(5), 609–617. https://doi.org/10.1007/s00038-015-0686-7

Howe, S. (2020). Mental health update: Recognizing and treating depression in primary care. *Clinical Advisor, 23*(3), 13–27, 7p.

Humes, K. R., Jones, N. A., & Ramirez, R. R. (2011). *Overview of race and Hispanic origin: 2010: 2010 census briefs.* www.census.gov/prod/cen2010/briefs/c2010br-02.pdf

Indian Health Service (Ed.). (2018). *Indian health disparities.* https://www.ihs.gov/newsroom/factsheets/disparities/

Indian Health Service. (n.d.). *Ambulatory nursing.* https://www.ihs.gov/dper/planning/rrm-references/ambulatory-nursing/

International Council of Nurses. (2018). *Health of migrants, refugees and displaced persons: Position Statement.* https://www.icn.ch/sites/default/files/inline-files/PS_A_Health_migrants_refugees_displaced%20persons.pdf

International Organization for Migration. *UN Migration.* (n.d.). *Key migration terms.* https://www.iom.int/key-migration-terms

Knight, K., Kenny, A., & Endacott, R. (2016). From expert generalists to ambiguity masters: using ambiguity tolerance theory to redefine the practice of rural nurses. *Journal of Clinical Nursing, 25*(11–12), Journal Article UI:27139173. https://doi.org/10.1111/jocn.13196

Lopez, G., Bialik, K., & Radford, J. (2018). *Key findings about US immigrants. Pew Research Center.* https://www.pewresearch.org/fact-tank/2018/11/30/key-findings-about-u-s-immigrants/

National Congress of American Indians. (n.d.). *Tribal nations and the United States: An introduction.* National Congress of American Indians. http://www.ncai.org/about-tribes

National Institute on Drug Abuse. (n.d.). *Screening tools and prevention.* https://www.drugabuse.gov/nidamed-medical-health-professionals/screening-tools-prevention

Norris, T., Vines, P., & Hoeffel, E. (2012). *The American Indian and Alaska Native population: 2010.* https://www.census.gov/prod/cen2010/briefs/c2010br-10.pdf

Peeler, A. W. (2019). Strategies for cost saving through social determinants of health. *Journal of Healthcare Management, 64*(4), 222–230. http://dx.doi.org.proxy.library.emory.edu/10.1097/JHM-D-19-00113

Ritter, L. A., & Graham, D. H. (2017). *Multicultural health.* Jones and Bartlett.

Substance Abuse and Mental Health Services Administration. (n.d.). *US Department of Health and Human Services.* https://www.samhsa.gov/

Substance Abuse and Mental Health Services Administration, Centers for Disease Control and Prevention, Indian Health Service, & Centers for Medicare and Medicaid Services. (2009). *Culture card: A guide to build cultural awareness: American Indian and Alaska Native.* www.SAMHSA.gov/shin

Trauma Resource Center. (n.d.). https://www.traumaresourceinstitute.com/home

UNHCR The UN Refugee Agency. (1969). *OAU convention governing the specific aspects of refugee problems in Africa.* https://www.unhcr.org/en-us/about-us/background/45dc1a682/oau-convention-governing-specific-aspects-refugee-problems-africa-adopted.html

UNHCR The UN Refugee Agency. (1984). *Cartagena declaration on refugees.* https://www.unhcr.org/en-us/about-us/background/45dc19084/cartagena-declaration-refugees-adopted-colloquium-international-protection.html

UNHCR The UN Refugee Agency. (n.d.). *Convention and protocol related to the status of refugees.* https://cms.emergency.unhcr.org/documents/11982/55726/Convention+relating+to+the+Status+of+Refugees+%28signed+28+July+1951%2C+entered+into+force+22+April+1954%29+189+UNTS+150+and+Protocol+relating+to+the+Status+of+Refugees+%28signed+31+January+1967%2C+entered+into+force+4+October+167%29+606+UNTS+267/0bf3248a-cfa8-4a60-864d-65cdfece1d47

United Nations guiding principles on internal displacement (2nd ed.). (2004). https://www.brookings.edu/wp-content/uploads/2016/07/GPEnglish.pdf

U.S. Department of Health and Human Services. (2014, September). *About healthy people.* https://www.cdc.gov/nchs/healthy_people/hp2020.htm

U.S. Department of Health and Human Services, Office of Minority Health. (n.d.). *CLAS & CLAS standards.* https://minorityhealth.hhs.gov/omh/browse.aspx?lvl=2&lvlid=53

U.S. Food and Drug Administration. (n.d.). *Drug trials snapshot report 2016.* https://www.fda.gov/Drugs/InformationOnDrugs/ucm541105.htm

Wesson, D. R., & Ling, W. (2003). The Clinical Opiate Withdrawal Scale (COWS). *Journal of Psychoactive Drugs, 35*(2), 253–259.

World Health Organization. (2016). *Social determinants of health.* http://www.who.int/topics/social_determinants/en

UNIT 5

Advancing Ambulatory Care Nursing

15

Ambulatory Care: Educating the Next Generation

Linda A. McCauley and Caroline Varner Coburn

PERSPECTIVES

"Health networks now replace hospitals as the prime structure for 21st Century health care. Nurses can no longer anchor learning and practice in previous, now nonrelevant, clinical models located only in acute care. The contemporary nurse must be grounded in the continuum of health whose primary focus is found in the community and the continuum of care. This is the centerpiece of nursing value going forward; it's time now for nurse leaders to embed this reality inside the journey of nurse education, practice, and leadership. Indeed, this is the predominant work of our time."

Tim Porter-O'Grady, DM, EdD, ScD (h), APRN, FAAN, FACCWS, Senior Partner, Tim Porter-O'Grady Associates, an international healthcare consulting firm.

LEARNING OBJECTIVES

Upon completion of this chapter, the reader will be able to:

1. Describe current and workforce needs in ambulatory care nursing.
2. Identify the core competencies in ambulatory care nursing.
3. List issues that educators need to consider in assessing the adequacy of their curricula.
4. Describe challenges of integrating ambulatory care content into existing nursing programs.

KEY TERMS

Advanced practice nurses
Baccalaureate nurses
Interprofessional education
NCLEX-RN examination
Nursing curriculum
Nursing workforce
Population health nursing
Public health nursing
Role transition

Preparing Nursing Students for Ambulatory Roles of the Future

Healthcare reform will expand opportunities for all levels of registered nurses (RNs) in ambulatory care. **Advanced practice nurses** are recognized as having key roles in managing panels of individuals within a team-based care model, and doctorally prepared nurses with advanced education in population health will lead in evaluating the efficiency of new care models and testing new approaches to care. The number of nurses in doctor of nursing practice (DNP) programs has increased dramatically in the last decade (Redman et al., 2015). However, the team-based approach to ambulatory care also requires that baccalaureate-prepared nurses assume multiple complex roles in ambulatory care including managing individuals with chronic disease using protocols, such as titrating blood pressure medication and adjusting diabetes medication, leading complex care management teams for individuals with multidiagnoses, and coordinating care between ambulatory care practice and the other components of the healthcare system (Lamb et al., 2015).

In recent years, the national outlook for the supply of RNs has improved; however, there are cautionary aspects to this data. These include regional variabilities and uncertainty as to future projections of workforce retirement (Auerbach et al., 2017). The need to increase the number of new RNs continues to be an issue for nursing schools, even in the presence of increased enrollment and new online programs. An additional element in the landscape of RN education is the changing role of the RN in primary and ambulatory care. RNs are well positioned to take the lead in addressing critical needs in U.S. healthcare, but addressing these needs will require both adequate workforce and adequate education.

Although the evidence is limited, there appear to be barriers in educating prelicensure nursing students in ambulatory care. These barriers exist both within schools of nursing education and within the sites for which students are being prepared. The main barriers are the following:

1. Lack of faculty buy-in
2. Logistical challenges coordinating with ambulatory care and community-based teaching sites
3. Lack of high-level RN role models in ambulatory care
4. Cost of RN salaries and benefits
5. Gaps and deficiencies in the education of RNs in ambulatory nursing (Bauer & Bodenheimer, 2017; Wojnar & Whelan, 2017)

This chapter describes the major challenges and opportunities for nursing educators to provide learning experiences that prepare **baccalaureate nurses** to function at optimal levels in ambulatory care.

Current Practice Patterns

Historically, primary care was delivered by physicians in private practice to a small panel of individuals; they had few employees, most often medical assistants (MAs) or nurses, who primarily performed patient triage and clerical tasks. Current practice size is increasing. The percentage of physicians in practices of more than 50 employees grew from 3% in 2001 to 36% in 2011 (Welch et al., 2013). These larger practices in which physicians and advanced practice providers care for large panels of individuals will have the resources to hire and train a larger RN workforce to serve as care managers, especially chronic disease managers. Additionally, as rates and length of hospitalizations decrease, more complex individual management will take place outside of hospital settings.

In March 2004, there were 2.9 million RNs in the United States. In 2017, there were 3.7 million (AAACN, 2017). According to data from the Bureau of Labor Statistics (BLS), in 2016 18% of RNs worked in ambulatory care, which includes physicians' offices, home healthcare, and outpatient care centers. This number is potentially higher because ambulatory care nurses may also be represented in the BLS category of government (eg, military, veterans), accounting for 5% of RN jobs. The BLS also estimates that RN employment will increase 12% from 2018 to 2028, with the fastest part of this increase being in outpatient care centers (Bureau of Labor Statistics, 2016).

Within ambulatory care, RNs can increasingly be expected to find roles in chronic disease management, health education, wellness, and care coordination in ambulatory and primary care settings (Smolowitz et al., 2015). During 2015, an estimated 990 million visits were made to outpatient physician offices, 53% of these visits being in primary care; this does not include the 126 million visits made to hospital-based outpatient offices, for over one billion ambulatory care visits (National Ambulatory Medical Care Survey, 2015).

These data support the conclusion that medical care is increasingly being delivered outside of the hospital setting and that nurses have been responding and will continue to respond to this need. Much of this need and increase is in the primary care setting of ambulatory care, where the effectiveness of nurses in ambulatory care has been supported in many studies. One extensive review found that nurse-led care resulted in at least equal outcomes in the specific areas of "HRQoL (health-related quality of life), symptom burden, self-management and disease-specific clinical targets compared to physician-led care for managing chronic conditions" (Chan et al., 2018, p. 79).

Additionally, the introduction of Medicare fee-for-service add-on payments for RN functions such as wellness visits and chronic disease management services is producing extra revenue to support RNs on primary care teams (Basu et al., 2015), adding to the potential for increase in this workforce. Further discussion of the RN role in primary care and as part of the national workforce can be found in Chapters 2 and 10, respectively.

New Roles

The American Association of Colleges of Nursing's (AACN) *Essentials of Baccalaureate Education for Professional Nursing* (2008) states that the professional roles of the baccalaureate generalist nurse include being a provider of care, as well as the designer, manager, and coordinator of care. Thus, nursing practice includes the direct care of the sick in and across all environments and the provision of health promotion, clinical prevention, and population-based healthcare. Although the *Essentials* clearly delineate competencies needed to work in ambulatory care, few new-to-practice RNs seek ambulatory care positions as their first employment avenue. Historically, hospitals were seen as the setting that would best prepare nurses for their future practice, and working as a medical surgical nurse was viewed as the desired preparation for transitioning to out-of-hospital settings.

Additionally, many ambulatory out-of-hospital settings would hire only nurses who had hospital employment experience. This preference was often based on the need to have experienced nurses who could respond to an emergency in an ambulatory care setting, whether in a school, workplace, home, or clinic. Hospitals were seen as the environment in which to best hone one's skills in procedures and to be exposed to the largest number of individuals with different diagnoses in the shortest time. The argument could be made that this benefit was gained, at least in part, because hospital stays were longer and nurses could see more of the full trajectory of individuals' illness and recovery. Longer hospital stays also allowed more time for assessment of the resources needed to support recovery, individual and family comprehension of care plans and goals, and referrals to support services that would begin during the hospitalization.

In today's healthcare world, however, the majority of new-to-practice RNs who choose a hospital employment setting, often in critical care, are providing care for individuals with complex immediate needs who spend the briefest possible time in the acute care setting. As a result, the in-hospital setting often provides less RN preparation for transition to the ambulatory setting than it may have done in the past.

Although the assumption may persist that critical care experience is necessary prior to working in ambulatory care, more recent evidence indicates that this is not the case and that nurses who transition from acute care to ambulatory care actually require additional support for successful transition (Allen, 2016). Medical education has long recognized that although educational rotations through all types of clinical services provide the breadth of exposure for new physicians, practice in acute settings such as critical care is not a prerequisite for specializing in primary care medicine.

As rates of hospitalization decrease, studies in the United States and other countries point to a slow increase in the number of RNs working in ambulatory care and primary care settings (AIHW, 2013; Palumbo et al., 2017). However, this increase and the need for additional nurses may not be best met through transfer from acute to ambulatory care but may be an opportunity for schools of nursing to increase the number of new graduates entering that field. Several factors work against the traditional route of acute care RN moving to ambulatory care. For newer nurses, transitioning into ambulatory care settings from acute care settings is not always seen as a positive career move and may be associated with perceived skill loss, lower wages, and fewer professional opportunities compared to employment in acute care settings (Curtis & Glacken, 2014; Halcomb et al., 2016).

For more experienced nurses, the reasons for moving to ambulatory care may have more to do with lifestyle than professional interest. In a study of Australian nurses, the primary reasons provided for transitioning to employment in primary care settings were work satisfaction, better hours, and work–family balance. It is noteworthy that some of the nurses had little understanding about the roles in ambulatory care (McInnes et al., 2015).

In a review of the literature of the transition of nurses from acute care to primary/ambulatory settings, Ashley et al. (2016) identified the major barriers or enablers in the transition to be relevant educational preparation, skills development, access to continuing education, and availability of support systems. The review of the literature also points to the need for more research on roles in ambulatory care and predictors of successful transition to ambulatory practice (Wojnar & Whelan, 2017).

Although it is clear that healthcare reform will increase the need for more RNs in ambulatory settings, the evidence that RNs are moving from hospitals into ambulatory settings is limited.

The greatest proportional increase in nurses was seen among associate degree (AD)-prepared nurses (34% to 48%), suggesting that baccalaureate-prepared nurses are not fully gravitating toward ambulatory employment opportunities (Palumbo et al., 2017). This is particularly concerning because AD-prepared nurses, the largest proportion of the **nursing workforce** in many regions of the country, typically do not have the coursework to prepare them to work in population health-focused settings or in settings outside of traditional acute or long-term care. As noted by Fraher et al. (2013), "Because of sheer numbers … it is nurses who are arguably in the most pivotal position to drive system change" (p. 1813). However, they also note that role changes are rapidly occurring in other healthcare jobs such as licensed practical nurses (LPNs) and MAs.

In summary, the state of nursing in ambulatory care is in flux. Experienced RNs who transition from acute care because ambulatory care is perceived as less challenging are often finding that is not the case. However, in many settings new graduates do not see the potential for RNs to practice at the top of their licensure, which makes the field less appealing to them. Roles are blurred between RNs, LPN/LVNs, and MAs, creating further challenges to recognizing the contributions of RN education to the ambulatory care setting. Because many schools of nursing provide limited clinical experience in ambulatory care for their students, they also may contribute to the emphasis on acute care employment for new RN graduates.

Despite these challenges, it has been noted that "the transformation of primary care creates favorable conditions for growth in the number of RNs, with their likely role focused on elements of the chronic care model such as chronic care management, the management of complex, high-utilizing patients, and the coordination of care among hospital, long-term care, ambulatory care, and home" (Bauer & Bodenheimer, 2017, p. 630). Nursing schools, especially those connected with academic health systems, are well positioned to provide the resources needed to address these system-wide changes and challenges through educational and collaborative offerings.

Ambulatory Care Practice Arenas

To fully support the educational preparation of Bachelor of Science in Nursing (BSN) students, it is important to have an understanding of the many subspecialties and practice patterns that currently make up the specialty of ambulatory care. Similar to the many subspecialties that exist under the umbrella of medical–surgical nursing, ambulatory care nurses have the opportunity to practice in a wide variety of settings. The topics mentioned here are discussed more fully in other areas of this book; this inclusion is simply an overview of the knowledge and skill areas needed to prepare students for ambulatory care education. In this context, examples are provided when applicable comparisons can be made between ambulatory and acute care settings.

Care Coordination and Transition Management

Care Coordination and Transition Management (CCTM) is arguably one of the ambulatory care concepts that informs every practice setting. It can be exemplified in all areas of didactic content, from primary care to oncology to same-day surgery. In a nursing education context, care coordination should be introduced both as a topic with specific elements of expertise and as one that applies to all aspects of healthcare, both acute and ambulatory. The elements of CCTM are detailed in a separate chapter of this book, including content that should clearly present CCTM in nursing curricula as a specialty with specific knowledge and skills.

Additionally, in the context of nursing education, the skills and knowledge needed for CCTM in ambulatory care can be compared with similar skills needed in acute care. For instance, comparing outpatient care coordination for an individual with cancer needing multiple tests and treatments with that of a new postoperative in-hospital patient can give students a frame of reference for application of existing knowledge to a new setting.

Nurse-Led Care

The concept of nurse-led care also transcends any single ambulatory care setting, but, unlike care coordination, it is less applicable to the acute care comparison. In ambulatory care, RNs may apply standing orders and treatment guidelines to provide services such as health and wellness assessment, chronic disease management, and primary care for specialty populations, such as the incarcerated, school clinics, and public health.

Clinical outcomes for nurse-led clinics in a variety of settings have been shown to be equal to or better than standard or physician-led care. Although this comprehensive literature review included all levels of nurses in multiple countries, including nurse practitioners, there were examples of RN-level nurses successfully managing complex care under appropriate protocols (Chan et al., 2018). In addition to providing quality care, nurse-led clinics allow RNs to work at the top of their licensure, an important component in the evolution of ambulatory care nursing.

Primary Care

The primary care setting arguably provides the RN with the greatest potential for full scope of practice. The elements of care coordination described previously are especially valuable in the primary care population of individuals with complex care needs. Additionally, RNs in high-level primary care practices are able to independently manage patients under specified protocols for reimbursable items such as annual wellness visits and nurse visits for chronic diseases (Flinter et al., 2017).

Outpatient Treatment Centers

Many baccalaureate programs offer little to no opportunity for students to rotate through the operating room, so the clinical and didactic content for same-day or outpatient surgery may include concepts that are either new to students or have not been presented since their first semester fundamentals course. In ambulatory care didactic, students may be reminded of the concepts of sterile technique, but in a broader setting than simply opening a sterile dressing tray. In addition to day surgery, this content also applies to other short-term treatment areas such as infusion centers, transplant centers, and hemodialysis.

All of these areas generally require the use of hands-on skills to a greater extent than areas such as primary care and are often perceived as being more satisfying to the novice or undergraduate nurse. It is both a clinical and a didactic challenge to help the student understand that fewer physical clinical interventions such as telehealth and behavior change activities are equally important for excellent health outcomes.

Specialty Populations

The multitude of specialty populations, not to be confused with medical specialties, discussed next, are fully described in Chapters 13 and 14. Examples of these populations include pediatrics, geriatrics, prisoners, students, the underserved (homeless, refugee, immigrant), and women (maternity or general women's health). For any of these populations, the most important concept is one of perspective. In the didactic setting, there will be little new actual content about the challenges, health issues, and treatment modalities for these populations. The ambulatory care difference is one of locus of control, as discussed in Chapter 1, and application of principles of care coordination and socioeconomic determinants of health.

Medical Specialties

As noted previously, the academic emphasis on RN role in medical specialties is primarily one of perspective rather than new knowledge: understanding that the locus of control resides with the individual. Using an example of heart failure, the treatment concepts may be similar to those in acute care. However, for students new to ambulatory care it may not be intuitive that in ambulatory care an additional part of the RN role includes conducting a detailed review of diet and medications as well as addressing financial, emotional, and support challenges that may have an impact on successful treatment.

In medical specialty areas of ambulatory care, the RN arguably plays the most comprehensive role of care coordination, facilitating care between the specialty and primary care and coordinating treatments and medications for other medical issues that may affect the individual's treatment.

Home Health

Home health is a growing field for RNs, both as practitioners and as entrepreneurs, and is an important didactic content area for ambulatory care nursing. Baccalaureate students may have in-home exposure to individuals through a population health course, but the ambulatory care perspective emphasizes intervention and maximizing individual independence, rather than observation or assessment only.

Public Health

One distinction between **public health nursing** and ambulatory care has been that interventions in public health are applied at a population rather than at an individual level. However, public health nurses certainly practice in clinics that provide individual care, and the roles often become somewhat blurred. The word "population" may also contribute to confusion. Within an ambulatory practice, population may refer to those with specific diagnoses, or even all individuals in the practice. In terms of maximizing impact on healthcare, students are taught that the most effective target population is the one classified as rising risk, regardless of the specific diagnosis. However, in quality improvement terms, population may refer to individuals with hypertension who are the focus of a specific project. In public health nursing, a population of interest may be those in a specific demographic profile or a particular geographic location.

For purposes of clarity in ambulatory care curriculum, the emphasis should remain on individual care. The individual may be classified in more than one type of population group, but the intervention remains at the individual level, tailored to that specific individual, rather than the classic public health intervention at a higher level of population group.

Educational Curricula and Practicums to Support Ambulatory Nursing Preparation

The core competencies for RNs in ambulatory settings include a range of content including care coordination, quality and safety, interprofessional practice and teamwork, and public/**population health nursing** (Flinter et al., 2017; Haas et al., 2013, 2019; Wagner et al., 2017). All of these competencies are enacted in the context of team-managed care. **Interprofessional education** also gives new-to-practice RNs the skills and attitudes to function in a team environment.

The American Academy of Ambulatory Care Nursing (AAACN) developed a core curriculum for ambulatory nursing (Laughlin, 2018) with a strong focus on all of these areas as well as separate certifications for RNs. The ambulatory care core curriculum offers a foundation for undergraduate course content and makes available resources to provide students with a fundamental understanding of the knowledge and skills required in this field.

The *BSN Essentials* also includes the competencies listed previously. However, in most schools of nursing, these competencies are more frequently measured and evaluated in acute rather than ambulatory care settings. An additional challenge lies in the clinical setting. Acute care settings allow faculty to supervise six to 10 students rotating on an in-hospital unit, whereas students in ambulatory settings are more likely to be separated from other students and working more with the team delivering care in the ambulatory site. These differences in the educational milieu require innovation in teaching methods to ensure that students have the opportunity to demonstrate the required competencies in an ambulatory site.

To prepare nurses of the future who can effectively practice in ambulatory care settings and integrate care coordination, quality and safety, interprofessional practice, and population health, faculty will need to create innovative academic practice partnerships and master new technologies, such as high-definition simulation and virtual communities, to enhance student learning outcomes (Fortier et al., 2015). This challenge will include making an educational shift from an illness-based, acute hospital model to a community and population health-based model, caring for individuals across the care continuum (Shaffer et al., 2018).

Baccalaureate Curriculum Considerations

Several authors have outlined the major changes that need to occur in nursing education to prepare nurses to practice effectively in an ever-changing healthcare system (Bauer & Bodenheimer, 2017; Bouchaud et al., 2017; Coburn, Gilland, Owen, et al., 2018; Shaffer et al., 2018). More Americans have access to healthcare services than ever before, increasing the volume of services and the need for more RNs, particularly RNs engaged in innovative care models and community-based services aimed at reducing cost and inefficiency. Of particular importance are aging adults with more chronic illnesses, comorbidities, and functional impairments.

BOX 15.1 Questions to Consider When Designing Ambulatory Care Curriculum

1. Is the curriculum designed to foster mastery of core knowledge and competencies in ambulatory settings, whether taught in stand-alone courses or integrated throughout the curriculum?
2. Do faculty have sufficient educational and experiential preparation in ambulatory care nursing and/or population health?
3. Are the teaching/learning methods and technologies appropriate for student learning, and are the core concepts and learning experiences arranged in a sequential, leveling manner?
4. Is the content appropriate for the RN generalist level rather than for advanced practice?
5. Are there opportunities for education-service collaboration and mentoring?
6. Are there opportunities for interprofessional learning and practice?

This system change in healthcare will require nurses who are comfortable working with teams and technology, including telehealth modalities by which individuals are monitored at home and through which RNs can quickly intervene to make adjustments to diet, fluid intake, medications, and physical activity. Educational programs must focus on critical thinking, ethical approaches, and judgment skills to accommodate these innovations (Bouchaud et al., 2017; Brennan & Sullivan-Marx, 2012).

Several questions are important for all educators to consider in assessing the adequacy of their curriculum in addressing ambulatory care competencies. These are noted in Box 15.1.

Complex Care Management Curriculum

The complexity of population-based nursing is different than that seen in acute care but is no less demanding of high levels of critical and analytical thinking. Undergraduate programs need to adjust to this reality. Faculty may need to examine the extent to which the curriculum they are delivering delineates between public health nursing, population health, and ambulatory care nursing and how the knowledge and skills are similar or different (RWJF, 2017).

The highly technical acute care nursing courses are often viewed as the most rigorous and demanding in the curriculum, reflecting the need for rapid response to changing physiologic signals that could represent a life or death situation for an individual. However, undergraduate students may have rotations in ambulatory settings and care for or manage comparable physical and socially complex situations. The practicum experiences may focus on health promotion, screening, or health education, as well as community outreach, behavioral health and mental health, primary care/population health such as chronic disease prevention and control, and healthy lifestyles such as substance use conditions. Students may have the opportunity to participate in care coordination for an individual and their family and/or experience team-based care delivery working with both healthcare providers and colleagues from community organizations. The learning opportunities and knowledge and skills that are required in ambulatory care are as rigorous and demanding as those needed in acute care.

One way to address the need for content on complex care in the ambulatory setting is by assessing and evaluating current didactic and clinical courses. In many curricula, it is not feasible to provide a separate course on ambulatory care nursing, and population health or public health courses may seem to have no relationship to the acute care setting. However, integrating these areas can both provide needed content and help students understand the continuum of care, both acute and ambulatory.

For example, courses that include acute and chronic health conditions, and rotations on medical/surgical units within a hospital, should include content that describes skills in coordinating care and managing transitions needed to prevent rehospitalization and the role of the interprofessional care team to ensure a seamless transition from the hospital to community-based care. Students should understand issues of health literacy and the social determinants of health that affect individuals' ability to access the services needed to ensure recovery once at home and the financial resources to purchase medication or adequate food to ensure healing and recovery. Teaching about CCTM should replace discharge planning in the **nursing curriculum**, emphasizing that teaching an individual and ensuring that they understand instructions is only a small and insufficient component of care coordination. Additional topics to consider for incorporation of ambulatory care content include the following:

- The role of the ambulatory care nurse
- Quality and meaningful measurement of nursing in ambulatory care
- Mental health and substance abuse certification
- Incorporating an interprofessional Team Strategies and Tools to Enhance Performance and Patient Safety Program (TeamSTEPPS)
- Acquiring motivational interviewing skills
- Developing health coaching skills

Completing a self-assessment of unconscious bias (AAACN, 2017; Shaffer et al., 2018; Start et al., 2016).

Clinical Experience

Providing students with clinical rotations in ambulatory care is critical to building clinical reasoning skills and empowers students in a variety of activities in the context of the interprofessional team. For example, nurse-led visits enable students to make more clinical decisions, contribute to team-based care, offer covisits, provide chronic care management visits, and employ knowledge and skills to care individuals with complex healthcare needs. Students need exposure to ambulatory care settings in which nurses exemplify the roles of coordinating care and managing transitions. In contrast to acute care settings, community centers, ambulatory care centers, and senior centers, as well as long-term care and rehabilitation centers, will be the major settings where the delivery of healthcare, care coordination, and transition management will occur.

Many of these ambulatory care settings have a wealth of learning opportunities and require support in integrating educational practice into their delivery of care. Concentrated effort and academic practice partnerships will be necessary to locate and support student learning at new clinical sites. Schools of nursing will need to seek out ways to partner with ambulatory care organizations (both practice-based and accountable care organizations) with RNs in a variety of roles from in-person individual and group visits to telehealth and remote monitoring visits, and home visits, to population health risk stratification, data analytics, value-based purchasing, and quality and safety (Salmond & Echevarria, 2017).

These partnerships can also support innovative strategies for faculty development and contribute to effective student teaching and learning strategies (Fortier et al., 2015). To facilitate the transition from an acute care setting to the community, RNs in academia or in partnership with other healthcare professionals, community leaders, business leaders, and elected and nonelected officials will need to design and pilot new programs to benefit communities, thus contributing to healthier populations and the forging of new partnerships (Rapin et al., 2015). The benefits are multiple: students acquire needed experience, communities are enhanced, and ambulatory sites are provided with the potential for new graduate employees.

An essential part of a successful clinical partnership is effective preceptorship. Because, as noted previously, ambulatory care does not support the traditional setting of one clinical instructor for six or more students, there is a great need for RN preceptors in the clinical setting. However, this is a new outreach for many schools, and there is often little infrastructure to support ambulatory care preceptors. In response, schools of nursing must assess and evaluate the challenges and needs that are unique to the ambulatory care setting. This also offers schools of nursing the opportunity to reevaluate traditional roles of clinical preceptors and, in a sense, start afresh in a clinical environment free of preconceived ideas as to the role and responsibilities of student nurse preceptors.

In traditional units within a hospital, the clinical instructor is part of the school of nursing and is directly responsible for the students; furthermore, the impact on nursing time for hospital employees is minimized. In contrast, few ambulatory care sites can accommodate more than two students, requiring that the RNs in those areas be preceptors, even though there may be a faculty member who makes site visits. The resulting impact on the RNs and the system is greater than in a hospital setting. In order for this to succeed, it is important for all involved institutions to understand and support the commitment.

The ambulatory care RN preceptor is most effective when fully supported by the academic institution. This includes clear communication about the level of experience and competencies that should be expected of the student and the clinical goals of the rotation. Preceptors should be provided with resources on effective preceptorship, including an environment in which students are encouraged to ask questions and seek answers. Because the pace of care in ambulatory settings may be erratic, preceptors benefit from suggestions concerning ways to keep students engaged in learning during slower clinical times. This type of preceptor support requires the academic institution to maintain clear communication with its clinical partners in order to assess preceptor needs and share its expertise in learning theories and competencies.

Even with competent preceptors, an additional clinical challenge is providing experiences for students that consistently supply the appropriate level of critical thinking and clinical judgment. Although there are exemplars of schools of nursing offering undergraduate direct experience in team-based ambulatory care, more can be done (Wojnar & Whelan, 2017). In addition, until sufficient numbers of RNs are in positions in which they function to the full extent of their education and fully utilize the skills needed for the healthcare systems of the future, simulation activities may be needed to demonstrate the complexity of the care to be provided.

Although there are few examples of simulation specifically designed for ambulatory care content, Badowski (2017) described virtual simulated care coordination rounds for an acute care setting that were integrated into an AD nursing curriculum. The designers used the National League for Nursing's (NLN) Advancing Care Excellence (ACE) unfolding cases (NLN Center for Excellence in the Care of Vulnerable Populations, n.d.) to illustrate healthcare quality for vulnerable populations. This component of an online course engaged students in activities associated with care coordination including teamwork, communication, and shared knowledge, in an acute care setting.

In another university ambulatory care course in a baccalaureate program, live human simulation was used to prepare students for the differences in skills and knowledge needed in the ambulatory setting (Coburn, Gilland, et al., 2017). This simulation was constructed to mimic an outpatient setting as closely as possible and emphasized the specific ambulatory skills of telehealth and chronic care management.

Strong clinical experiences and support for preceptors may be the most significant challenges for ambulatory care curriculum. Both high-quality simulation and preceptor education, as described in the case study, can contribute to the success of this essential part of student education. However, until more robust academic practice partnerships are developed in ambulatory care, schools of nursing will be challenged to find rotation sites and preceptors that provide rich environments for teaching all the roles of ambulatory care nursing.

Educational Innovations

Nursing curricula should be revised to introduce students early to the community systems in which individuals and families live and not overemphasize the bedside skills needed only in hospital settings. One example of this paradigm is illustrated by population health curricula with progressive content, in which students are introduced to basic content, skills, and tools necessary for success in primary care followed by application of those skills. They follow this up with a full semester of immersion in healthcare in the community. In their final semester, students are expected to apply what they have learned related to care coordination, critical thinking, and ethical and clinical judgment and to focus on leadership skills in action in a variety of clinical settings, including those based in the community. Students exposed to this integrated curriculum graduate prepared to explore employment opportunities in primary care, home healthcare, schools, and occupational settings (Brennan & Sullivan-Marx, 2012).

Other possibilities for educational innovations to prepare the ambulatory care teams of the future include the following:

- Rotations of interprofessional students to community-based ambulatory care sites. As part of a team, students conduct needs assessments, complete projects around social and economic determinants of health, and undertake quality improvement projects. Nursing students may be paired with students from other disciplines such as medicine, pharmacy, and physical therapy.
- Development of basic data analytic skills using deidentified data. Students need to experience the entire power of the electronic health record systems to examine the data not only on specific individuals but also on specific populations. Faculty should be encouraged to use real-world data in their curriculum.
- Providing BSN-prepared nurses with **role transition** and/or immersion experiences that allow them to move seamlessly from their educational programs into ambulatory settings, including complex community systems and organizational structures, where they can apply leadership, skills, and decision-making in the provision of care, healthcare team coordination, and the oversight and accountability for care. This can provide opportunities for interprofessional team practice to demonstrate their leadership and communication skills.
- Enabling the expansion of BSN programs' traditional major focus on quality and safety in the care of individuals in hospital settings to incorporate a focus on ambulatory settings.

Quality and safety is an additional important area of study in preparing students and RNs who are new to ambulatory care. The issues specific to ambulatory settings can be complex given the lack of direct control of the individual's environment, including slip/fall factors in the home; poor driving skills in an elderly individual; or lack of supervision of medications, meals, and ambulation outside of the clinical setting. Social determinants of health also play a much larger role in predicting the safety and quality of home-based care.

New-to-practice RNs have the education and training to apply concepts of quality and safety using structure, process, and outcome measures; however, they may need experiential learning to apply these concepts and identify factors that create a culture of health and safety and caring outside of the hospital setting.

Measuring Critical Thinking and Decision-Making in Ambulatory Care

Palumbo et al. (2017) point out that the National Council Licensure Examination-Registered Nurse (NCLEX-RN) examination, for entry into professional nursing practice, tests for competency in common practice settings but has historically emphasized acute care situations. Different skill sets are needed for nurses practicing in settings focused on ambulatory care and population health management. In 2012, the National Council of State Boards of Nursing (NCSBN) evaluated salience of the examination: Was it measuring the right things? Given the rapid increase in knowledge and technology, nurses and other health professionals can no longer memorize all the knowledge needed to care effectively for individuals and populations.

Although nurses will always learn skills and memorize facts, it is more important that they be able to access the knowledge they need to apply their critical thinking and decision-making skills. The **NCLEX-RN examination** will continue to revise, using a *Clinical Judgment Model* framework to test different components of the process of an initial encounter, assessment, forming hypotheses, prioritizing them, and taking action. This assessment of higher order functioning will be critical for public safety and essential to delivering care that extends beyond the walls of a hospital. The core competencies of ambulatory nurses could serve as perfect frameworks for the development of test items that go beyond memorization and instead reflect problem identification and prioritization and recognizing actions that are within the scope of practice for professional nursing.

Transition to Practice in Ambulatory Settings

If schools of nursing develop educational programs that provide students with the opportunity to demonstrate competencies in ambulatory nursing, then, optimally, their transition to practice will be such that they feel competent and satisfied in their employment positions. The NCSBN conducted a study of the factors that promote the successful transition of a new nursing graduate into practice (NLN Center for Excellence in the Care of Vulnerable Populations, n.d.). One part of the NCSBN study focused on the feasibility of implementing a transition to practice residency program in nonhospital settings. Sites, including nursing homes, public health, and home health agencies, were recruited to participate in the study, and 23 facilities hired 48 new nurses who were enrolled in the study between April 1, 2012, and October 31, 2012. The study compared NCSBN's Transition to Practice program with the control group, which used sites' existing onboarding orientation programs. Results presented on competency assessment, reports of errors and safety practices, work stress, job satisfaction, and retention showed that transition to practice programs have the potential for improving outcomes in nonhospital settings, but more evidence is needed.

As the importance of RN residency programs becomes more evident, support for those programs has also grown. The AAACN has developed the Ambulatory Care Registered Nurse Residency Program, which provides content and a guide for implementation (Levine, 2017; More, 2017). As support and resources grow, ambulatory care centers are implementing RN residency programs that match the rigor of those in the acute care setting (Gilland et al., 2019).

Certification and Certificate Programs

Certification programs are offered in Ambulatory Care Nursing (American Nurses Credentialing Center) and in CCTM (American Association of Ambulatory Care Nursing through the Medical-Surgical Nursing Certification Board). Additionally, academic centers are offering certificate programs in areas such as care coordination and clinical case management.

Development of certificate programs is an appropriate way for schools of nursing to contribute to the field of ambulatory care nursing; it leverages the strengths of academic institutions to provide RN workforce development. This, in turn, will help to elevate the role of the RN in this rapidly growing specialty.

Summary

The healthcare landscape of the United States is changing focus toward that of ambulatory care, and nursing is well positioned to address the growing need for care expertise for individuals with complex health issues. The majority of this care will not happen in acute care settings, which has been the traditional focus for prelicensure education, but rather in ambulatory settings. Although the focus of prelicensure nursing education has traditionally not been ambulatory care, many of the core competencies such as care coordination, transition management, and interprofessional collaboration are basic to nursing education. These concepts provide new graduates with content that can be applied to a range of ambulatory settings, but full competence requires intentional change to nursing curricula and postgraduate education.

Ambulatory care nursing concepts can be integrated into existing curricula as described previously or implemented within a separate course that incorporates population health and ambulatory care. However, clinical experience is a greater challenge in the ambulatory care setting than in traditional hospital units, and simulation may be an important adjunct to site-specific rotations.

Postgraduate education is an important part of maximizing the impact and effectiveness of the RN workforce. RN residency has been well documented as a valuable tool in postgraduate education for acute care and ambulatory care settings. Other continuing education options for ambulatory care include a variety of certifications and certificates, which may also position nurses for advanced degrees.

Addressing the need for visibility and competence in ambulatory care nursing requires commitment by the nursing education and practice communities. It is incumbent on educators to provide students with the knowledge and clinical experience that will allow them to apply the foundational content of nursing education in an ambulatory setting and to flourish in this changing environment.

Case Study

Mr. Johnson is an experienced RN holding a BSN and has worked for 3 years in a primary care clinic affiliated with a large academic health center. He has never served as an educational preceptor before and has been assigned to that role for undergraduate nursing students enrolled in a course on ambulatory care who will rotate through his clinic in the upcoming semester.

The unit manager is supporting Mr. Johnson in this new role by providing 2 hours of orientation on being a preceptor. This orientation includes an overview of learning styles for different generations and types of learners, learning objectives for the students rotating in his clinical area, the student clinical expectations, and the clinical evaluation form to be submitted to the students' course instructor.

At the end of the semester, his student evaluations included negative comments such as the following: "I thought I was doing fine until the end of the rotation. Mr. Johnson never told me that he was not happy with my work, but I got a terrible evaluation." "There were times when there was very little to do and I found it boring." "Mr. Johnson made me nervous when he would ask a lot of questions about what I knew, so that sometimes I couldn't remember things I actually could have answered."

Consider the following questions based on the student evaluations:

1. What educational content might be added to the preceptor's workshop?
2. How should orientation content be presented in a way that helps the preceptor apply the concepts?
3. What are other ways to support a new preceptor?

After the first semester and on receiving student evaluations, the school made the following changes to the preceptor support program:

- Addition of content on evaluation of students, including both formative and summative components.
- Tips for ways to provide constructive criticism and an activity to apply those principles.
- Tools for ways to support student learning in the clinical area, such as the "5-minute preceptor" and suggestions for handling "downtime."
- Providing a toolbox of activities that build on the overall competencies of ambulatory care. Nursing students can complete the activities when not working with individual patients.
- A midsemester check-in meeting between the preceptor and nursing education director to discuss any challenges or needs.

Key Points for Review

- The changes in U.S. healthcare provide both the need and the opportunities for RNs to support the care of individuals outside the acute care system.
- Traditional nursing education has focused primarily on the acute care setting, but this focus is beginning to shift toward greater emphasis on ambulatory care.
- Including ambulatory care content in nursing curricula requires incorporating new concepts, applying old concepts to new settings, and providing rich clinical experience.
- An important part of sustaining the impact of RNs in ambulatory care is the creation and support of certifications and residency programs.

REFERENCES

Allen, J. W. (2016). Transitioning the RN to ambulatory care. *Nursing Administration Quarterly, 40*(2), 115–121. https://doi.org/10.1097/NAQ.0000000000000151

American Academy of Ambulatory Care Nursing. (2017). *The role of the registered nurse in ambulatory care*. American Academy of Ambulatory Care Nursing.

American Association of Colleges of Nursing. (2008). *Essentials of baccalaureate education for professional nursing*. American Association of Colleges of Nursing.

Ashley, C., Halcomb, E., & Brown, A. (2016). Transitioning from acute to primary health care nursing: An integrative review of the literature. *Journal of Clinical Nursing, 25* (15–16), 2114–2125. https://doi.org/10.1111/jocn.13185

Auerbach, D. I., Buerhaus, P. I., & Staiger, D. O. (2017). How fast will the registered nurse workforce grow through 2030? Projections in nine regions of the country. *Nursing Outlook, 65*(1), 116–122. https://doi.org/10.1016/j.outlook.2016.07.004

Australian Institute of Health and Welfare. (2013). *Nursing and midwifery workforce 2012*. National Health Workforce Series No. 6. Cat. No. HWL 52. http://www.aihw.gov.au/publication-detail/?id=60129545333&tab=2

Badowski, D. M. (2017). Virtual simulated care coordination rounds for nursing students. *Nursing Education Perspectives, 38*(6), 352–353. https://doi.org/10.1097/01.NEP.0000000000000133

Basu, S., Phillips, R. S., Bitton, A., Song, Z., & Landon, B. E. (2015). Medicare chronic care management payments and financial returns to primary care practices: A modeling study. *Annals of Internal Medicine, 163*(8), 580–588. https://doi.org/10.7326/M14-2677

Bauer, L., & Bodenheimer, T. (2017). Expanded roles of registered nurses in primary care delivery of the future. *Nursing Outlook, 65*(5), 624–632. https://doi.org/10.1016/j.outlook.2017.03.011

Bouchaud, M., Brown, D., & Swan, B. A. (2017). Creating a new education paradigm to prepare nurses for the 21st century. *Journal of Nursing Education and Practice, 7*(10), 27–35. https://doi.org/10.5430/jnep.v7n10p27

Brennan, A. M. W., & Sullivan-Marx, E. (2012). The paradigm shift. *The Nursing Clinics of North America, 47*(4), 455–462. https://doi.org/10.1016/j.cnur.2012.09.001

Bureau of Labor Statistics. (2016). *Registered nurses: Work environment*. https://www.bls.gov/ooh/healthcare/registered-nurses.htm#tab-3

Chan, R., Marx, W., Bradford, N., Gordon, L., Bonner, A., Douglas, C., Schmalkuche, D., & Yates, P. (2018). Clinical and economic outcomes of nurse-led services in ambulatory care setting: A systematic review. *International Journal of Nursing Studies, 81*, 61–80. https://doi.org/10.1016/j.ijnurstu.2018.02.002

Coburn, C. V., Gilland, D., Owen, M., & Amar, A. (2018). Ambulatory care education: Preparing nurses for the future of healthcare. *Nurse Education Today, 66*, 79–81. https://doi.org/10.1016/j.nedt.2018.03.015

Coburn, C., Gilland, D., & Stahl, K. (2018). High-fidelity simulation in an undergraduate ambulatory care nursing course. *Nursing Education Perspectives, 41*(1), 54–56. https://doi.org/10.1097/01.NEP.0000000000000427

Curtis, E. A., & Glacken, M. (2014). Job satisfaction among public health nurses: A national survey. *Journal of Nursing Management, 22*(5), 653–663. https://doi.org/10.1111/jonm.12026

Flinter, M., Hsu, C., Cromp, D., Ladden, M., & Wagner, E. (2017). Registered nurses in primary care: Emerging new roles and contributions to team-based care in high-performing practices. *Journal of Ambulatory Care Management, 40*(4), 287–296. https://doi.org/10.1097/JAC.0000000000000193

Fortier, M. E., Perron, T., Fountain, D. M., Hinic, K., Vargas, M., Swan, B. A., & Heelan-Fancher, L. (2015). Health care in the community: Developing academic/practice partnerships for care coordination and managing transitions. *Nursing Economic$, 33*(3), 167–175, 181.

Fraher, E. P., Ricketts, T. C., Lefebvre, A., & Newton, W. P. (2013). The role of academic health centers and their partners in reconfiguring and retooling the existing workforce to practice in a transformed health system. *Academic Medicine, 88*(12), 1812–1816. https://doi.org/10.1097/ACM.0000000000000024

Gilland, D. G., Muirhead, L. M., Toney, S., & Coburn, C. V. (2019). Building a workforce pipeline: Development of an ambulatory nurse residency program. *Nursing Management, 50*(7), 32–37. https://doi.org/10.1097/01.NUMA.0000558520.60241.1f

Haas, S., Swan, B. A., & Haynes, T. (2013). Developing ambulatory care registered nurse competencies for care coordination and transition management. *Nursing Economics, 31*(1), 44–49, 43.

Haas, S., Swan, B.A., & Haynes, T. (2019). *Care coordination and transition management core curriculum* (2nd ed.). American Academy of Ambulatory Care Nursing.

Halcomb, E., Stephens, M., Bryce, J., Foley, E., & Ashley, C. (2016). Nursing competency standards in primary health care: An integrative review. *Journal of Clinical Nursing, 25*(9–10), 1193–1205. https://doi.org/10.1111/jocn.13224

Lamb, G., Newhouse, R., Beverly, C., Toney, D. A., Cropley, S., Weaver, C. A., & Task Force Members. (2015). Policy agenda for nurse-led care coordination. *Nursing Outlook, 63*(4), 521–530. https://doi.org/10.1016/j.outlook.2015.06.003

Laughlin, C. B. (2018). *Core curriculum for ambulatory care nursing* (4th ed.). American Academy of Ambulatory Care Nursing.

Levine, J. (2017). Transition to practice—Part 1: Implementing an ambulatory care registered nurse residency program, the importance of a structural framework. *Nursing Economics, 35*(5), 267–271.

McInnes, S., Peters, K., Hardy, J., & Halcomb, E. (2015). Clinical placements in Australian general practice: (Part 1) the experiences of pre-registration nursing students. *Nurse Education in Practice, 15*(6), 437–442. https://doi.org/10.1016/j.nepr.2015.04.003

More, L. (2017). Transition to practice—Part 2 Implementing an ambulatory care registered nurse residency program: Competency—It's not just a task. *Nursing Economics, 35*(6), 317–321.

NLN Center for Excellence in the Care of Vulnerable Populations. (n.d.). http://www.nln.org/centers-for-nursing-education/nln-center-for-innovation-in-education-excellence/institute-for-the-care-of-vulnerable-populations

Palumbo, M. V., Rambur, B., & Hart, V. (2017). Is health care payment reform impacting nurses' work settings, roles, and education preparation? *Journal of Professional Nursing, 33*(6), 400–404. https://doi.org/10.1016/j.profnurs.2016.11.005

Rapin, J., D'Amour, D., & Dubois, C. A. (2015). Indicators for evaluating the performance and quality of care of ambulatory care nurses. *Nursing Research and Practice, 2015*, 861239. https://doi.org/10.1155/2015/861239

Redman, R. W., Pressler, S. J., Furspan, P., & Potempa, K. (2015). Nurses in the United States with a practice doctorate: Implications for leading in the current context of health care. *Nursing Outlook, 63*(2), 124–129. https://doi.org/10.1016/j.outlook.2014.08.003

Robert Wood Johnson Foundation. (2017). *Catalysts for change: Harnessing the power of nurses to build population health in the 21st century*. Robert Wood Johnson Foundation.

Rui, P., & Okeyode, T. *National Ambulatory Medical Care Survey: 2015 State and National Summary Tables*. Available from http://www.cdc.gov/nchs/ahcd/ahcd_products.htm

Salmond, S., & Echevarria, M. (2017). Healthcare transformation and changing roles for nursing. *Orthopedic Nursing, 36*(1), 12–25. https://doi.org/10.1097/NOR.0000000000000308

Shaffer, K., Swan, B. A., & Bouchaud, M. (2018). Designing a new model for clinical education. *Nurse Educator, 43*(3), 145–148. https://doi.org/10.1016/j.outlook.2014.08.004

Smolowitz, J., Speakman, E., Wojnar, D., Whelan, E.-M., Ulrich, S., Hayes, C., & Wood, L. (2015). Role of the registered nurse in primary health care: Meeting health care needs in the 21st century. *Nursing Outlook, 63*(2), 130–136. https://doi.org/10.1016/j.outlook.2014.08.004

Start, R., Matlock, A. M., & Mastal, M. (2016). *Ambulatory care nurse-sensitive indicator industry report*. American Academy of Ambulatory Care Nursing.

Wagner, E., Flinter, M., Hsu, C., Cromp, D., Austin, B., Etz, R., Crabtree, B., & Ladden, M. (2017). Effective team-based primary care: Observations from innovative practices. *BMC Family Practice, 18*(13), 1–9. https://doi.org/10.1186/s12875-017-0590-8

Welch, W. P., Cuellar, A. E., Stearns, S. C., & Bindman, A. B. (2013). Proportion of physicians in large group practices continued to grow in 2009–11. *Health Affairs (Project Hope), 32*(9), 1659–1666. https://doi.org/10.1377/hlthaff.2012.1256

Wojnar, D., & Whelan, E. M. (2017). Preparing nursing students for enhanced roles in primary care: The current state of prelicensure and RN-to-BSN education. *Nursing Outlook, 65*, 222–232. https://doi.org/10.1016/j.outlook.2016.10.006

16

Infrastructures That Support Ambulatory Professional Nursing Practice

Noreen Bernard, Sharon Pappas, Carrie McDermott, and Roy L. Simpson

PERSPECTIVES

"Bringing new graduates into ambulatory care is a logical approach to address the approaching shortage; however, this has not been the case. It is not customary for new graduates to gain competency in ambulatory nursing skills in pre-license education. This, coupled with an often-inadequate orientation suggests the need [for] comprehensive RN residency programs to allay the fears of the new graduates and current staff."

June Levine, MSN, RN AAACN

LEARNING OBJECTIVES

Upon completion of this chapter, the reader will be able to:

1. Articulate the infrastructures needed to support ambulatory professional nursing practice.
2. Describe key elements of a positive practice environment.
3. Discuss professional governance in an ambulatory setting.
4. Name elements of a professional practice model.
5. Recognize the role of residencies in ambulatory nursing.
6. Identify the role of informatics in ambulatory nursing.
7. Evaluate elements of ambulatory professional development.
8. Explain the role of ambulatory nurse residency programs.

KEY TERMS

Ambulatory medical record (AMR)
Electronic medical record (EMR)
Nurse residency program (NRP)
Professional governance
Professional practice environment
Professional practice model (PPM)
Quality and Safety Education for Nurses (QSEN)

Nursing as a Profession

The role of the nurse in any setting includes understanding the meaning of the experience health or illness has on an individual and facilitating those processes and outcomes important to meet the individual's expectations. The important intersections necessary to meet this requirement involve the nurse in the role of following the directives of others such as physicians, supervisors, or regulators, while providing care to individuals who benefit from the care of a nurse. The nurse must actualize these unique contributions for the benefit of individuals. However, both colleagues and individuals often overlook aspects of the work of nursing. Frameworks and structures make nursing work visible by defining the practice role of nurses and describing their individual and team accountabilities to individuals and the organization.

The discipline of nursing evolved across more than a century. Nursing was first viewed as simply something women did in their traditional caregiver role. Today, the practice of nursing is guided by theory and practice models with integration of education, practice, and research to advance nursing science (Shaw, 1993). To further expose nursing's uniqueness, clear definitions of nursing that articulate the autonomy and accountability of professional nurses come from professional nursing groups and organizations as they respond to evolving societal needs. The American Nurses Association (ANA) states "nursing is the protection, promotion, and optimization of health and abilities, prevention of illness and injury, alleviation of suffering through the diagnosis and treatment of human response, and advocacy in the care of individuals, families, communities, and populations" as part of the ANA social policy statement (ANA, 2003).

The Future of Nursing (FON) report finalized in 2010 describes the expanding role of the nurse to be visible across the full spectrum of care including management of chronic disease and prevention of disease (Future of Nursing, 2011). These evolving concepts have served as an important foundation for the development of the specialty of ambulatory nursing practice because the nature of managing and preventing disease most often occurs outside a hospital. The American Academy of Ambulatory Care Nursing (AAACN) believes that professional ambulatory care nursing is a complex multidimensional specialty practice of nursing that has components of independent and collaborative practice (AAACN, 2018).

Ambulatory nursing care shares much in common with acute care nursing such as wellness promotion, assistance in management of chronic illness, and supporting individuals at the end of life. These are all common elements of nursing practice and confirm nursing as a unique discipline. The specific differences for the ambulatory nursing specialty lie in the scope of ambulatory nursing practice and in the sites and mechanisms of care delivery that span beyond solely in-person care to also integrate technology and telephonic management of individuals including management of individuals across a lifetime (AAACN, 2018).

As our healthcare system transforms, the role of nursing transforms as well to call on the wisdom, expertise, knowledge, and compassion of nurses to meet healthcare needs. The purpose of this chapter is to describe important infrastructures that expose and optimize the uniqueness of nursing practice and the contributions of professional nurses to individual care. The infrastructures that support professional ambulatory nursing practice include the **professional practice environment** (PPE) guided by a **professional practice model (PPM)** and shared governance along with the reinforcement of ambulatory nursing practice by the **ambulatory medical record (AMR)** and professional development including the role of nurse residencies. These structures cannot exist in isolation and must be aligned and integrated to create the desired infrastructure for professional ambulatory nursing practice.

The Context of the Care of Individuals

The importance of a PPE was discovered through an important study commissioned by the American Academy of Nursing in the early 1980s (McClure et al., 1983). Reacting to ongoing nursing shortages, the researchers studied organizations that had strong nursing recruitment and retention. They sought to identify the characteristics of the hospitals and the context of care that caused these hospitals to succeed. Some of the findings that are highly relevant today included:

- Strong nursing leadership that supports the practice of nursing
- Individual-centered philosophy of care guided by a PPM
- Nursing involvement in decisions about direct individual care
- Support for professional development
- Interprofessional collaboration

Over the decades since the original Magnet® study, researchers have confirmed the findings and further described PPE through programs such as the American Nurses Credentialing Center (ANCC) Magnet® recognition program and reports such as the FON. Many specialty organizations have applied the broader nursing findings to their specialty practice. The concepts of a PPE apply to ambulatory nursing and serve as the foundation for professional ambulatory nursing practice.

Leading a Professional Practice Environment

A PPE as the context of individual care begins with leadership. Nursing leaders are keenly aware of the importance of the work environment and its impact on nurses and thus on individual care. Leaders make sure clinicians can respond to individual and organizational needs through motivation, support, and encouragement to innovate and create by providing environments where they are physically and psychologically safe, informed by models that guide their practice, and relationships that inspire them to be professionals. In a study of new graduate nurses, Spence Laschinger et al. (2012) found that a supportive practice environment predicted work engagement to support retention and well-being of nurses. These findings are consistent with the evidence from the original Magnet® study about clinical nurses. These environments require leadership qualities that transcend the historical role of leaders who led from a transactional framework of emphasizing rules and task completion to leaders who are transformational. Transformational leaders generate excitement and motivation, they ask questions that stimulate intellectual development, and they influence others through modeling the behaviors they want to see.

Leaders are the keepers of the individual care culture. The leaders' style and ability to close the gap between vision for practice and current state of practice define the success of the leader. Both the vision and the path to achieve the vision are often described by structures such as the PPM and the decision-making and are reinforced by the mechanisms that support nursing practice and professional development. The PPE, specific to nursing, demonstrates how to value and advance the discipline of nursing. It is defined "as an organizational culture that advances the clinical practice of nurses and other health professionals by ensuring unity of purpose and organizations alignment" (Ives Erickson, 2012, p. 9).

In Figure 16.1, a practice environment conceptual framework developed by Jeannette Ives-Erikson (2012), chief nurse executive at Massachusetts General Hospital, provides a representation of the dynamic interactions within a PPE.

The interrelationship between elements necessary for a PPE and the existing organizational characteristics is depicted structurally as a path to culture change. The elements represent the four areas of influence that come from a shared understanding from within the environment

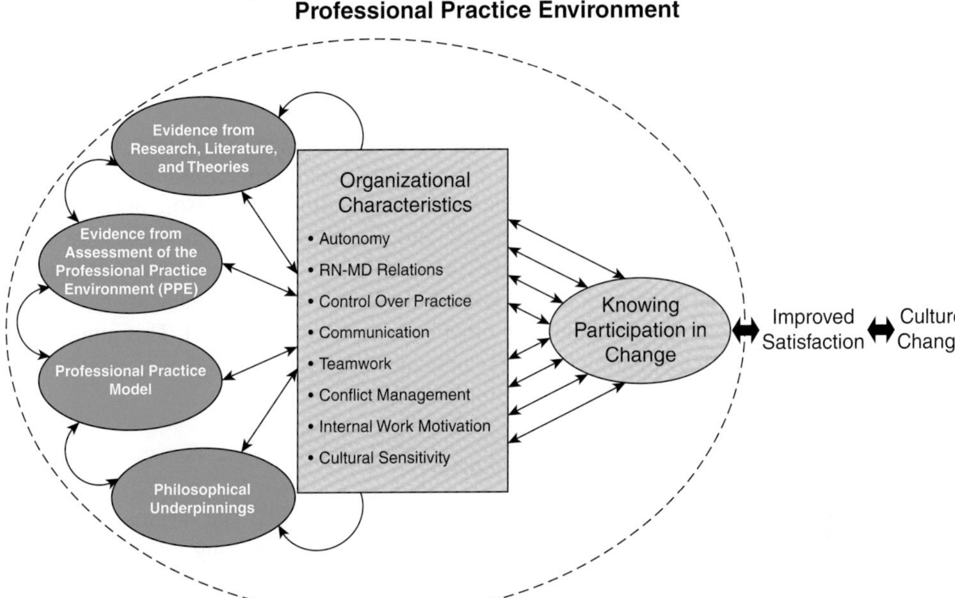

FIGURE 16.1 Interactions within a professional practice environment. This representation was developed to demonstrate the interrelationships between the elements necessary to improve the professional practice environment. The graphic incorporates four areas of influence that result in shared understanding between constituents in the environment of care that have the potential power to improve the environment in which they practice. (From Ives Erickson, J. [2013]. Influencing professional practice at the bedside. In J. Ives Erikson, D. A. Jones, & M. Ditomassi [Eds.], *Fostering nurse-led care* [p. 5]. Sigma Theta Tau.)

that have the potential to improve the environment in which nursing practice occurs. The four areas of influence include the following:

1. The philosophical underpinnings or a basis for nursing practice where nurses answer the question of who they are as a nurse;
2. The PPM that serves as a framework for professional practice;
3. Evidence from research, the literature, and theories where leaders ensure nurses develop, support, and utilize evidence to inform and influence the delivery of quality and safe care; and
4. Evidence of nurse perceptions from concurrent assessment of the effectiveness of the PPE (Ives Erickson, 2013, p. 5).

Professional Practice Model

A Professional Practice Model is a structure that describes the contributions of nursing practice within a specific organization or practice area. The structure most often describes the context of the nurse relationship with the individual, to their own practice, to the roles of other clinicians in contributing to the individual care plan, and to the organization (Ives Erickson & Ditomassi, 2011). Most practice models are based on a theory and are designed to evolve as an essential description of how nursing is practiced and individual care provided, the nursing and organizational relationships, and the organizational concepts. The model also grounds and aligns nurses with the purpose they serve. The model serves to make nursing work visible through describing the path for achieving outcomes. For PPMs to be real and effective, the clarity of the clinical and leadership skills required must be explicit. Nurses must understand the intent of the model and see it used in order for it to be fully actualized and useful (Ives Erickson & Ditomassi, 2012). When leaders embrace this modeling, such as in Magnet® organizations, nurses can describe the meaning of the model and discuss how models are developed, implemented, and evaluated regularly. This process maintains the meaningfulness of the model to clinical nurses.

PPMs are developed from within organizations with guidance from evidence on the necessary components to nursing practice. Often a qualitative process is convened, which through the involvement of clinical nurses, the individual relationship, nursing practice, the team relationships, the purpose of nursing practice, and organizational relationships are developed and described. If a PPM has been in place, the same process can be used to evaluate and expand on concepts of an existing model (Cobb et al., 2018). Next, mechanisms are needed in order to make decisions and guide nursing practice according to the PPM. This guidance of practice plus a process for evaluating the PPE can be accomplished through a dynamic and supportive nursing governance structure.

Professional Nursing Governance

Professional governance is an essential element of a PPE. The origins of this practice of a shared nonhierarchical structural framework for decision-making related to nursing practice come from a desire for a mechanism to support and establish that nurses make decisions about professional nursing practice. This oversimplification of the concept served as the beginning of contemporary models of shared governance that serve as a mechanism for nurses to work collaboratively to accomplish important activities that support clinical nursing practice such as development of standards, management of individual outcomes that tie directly to nursing practice, and advancement of nursing science (McDonagh, 1990). Shared governance in its support of a PPE aligns with the Magnet® model component of structural empowerment and includes the support of nursing ownership of practice, nurse engagement, role development, professional development, and a positive practice environment (ANCC, 2017).

Healthcare is evolving, and growing financial pressures from increasing costs of operations and stagnant to declining reimbursement are common. Nurses are a significant cost to healthcare systems occupying a large percentage of a typical hospital operating budget, and these pressures require a demonstration of the clinical and financial impact of nurses on individual care. Especially in ambulatory practice environments, the importance of describing the professional nursing role and its impact on individual outcomes is essential. The importance of a nursing professional identity, role accountability, and interprofessional interface must be explicit and evolve to meet the needs in the practice setting including clinical performance expectations and individual engagement (Clavelle et al., 2016). The disciplines must specifically define their roles, relationship, and distinct contribution as part of an aggregated professional team. In addition, although nursing is affirmed as a profession, individuals must demonstrate this professional status behaviorally through the discipline-specific ownership of practice, quality, competence, and management of the requisite knowledge of nursing. The evolving concept of shared governance takes on new meaning in a practice environment where individuals need and deserve the best of all disciplines when they receive their care. Healthcare has grown in complexity and the herculean effort of one team member directing the work of every member of the team is no longer effective. These shifts require an advancement of the concept of shared governance to one of professional governance, which builds on the conceptual foundation of shared governance and is characterized by the attributes of accountability, professional obligation, collateral relationships, and decision-making (Clavelle et al., 2016).

In an ambulatory practice setting where roles can be blurred, interprofessional governance works because there is a table where all members collaterally participate and the expectation is that all are clear about their role, contribution, and the value each brings to that table

(Porter-O'Grady, 2017). Governing from inside, one discipline falls short of how ambulatory care is provided and is often accelerated through the interprofessional approach as long as the scope of each discipline is optimized. Models for professional governance take on many forms, and the essential elements of professional governance include ownership of professional practice and accountability for the outcomes of that discipline's practice. Commonly, these councils are interprofessional and should maintain clarity of the outcomes that are accomplished as a team and the outcomes largely related to nursing practice. This is important in order for appropriate interventions that are both discipline specific and within the scope of practice can be applied where improvement is needed. Improvement in individual outcomes is core to the work of a council where members evaluate their own practice protocols through using current evidence to guide changes. Councils are a structural format that demonstrates discipline-specific ownership of practice, quality, and competence and discipline-specific knowledge management (Joseph & Bogue, 2016).

Reinforcing Ambulatory Nursing Practice Through the Ambulatory Medical Record

Moving the documentation of individual care from traditional paper-based documents to **electronic medical records (EMRs)** and AMRs has the potential to change individual care as we know it today. Making the details of individual care decisions, communications, and interactions available for big data analysis could prompt nursing to make emboldened choices that accelerate the standard of care significantly. As a result, the effectiveness of individual care could improve as outcomes become more predictable. Finally, knowing which processes and protocols yield optimal results could hold down costs as less-effective practices are phased out.

The AMR serves to reinforce evidence-based standard care to accelerate improvement in individual outcomes. Electrifying the medical record could propel nursing over the precipice of information into the nirvana of large-scale research. With massive amounts of digitized individual records available for analysis, big data may be able to help nursing determine the monetary value of the critical thinking it brings to individual care, which is one of the goals of a PPE.

Government-Mandated Electronic Individual Records

When the government-mandated EMRs and AMRs, the requirement was designed to move physicians from traditional paper-based medical records to a semi-standardized digital or electronic format that could be shared between and among healthcare providers. This operational shift, it was thought, would streamline communications across the continuum of care, improve outcomes, and bring down costs.

Typically, an EMR includes an individual's medical history, limited social history, current and past diagnoses, treatment plans, immunization details, known allergies and medical images, as well as lab and test results. Authorized providers apply evidence-based tools to this data to make individual care decisions. EMRs were created to automate and streamline communication and workflows between and among providers. Not only can authorized users access EMRs in real time, but also these documents go beyond the boundaries of a single provider's view to include care across the traditional boundaries of provider, location, and time.

With the advent of the EMR, individual charts became electronic repositories of individual care interactions and outcomes. They became living, breathing documents that are updated across the continuum of care. At least, that was the vision that propelled EMRs into the spotlight. Reality, however, is different and, in some cases, very different.

Differences Between Electronic Medical Records and Ambulatory Medical Records

The differences between EMRs and AMRs relate not just to the volume of information they contain but the number of clinicians who contribute to the record and the workflows that support information as well. For example, in acute care settings, physicians and nurses dominate the provider and clinician types that add data to EMRs. Although they also make entries onto AMRs, several additional types of clinical staff, including medical assistants, licensed practical nurses (LPNs), and advanced practice providers, as well as nonclinical staff update AMRs.

Second, although the EMR contains information about surgical care requiring at least an overnight stay in an acute care hospital, the AMR captures information about care given in nonhospital settings such as urgent care clinics, physicians' offices, and telephonic or in-home care. Ambulatory care usually involves different and often independent providers who work in concert with one another. This further strengthens the requirement for the AMR to serve in an information-integrating role to facilitate the coordination of care. For example, ambulatory care decisions depend heavily on information from referring physicians, pharmacies, outside medical consults, external laboratories, and imaging centers, and the AMR becomes a central repository for communication and documentation of care-related decisions.

Another major difference between an EMR and an AMR focuses on location-specific workflows—that is, the way information moves through the type of setting where individual care is delivered. For example, whereas urgent care clinics' workflows vary from those found inpatient and outpatient surgery centers, including workflows in the same setting, a physician's office workflow can vary based on specialty.

Additionally, information moves through an ambulatory facility much differently than it flows through an acute care operation. By thinking of an ambulatory setting as a "service node" in a larger healthcare delivery ecosystem, one can see why the variation exists. In many situations, these differences call for two totally different EMR/AMR products, each tailored to accommodate the specific operational workflows of the ambulatory or acute care setting where they are used.

As providers across the continuum of care continue to affiliate and consolidate, many hospitals are acquiring ambulatory care facilities and requiring that these operations replace their existing, web-based EMR/AMR software (often hosted offsite) with the acquiring organization's existing EMR solution. This strategy sometimes results in unintended consequences such as variation in the degree of information sharing, considering that some hosted, web-based EMRs/AMRs (popular in ambulatory facilities) have less interaction with external resources, such as laboratories, pharmacies, and imaging centers, compared to the high interactions hospital EMRs have with internal, clinical departments (Jamoom et al., 2016). In addition, hosted, web-based EMRs can be updated and maintained faster and more easily than EMRs that are integrated with comprehensive hospital-wide information technology systems. The episodic nature of AMRs generally makes the content in these electronic documents less dense and easier to manage than the data found in EMRs.

The Promise of a Universal Health Record

For the EMR to deliver on the promise of becoming a universal health record, integration of varying EMR and AMR formats is needed along with ubiquitous secured connectivity. Integration is an expensive proposition and one that the federal government is underwriting to some degree. The 2009 Health Information Technology for Economic and Clinical Health Act (HITECH, 2009) set out to bring healthcare providers "into the tent" by demonstrating their "meaningful use" of a certified EMR. Providers meeting the requirements of Stage 1 of that certification received financial incentives that could be used to defray the cost associated with implementation and maintenance of EMRs.

In addition, The Joint Commission embraced EMRs by mandating electronic documents collect data to show compliance with the accreditor's 2018 National Individual Safety Goals® (TJC, 2018). In the future, hospital EMRs will need to be re-architected to collect the data needed to improve:

- individual identification,
- communication between departments and during handoffs,
- the safe use of medications,
- infection control,
- medical reconciliation during transitions of care, and
- suicide prevention efforts.

In many cases, checklist-driven documentation, which will be built into the new EMR software for hospitals, will help providers achieve their performance in these critically important individual care areas.

In the future, new data collection requirements will emerge on a regular basis to expand the content and scope of EMRs, complicating an already complex data collection effort. For example, with the current national opioid crisis, there is a critical need to better understand the ordering patterns and subsequent care requirements of this vulnerable population so that addiction intervention and prevention can occur (Palmer et al., 2015). These emerging requirements mean that the costly integration already achieved for EMRs will require another expensive revision to accommodate the expanding scope of EMR/AMR data. Future shifts in data collection and communication protocols will drive up the implementation, integration, and training costs associated with EMRs/AMRs.

For those using EMRs in ambulatory settings, hospital-focused documentation changes indicate a need for the AMR to more closely mirror the hospital EMR. This evolution will create portable data that can be easily integrated into hospitals' information technology systems, particularly individual care applications. EMR enhancements can also support functions such as telephonic care coordination so that providers have immediate access to all individual information irrespective of the setting where care was provided.

In an ideal world, healthcare providers' data collection and EMR usage would move toward a standardized design with intuitive navigation to ensure ease of use. Historically, however, EMR goals are misaligned, with some users desiring efficiency, some requiring comprehensiveness, and some focusing on financial functionality versus individual care function. Therefore, institutional and individual users of healthcare information technology have enthusiastically resisted standardization, which is counter to the desire for practice guided by evidence.

Nursing Input in Technology Selection

One way to minimize individual care disruption includes collaboration between software providers and clinicians to best represent individual care process. Specifically, nursing PPM guides nurses to have active involvement in decisions about professional practice. That knowledge, shared with software technologists, drives information systems design to model how care is provided, rather than requiring that individual care processes follow the format of information systems. Whether software design changes or not, it is critical that nurses lead selection of information technology that involves care of individuals.

Although nurses continue to be the largest EMR user population, the profession disappointingly has the least amount of influence on technology selection. Too often, important system selection decisions are delegated to committees heavily populated by physicians and business professionals from administration. Nursing's voice, if represented at all, becomes a small echo in the discussion. This occurs mostly because nurses lack the technical knowledge to participate in, let alone lead, these crucial selection efforts.

Large hospitals have a CNIO (chief nursing information officer) or CNO (chief nursing officer) with the needed expertise, whereas few, if any, ambulatory operations have such an equivalent. As a result, most EMR/AMR systems are evaluated and selected with little, if any, input from nursing. In the history of health information systems, few automation efforts encountered the resistance the EMR encountered. In fact, it was pressure from the federal government and payers that championed the effort and made the EMR the de facto care documentation format that it is today.

Electronic Medical Records and Ambulatory Medical Records: Vital to Innovation and Research

In the past, small sample sizes and an inability to extrapolate clinical findings to larger populations hampered the scope and subsequent value of nursing research, which is an important element of a PPE. More than a simple repository of individual care interactions, today's EMRs contain a treasure trove of clinical data that are available—often on a massive scale. The value of EMRs to nursing research cannot be overstated. Leading nursing schools can harvest EMRs from affiliated hospitals and ambulatory care operations, remove individual identifiers, and use this invaluable information to populate the massive databases crucial to nursing research. As a result, EMRs hold the power to change the scope and velocity of nursing research forever. Relational databases paved the way for the complex, multidimensional data analysis needed to quantify the value of nursing's critical thinking as a contribution to improved individual outcomes. Today's sophisticated data manipulation tools and massive, inexpensive computing power combine to form a basis for powerful, big data-driven nursing research that previously has never been possible.

One example of big data in action comes from Emory University's Nell Hodgson Woodruff School of Nursing in Atlanta, Georgia. A newly founded advanced data science center leverages the three components of big data needed to advance nursing science:

1. A data dictionary of research and activities related to research and its funding;
2. An educational database of more than one million individual records from the academic health system; and
3. Detailed biologic measurements for advancing precision healthcare and nursing research (Higgins et al., 2018).

Having access to large volumes of information is just the first step. To maintain the credibility of subsequent nursing research, an expert team of analysts is needed to make sense of all those numbers. At Emory's School of Nursing, three doctoral-prepared professionals including a statistician, a computer scientist, and a nurse make up the multidisciplinary team needed to perform complex analysis of the data. Before that activity can begin, however, the data must be aligned to the nomenclatures and taxonomies of practice as delineated by the ANA. Purposefully sampling the data to the same level of detail as that associated with a clinical trial prevents all data from being included in the analyses.

The unique contribution that the nurse on the team makes to the effort centers on understanding the science behind the nursing process and identifying and interpreting the various data sources through the eyes of a clinician. In addition, the nurse knows how the life cycle of data affects nursing practice and how to create evidence-based feedback loops for quality and practice. Finally, the nurse evaluates the intended and unintended biases of the process and integrates the ANA Code of Ethics for Nurses with Interpretative Statements, as well as the individual's bill of rights, into the analysis to give context to the data.

As academia and healthcare providers partner to conduct more big data-fueled analyses of nursing data, these multidisciplinary teams are accelerating the progression of data to information, then on to knowledge, and finally wisdom. Today, big data can enable nursing to take the lead to innovate and advance the profession at light speed. As a result, nursing may be able to reduce the time it takes for nursing research to reach the bedside.

Big Data Tracks Triple Aim Progress

The aspiration for better individual management within care setting and across the continuum of care was a key underpinning of the early vision for EMRs. The Institute for Healthcare Improvement (IHI) set out a Triple Aim—better care for individuals, better care for populations, and lower per capita costs—to optimize performance of the country's healthcare system (IHI, 2009). IHI's Triple Aim initiative was the outgrowth of a seminal article that advocated for taking a three-pronged approach to a quality-based effort for improving healthcare delivery worldwide (Berwick et al., 2008).

In the United States, this laudable goal becomes a tall order when multiple payers are involved, especially on the federal level, and healthcare consumers move from payer to payer—sometimes annually. This payer churn compromises, at best, and loses, at worst, the opportunity to aggregate performance data and determine improvement levels. The data contained in EMRs and AMRs, which hold the promise of being a source of truth if individuals remain in a single healthcare system, may be able to demonstrate the efficacy of existing and new individual care models when tested against actual individual outcomes.

The ability to quantify the value of ambulatory nursing lies within an EMR/AMR. Commonly, ambulatory nurse practitioners (NPs) serve as a clinical bridge between recently hospitalized individuals' discharge teams and the individuals' first follow-up clinic visits. This innovative use of NPs not only reduced hospital readmission for vulnerable populations but also decreased emergency room utilization. Quantifying the results of a nurse-based care delivery model within a large database of similar individuals can demonstrate that, in addition to improving individual quality of care, significant dollars of unreimbursed costs are avoided, highlighting the value of nursing. This valuable insight can only be discovered by using an extremely large individual sample, applying advanced nursing knowledge, and big data analysis. These three components are needed to answer the pivotal question, "Did nursing care provide value?"

Another opportunity to deliver on the Triple Aim develops through big data analysis to extrapolate the financial and administration transactions linked to individual healthcare providers via their national provider identifiers (CMS, 1996). Complex data analysis can track improved outcomes to the individual nurse or provider, giving nursing an opportunity to pinpoint individual care processes and steps that achieve improved outcomes and care efficiencies. The ability to answer questions about a nurse's ability to provide adequate individual surveillance, effective individual management, or achieve individual engagement forms the foundation elements of nursing practice that can influence education programming and improve clinical care.

Conclusions

Review of EMRs and AMRs enables large-scale nursing research, which can isolate and identify the clinical processes that most frequently produce improved outcomes. Once validated and quantified, nurses will have an opportunity to refine the standard of care and improve outcomes. Being able to minimize clinical variation through standardization is expected to not only improve outcomes but reduce costs as well.

In addition to feeding the massive databases needed for large-scale nursing research with real-world data, EMRs and AMRs also offer an electronic platform for documenting individuals' adherence to ongoing medical recommendations issued postcare, which is a future area of quality of care investigation. Capturing individual adherence data can offer valuable insight into the effectiveness of health-related interventions. Informatics as an essential infrastructure of ambulatory nursing professional practice will continue to grow and mature in the future.

The infrastructures that support professional ambulatory nursing practice include the PPE guided by a PPM and shared governance as well as the reinforcement of ambulatory nursing practice by the AMR and the science of informatics, along with professional development including the role of nurse residencies. These structures cannot exist in isolation of each other and must be aligned and integrated to create the desired infrastructure for professional ambulatory nursing practice.

Professional Development in Ambulatory Nursing

The lifelong learning of nurses is essential to ensure optimal professional practice. The development of competency-based professional development as a demonstration of technical, interpersonal, and clinical skills is measured through assessment of evidence-based knowledge, skills, and attributes (attitudes). The importance of competency evolved during the early formation of the nursing profession, prior to formalized nurse preparation in academic settings.

In 2011, the Institute of Medicine (IOM) clearly indicated the significance of nursing professional development by stating, "The nursing profession must adopt a framework of continuous lifelong learning that includes basic education, academic progression, and continuing competencies" (p. 213). Professional role expansion, advanced competencies such as systems thinking and quality improvement, and magnified public expectations of care value have created increased requirements for top of license nursing practice; therefore, the infrastructure of nursing learning and development as a key support for the practice environment is essential.

Current clinician development requires a multipronged approach, including university programs, advanced degrees, clinical learning sessions, training, simulation, certification, clinical residencies, fellowships, online courses, and conference/seminar/workshop attendance as examples. Professional learning is quantified and reported with nationally recognized continuing education units for use with licensure renewal, credentialing, and career advancement. Irrespective of the learning modality, nursing professional development is an expectation in all PPEs. The next section delineates the history, rationale, guiding evidence, business case, and the future of ambulatory professional development.

History of Ambulatory Nursing Professional Development

Formal infrastructures to support the ongoing development of professional nurses have instinctively been important to adequately provide clinical care and, over time, have become required by regulatory and professional bodies. Proof of proper training, licensure, ongoing education, training, and competence is an essential component to ensure adequate competency for the clinician's individual assignment (AAACN, 2018). Although historically academic education programs prepared nurses for clinical care delivery, as validated by national licensure, the advancement of ambulatory nursing to include advanced practice has required focused learning and development beyond the entry into practice educational level.

Ambulatory nursing professional development outside of the academic setting was formalized in 1976 with the first national workshop for ambulatory nursing directors and supervisors. The learning event was cosponsored by the American Group Practice Association (AGPA) in Alexandria, Virginia, and the Medical Group Management Association (MGMA) in Denver, Colorado. Over 100 participants engaged in discussions about organization, philosophy, leadership styles, nurses in ambulatory care settings, current health system developments, individual education, and expanded nursing roles (AAACN, 2018). The annual conference continues as a key national structural element of ambulatory nursing professional development. As the professional organization for ambulatory nursing, AAACN maintains important relationships with multiple professional organizations, highlighting the role of ambulatory professional development to advance nursing practice.

The expansion of ambulatory care provision to advanced practice nurses (APNs) launched in 1965 with the birth of the NP role in both America and Wales (Styles, 1990). The emergence of NPs coincided with the implementation of Medicare and Medicaid national health insurance plans for Americans over the age of 65 (Medicare) or for low-income citizens at the state level (Medicaid) (Timmons, 2016). The need to adequately provide care for all citizens supported the role of the independently licensed NP as the demand for clinical care exceeded existing physician supply. Societal care provision challenges were, and continue to be, a global challenge for all countries. The growth in NPs increased in the 1980s, slowed in the 1990s, and has grown rapidly since the execution of the IOM report and the implementation of the Patient Protection and Affordable Care Act (PPACA) (HHS, 2010; IOM, 2011). As the need for care providers has increased, professional development structures and academic preparation are now a required element of practice environments to ensure that care for all community members is delivered by competent nursing professionals.

Legislation for expanded nursing practice, which reflects the evolving state and national landscape, continues to drive the need for additional nursing professional development. NPs are now licensed as advanced practice registered nurses (APRNs) to reflect expanded responsibility and standardized national recognition. Professional development supports the capacity for APRNs to serve in primary care provider roles that deliver equally as good care as provided by physicians (Martinez-Gonzalez et al., 2014).

Role development, as a response to the advancement of nurse licensure and credentialing, has driven the presence of professional development as an expected structural element of a practice model. Learning opportunities that support the heightened nursing role include orientation, competency development, simulation, academic programs, certification, continuing education offerings, transition programs, and residencies/fellowships. Nurses can now function in expanded roles because of intentional professional development, promoting full utilization of the nurse's education and training in ambulatory settings (Allen, 2016).

Over time, the ANA, in partnership with professional organizations such as the ANCC, emphasized the salience of professional development, continuing education, and advancement of nursing practice through specialty certifications and nationally recognized competency development, because it promotes the portability of nursing skills across the nation (ANCC, 2018a). Professional nursing organizations have emphasized the importance of focused, specialty-based nursing professional development opportunities to drive excellence within specific clinical areas. Nationally recognized continuing education and certification now exists in most nursing practice areas.

The Rationale for Professional Development

A key structural element of a PPE is professional development. Within ambulatory care settings, the practice model relies on nurses to function at the top of their licensure for delivery of cost-effective, high-quality healthcare. In order for nurses to maintain evidence-based practice and prepare for expanded roles, ongoing professional development is key. Current and future ambulatory nursing roles include nurse-led clinics, primary care provision, telehealth, mobile health, clinic and practice settings, and virtual nursing. Professional development, therefore, ensures contemporary knowledge, skills, competencies, and attributes necessary for exemplary ambulatory professional practice in roles that produce high-value and safe nursing care.

Preparation for clinical competence in ambulatory settings requires ongoing professional development through activities that promote learning and advancement of the role, including:

- Professional conference attendance and presentations;
- Internal educational sessions;
- Specialty certification;
- Peer-to-peer education;
- Orientation;
- Preceptorships and mentoring;

- Transition to practice programs; and
- Clinical career ladders (Allen, 2016).

Increased individual and organizational professional responsibility for transforming the healthcare environment increases the public expectations of nurses' abilities, the addition of new competencies, and the demonstration of evidence-based nursing practice. For example, utilization of competency-based orientation programs to transition nurses from the inindividual setting to the outindividual setting is essential for any ambulatory healthcare organization (Allen, 2016). Thus, professional development is a key structural element of a fully actualized PPE (Ives Erickson & Ditomassi, 2011).

Importance of Professional Development

Ample evidence exists to demonstrate the importance of professional development as an essential component of any PPM. A clearly defined framework helps nurses visualize the conceptual model of a professional environment and how they fit into the organization and where they can make meaningful contributions. Professional development ensures the advancement of clinical and leadership competencies as a key priority (Ives Erickson & Ditomassi, 2011). High-performing organizations in all care settings rely on solid professional development elements. With the rapid growth of nursing roles in ambulatory care, organizations need to ensure adequate and ongoing role preparation. Historical professional development models focused on the use of resources within the immediate environment. Currently, educators in practice settings leverage internal expertise and resources as well as the resources from professional organizations. In the future, care settings and academic partners will work collaboratively to design and implement integrated, innovative professional development structures and processes (Bernard & Martyn, 2018).

Professional development in ambulatory practice environments considers the learning needs of nurses from prelicensure through experienced careerists who desire to practice in an ambulatory setting. Embedment of Benner's (1984) novice to expert model as a key ensures the right learning at the right time to promote effective professional development. Within the model, nurses develop from a novice level to advanced beginner to competent to proficient and, finally, to an expert level of knowledge and skills. A combination of intellectual training, technical competency development, and synthesis of practice experience promotes advancement of clinical expertise (Benner, 1984). Both ambulatory registered nurses (RNs) and APNs have vital responsibility to stay abreast of the newest clinical and leadership evidence to maintain licensure, credentials, and delivery of clinically excellent care. Evidence-based components of a professional development model include:

- Prelicensure academic content in ambulatory nursing;
- Student practicum and externship programs;
- Ambulatory **nurse residency programs (NRPs)**;
- Transition to ambulatory nursing residencies;
- Masters and doctoral academic preparation for APNs;
- APRN fellowships;
- Continuing education in state-required clinical areas such as pharmacology;
- Continuing professional education;
- Ongoing competency validation;
- Education and training on new products, devices, protocols, and care delivery;
- Meaningful orientation programs for ambulatory nursing; and
- Tailored ambulatory nursing leadership development.

Consistency and standardization in the development and delivery of any educational content is pertinent for organizations to measure the return on learning. The AAACN (2018) recommends a detailed, standardized, professional development structure for ambulatory nursing, which includes:

- Orientation planning, competency validation tools, and nurse educator resources;
- Organizational/systems role for ambulatory care nurse competencies;
- Clinical nursing practice competencies;
- Professional nurse role competencies;
- Telehealth nursing practice competencies;
- Core dimensions of the ambulatory care nursing staff educator;
- Planning for educational activities;
- Designing the learning environment and learner engagement;
- Evaluating learning effectiveness;
- Professional self-development; and
- Resources for transition to ambulatory care.

Comprehensive professional development contains multiple structural elements and considers the learning needs of individuals and clinical teams within the overall framework, ensuring competency-based approaches in all development offerings. In a fully actualized professional development model, an interprofessional approach to learning drives maximum teamwork and collaboration. Multiple teaching methods assist effective ambulatory professional development programming within the practice setting. Ambulatory nurse educators and clinical specialists possess the expertise in learning needs assessments, planning, delivery, and evaluation of education. Professional development models also address and integrate the Quality, Safety, and Education for Nurses (QSEN) competencies of individual-centered care, teamwork and collaboration, evidence-based practice, quality improvement, safety, and informatics into learning strategies (QSEN, 2018).

Outcomes of an effective ambulatory professional development model include mentoring, teaching, generating publications, conducting research and scholarly activities, and exemplifying individual care and family support (Ives Erickson & Ditomassi, 2011). Additionally, the actualization of the Triple Aim of improved clinical outcome measures, affordable healthcare, and improved community health demonstrates important outcomes of effective professional development (Berwick et al., 2008). In a study of ambulatory care nurses' top daily practice priorities, it was reported that the top five individual outcomes they influence during a typical day are (a) individual satisfaction, (b) interpretation of lab values and achievement of normal lab values, (c) prevention of complications, (d) correct level of medical treatment, and (e) reduction of anxiety levels (Rondinelli et al., 2014). Other identified priority nursing functions included assessment, triaging, coordination, initiation/evaluation of treatments and procedures, evaluation of individual/family education, establishing long-term health goals with the individual, and managing the plan of care (Rondinelli et al., 2014). Effective ambulatory professional development prepares and maintains nursing competency in these essential areas that support the daily nursing functions to drive measurable, clinical outcomes that demonstrate health improvement through advancement of the individual and team performance.

Examples of clinical outcomes affected by professional development include nurse-sensitive indicators of pain assessment and follow-up, depression screening, medication reconciliation, readmissions, hypertension, individual satisfaction, compliance with requirements such as immunization rates, and individual safety measures (AAACN, 2016). Ambulatory surgery centers have a set of outcomes specific to surgical care and safety. Within outindividual settings, professional development positively influences ambulatory practice volume measures, staffing, skill mix, and individual care hours by ensuring the requisite knowledge and skills to effectively manage the business of safe and effective clinical care.

The Business Case for Professional Development

Ambulatory nursing is the economic value at the gateway of the healthcare system. In recent decades, the healthcare system has recognized the growing need for increased access to care, much of which is met through ambulatory nursing. Evolving societal needs drive the need for innovative and unique care delivery models outside of the acute care setting, which nursing is able to provide. The shortage of medical providers since the 1960s supported the early development of the NP role as a cost-effective approach to meet the growing community health needs.

In 2010, national attention turned to healthcare reform as requisite to lowering the cost of healthcare delivery in the United States. The shift to pay-for-performance models and quantification of value as an outcome of reduced costs and increased quality provided a significant platform for nursing. The PPACA, enacted on March 23, 2010, launched healthcare insurance eligibility for an additional eight million Americans (Snavely, 2016). This expansion of healthcare coverage introduced new stressors on an already strained healthcare system. Combined with the projected growth in citizens over the age of 65 to reach 84 million and the reduction in working population paying into the Medicare funding, the mandate for cost-effective, accessible care is undeniable (Snavely, 2016).

A key tenet of the PPACA also included a shift from sick-care to well-care because proactively improving the health of communities has been shown to improve health outcomes in a far more affordable manner than the delivery of sick-care (HHS, 2010). Much of the well-care activities are contained in ambulatory settings and delivered by nursing. The economic shift from inindividual, acute care to outindividual, well-care signifies an opportunity for nursing to showcase the ability to achieve the Triple Aim outcomes of: (a) improved experience of care, (b) improved health of populations, and (c) reduced cost of healthcare (Berwick et al., 2008). Nurses contribute value in the provision of health services and as leaders/innovators in improving care delivery processes in practice environments through the use of evidence-based care interventions that coordinate care through a range of services from primary/ambulatory care, transitional care, and acute care (Lindrooth et al., 2015). Finally, the broadening of the scope of care for NPs increases access to care and reduces the cost of care provision, resulting in improved consumer welfare (Timmons, 2016).

Professional development subsequently is an important structural element to advance the competencies and scope of practice for ambulatory nurses and APRNs. Prelicensure ambulatory education, advanced academic preparation, specialty licensure/certifications, residencies, fellowships, and career development have emerged as key elements of the professional development necessary to achieve the national agenda. The business case for ambulatory nursing professional development is clear. Promotion of competent ambulatory nurses and APRNs ensures that the unmet needs of the community are realized in a value-based manner that results in healthier communities.

Quality and Safety Education for Nurses and Interprofessional Collaboration

Important components require consideration for the future of ambulatory nursing professional development. The actualization of **Quality and Safety Education for Nurses (QSEN)** competencies into the practice environment, relating learning to individual and workforce outcomes, shifting the culture to interprofessional learning environments, increased use of simulation, and focused attention on ambulatory nurse leader competency development, comprises the future priorities of top professional development models. Further, academic–practice partnerships will be required for optimum practitioner preparation.

Ambulatory care settings facilitate interprofessional learning opportunities. In a study of medical and nursing students in an interprofessional student placement experience, Saunders et al. (2018) reported that the blended clinical experience facilitated important learning opportunities that complemented the knowledge base of each profession. The future of ambulatory professional development requires the use of interprofessional learning for highest effectiveness and maximum effects for both the professional nurse and individual outcomes. The QSEN competency of teamwork and collaboration explicitly delineates the knowledge, skills, and attitudes of effective interprofessional team functioning, open communication, mutual respect, and shared decision-making. Future professional development models will also include competencies such as resilience and caregiver well-being as the fourth aim to drive QuadrupleAim outcomes.

One future priority is academic collaboration to establish primary care nursing education in prelicensure and nurse baccalaureate education as a routine standard. Nursing leaders and faculty will design both didactic and clinical learning experiences to advance preparation of nurses for ambulatory care roles (Wojnar & Whelan, 2017). The role of nurse leader preparation will begin in the academic setting and transition to continue in the practice setting, requiring that both academic and health system organizations provide structures for leadership development. Ambulatory nurse leader preparation will come into future focus because of the unique knowledge, skills, attributes, and competencies needed to lead clinical practice.

The American Organization for Nursing Leadership (AONL), formerly American Organization of Nurse Executives (AONE) set forth an evidence-based nurse leader competency model that includes unique ambulatory nurse leader competencies, such as care management, transitions of care, interprofessional communication, integrated delivery systems, provider relationships, and utilization/case management, in addition to the core leader requisite competencies of communication/relationship building, knowledge of the healthcare environment, leadership, professionalism, and business skills (AONL, AONE, 2015). Thus, professional education frameworks need to include specific leader-learning needs. In fully actualized professional development models, leadership development will occur in an interprofessional manner, with nurse leaders, business leaders, and physician leaders learning together to effectively lead the business of ambulatory care.

Other future professional development considerations include learning/development for partnership with nontraditional healthcare players such as the business sector. Health insurance companies will realign business strategies to create new healthcare products and services pricing, which will have significant operational implications for the industry. Ambulatory nurses need to learn how to effectively use data, quantify the value of their work and the affiliated outcomes, and leverage technology and artificial intelligence in the delivery of nursing services, all the while meeting the Triple Aim and adding the fourth aim of ensuring caregiver well-being (known as the Quadruple Aim). Ongoing learning and development, intentionally designed for maximum professional practice, will consider the knowledge, skills, attributes, and necessary competencies to deliver high-quality nursing care within the context of new business relationships. The future holds extensive opportunity for nursing, with professional development serving as the vehicle to migrate from the present state to the future state of ambulatory nursing care delivery.

Transition to Practice Nurse Residency Programs

The specific element of nurse residency programs highlights a salient component of professional development programming. The onset of ambulatory care nursing as the current and future priority for transforming healthcare requires specific success strategies. One such emerging structure is the advent of NRPs as a formalized method for preparing nurses for optimum professional transition into practice.

History of Residency Programs

The transition from graduated nurse to practicing nurse is a time of great stress for newly licensed registered nurses (NLRNs). With the increasing complexity of the healthcare system, the transition to competent professional is now even more challenging. Adapting to the nurse role and dealing with the realities of the nursing profession can be stressful and discouraging. Major challenges faced by NLRNs include delegation, prioritization, managing care delivery, decision-making, collaboration, conflict resolution, and self-confidence (Kramer et al., 2012). The challenges of this transition may prompt the NLRN to seek another position; they may even decide to leave nursing altogether.

With ever-increasing demands on our healthcare system, there is a need for highly trained nurses across the continuum of care, including ambulatory care, and we must rely on NLRNs to fill these critical vacancies. In 2010, Benner, Sutphen, Leonard, and Day called for radical transformation in nursing education, declaring that NLRNs were unprepared for the demands of the nursing workplace and suggested that there is a need for more emphasis on practice-based education (Benner et al., 2010). Research suggests that NRPs may be able to fill this need by easing the transition from student to practicing nurse (Goode et al., 2016). In 2011, the IOM recommended the implementation of structured NRPs for NLRNs, new APNs, and nurses transitioning to a new specialty area.

The IOM recommends that residency programs should also be developed for practice settings outside of acute care, including ambulatory care. Incorporating NRP into ambulatory care can yield numerous early benefits and impact practice in several ways, one being the ability to address the growing need for Bachelor of Science (BSN) RNs in ambulatory care by developing a pipeline of new nurses (Gilland et al., 2019). According to the American Academy of Ambulatory Care Nurses white paper, the need for an ambulatory NRP "when executed with a rigorous structure based on professional and specialty competencies, an ambulatory registered nurse residency program has a strong potential to transform the nursing profession and advance ambulatory nursing's contribution to leading change and advancing health" (Levine, 2014).

Costs of Turnover

In order to have enough nurses with the right skills, we must overcome workforce challenges such as staffing shortages and nursing turnover. Nursing turnover rates are high, especially among NLRNs. One study reported that 17.5% of NLRNs leave their position within the first year, and another reported that only 80% of NLRNs remained in the same position after 12 months (Kovner et al., 2014; Weathers & Raleigh, 2013). The cost of nursing turnover is estimated to be as high as $88,000 per RN, or 1.3 times the cost of the RNs' annual salary (Li & Jones, 2013). With the high costs of turnover and an ever-increasing need to rely on the newly licensed nurse to fill critical vacancies, it is paramount that healthcare organizations better manage the period of transition from nursing school to professional nurse.

Nurse Residency Programs

Nurse residency programs have emerged as an effective strategy for supporting the transition from advanced beginner to competent professional nurse. A structured transition to practice NRP is different from a traditional orientation. Orientation is paid instructional time focused on the requirements necessary to function in the role and usually includes a limited number of shifts with supervision by an experienced coworker (TJC, 2018). However, a transition to practice NRP is a structured set of formal and informal learning opportunities, typically lasting 6 to 12 months. These programs focus on developing professional nursing practice through reflection, small group activities, and formal presentations (Bleich, 2012). NRPs also have protected time for the nurse resident to attend scheduled learning activities. These programs rely on clinical immersion and a highly supportive preceptor program to facilitate the newly licensed nurse's transition from advanced beginner to competent professional.

Evidence supports the benefit and the need for NLRNs to complete a residency program. Participation in an NRP can increase NLRNs' self-confidence, competence, organization, and prioritization (Goode et al., 2013). Residency program participants report greater job satisfaction and enjoyment of work (Ulrich et al., 2010) and better socialization and integration onto the unit (Kramer et al., 2012). Crucially, NRPs have been shown to increase NLRN first-year retention rates to nearly 95% and decrease voluntary turnover rates (Goode et al., 2013). One study of transition to practice NRPs reported that these programs are also associated with decreased numbers of errors and fewer negative individual safety practices in NLRNs (Specter et al., 2015).

Evidence-Based Curriculum

Curriculum content for an NRP focuses on developing clinical leadership skills, clinical decision-making skills, quality and individual safety competencies, and the professional role of NLRNs. The literature suggests content on individual safety, clinical reasoning, communication and teamwork, individual-centered care, evidence-based practice, quality improvement, and informatics should be included in the NRP curriculum (Specter et al., 2015). Additional topics like delegation, managing conflict, and care coordination support leadership skill development. To support professional role development, content on ethical decision-making, end-of-life care, stress management, and cultural competence should be included. Topics on quality individual outcomes can include managing the changing individual condition, infection prevention, medication administration, pain management, fall prevention, and individual/family education (Vizient Inc, 2017).

Topics may be presented at monthly seminars where in-person participation is encouraged over self-paced or distance-accessible learning. Bringing the residents together monthly allows time for feedback and reflection. Participation in small group discussions and case studies allows residents to apply concepts, seek feedback, and reflect. One way to ensure the NRP curriculum is evidence based is to purchase one of the commercially available NRP programs. These programs offer an evidence-based curriculum, training, and support for the residency coordinator and routine evaluation of NLRNs and program outcomes.

A formalized, structured transition to practice NRP with support from the CNO and the leadership team can improve quality and safety practices, increase job satisfaction, reduce work stress, and decrease turnover in new graduates. The literature suggests that NRPs with characteristics delineated in Table 16.1 have optimal outcomes.

Advance Practice Registered Nurse Transition to Practice

The transition to practice for newly graduated APRNs is stressful, and there is little support for these newly licensed independent practitioners (Bush & Lowery, 2016; Barnes, 2015). In 2017, Martsolf, Nguyen, Freund, and Poghosyan reported that there were as few as 68 postgraduate NP residency programs, and in 2016 Barnes reported that only 33% of NPs surveyed received a formal orientation program in their first NP position. Reports of transition to practice programs for APRNs in the literature have demonstrated that structured education for role transition after graduation has a positive effect on job satisfaction (Bush & Lowery, 2016) and role transition (Barnes, 2015). It is possible that APRNs could benefit from structured transition to practice programs just as NLRNs have done. To support the need for evidence-based transition to practice programs, the ANCC (2018b) has published standards for accreditation of these programs for early career APRNs.

TABLE 16.1 **CHARACTERISTICS OF SUCCESSFUL NRPs**

Program Length	• Programs should be at least 9–12 months long. Increased job satisfaction, competence, confidence, and leadership scores measured in NLRNs can be improved by participation in an NRP, and better outcomes are associated with longer programs (Goode et al., 2016). • NLRN self-reported stress levels go up and job satisfaction levels go down at 6–9 months. The period from 6 to 12 months after entering the workforce appears to be a vulnerable time for NLRNs. However, by 12 months, the self-reported stress levels had decreased and job satisfaction had increased (Rush et al., 2013; Specter et al., 2015). • Extending the duration of the NRPs to at least 9–12 months allows the program to continue to support the NLRN through the more stressful time in the transition to practice.
Preceptors	• Programs should have a highly supportive preceptor program where the preceptor has a reduced clinical assignment for shifts worked with an NLRN. The NLRN and the preceptor are on the same schedule, and the preceptor shares an assignment with the NLRN. • The number of NLRNs for each preceptor is kept low and the NLRN has the same preceptor on most days. In one study of hospitals with high preceptor support, the NLRNs and their preceptors scored the NLRN competence levels higher when compared to NLRNs in hospitals with low preceptor support. • Work units in ambulatory setting can often be small groups, making a one-to-one preceptor assignment impossible. In order to create a highly supportive environment for the NLRN in ambulatory care, the residency coordinator or clinic manager may need to provide close follow-up with the NLRN in the ambulatory setting. • NLRNs are significantly more likely to be retained after the first year if they received high preceptor support. These results suggest that practice settings with a more supportive preceptor program will also see increased retention at 1 year and more competent NLRNs (Blegen et al., 2015).
Curriculum	• Program curriculum should include content on EBP and how to incorporate evidence into practice in order for the NLRN to lead change and promote the highest quality, safe individual care. • The residents should be encouraged to identify a topic for an EBP project that is relevant to their clinical area, independently or in small groups, seek out evidence from the literature, and implement a best practice recommendation. The completed projects are shared publicly through staff meetings, journal clubs, conferences, and poster presentations. • This project helps the NLRN learn the quality improvement process as well as develop experience with dissemination of knowledge through abstracts, posters, and presentations (Vizient Inc., 2017).
Specialty Areas	• Programs should include customization for specialty areas (Specter et al., 2015). One of the key elements of an NRP is the time allowed to apply concepts and technical skills learned and, over time, move through the stages of skill acquisition to become a competent professional. During this time, the NLRN is learning general concepts like clinical decision-making, leadership, and professionalism in tandem with the specialty-specific clinical skills. • Ambulatory care is a specialty that requires customization of the NRP. Concepts critical for an ambulatory care NRP include health promotion, managing acute illness, managing chronic conditions, individual and family teaching, and discussing care preferences at end of life (Vizient Inc., 2017). The NRP should consider the NLRN strengths and interests in the progression of the program.

Note. EBP = evidence-based practice; NRP = nurse residency program; NLRN = newly licensed registered nurse.

The Future of Nurse Residency Programs

As noted in Table 16.1, there is growing evidence to support that structured, evidence-based NRPs can improve NLRN retention, satisfaction, competence, confidence, and leadership and may have a positive effect on individual safety (Goode et al., 2016). In light of this growing evidence, it is expected that the use of NRPs will continue to expand. Reports of ambulatory NRPs are rare. AAACN surveyed over 300 of its members and only 10% of respondents indicated the presence of a residency program (AAACN, 2014). In comparison, almost 48% of hospitals report having an NRP (Barnett et al., 2012). In 2014 the AAACN published a white paper making the case for ambulatory NRPs, and in 2018 the American Academy of Nursing issued a policy statement recommending that all NLRNs be required to complete a residency program as a condition of employment. Other recommendations include requiring accreditation of NRPs in an effort to ensure curricular standardization, including content on how to incorporate evidence into practice, and collaborating with an academic partner because NRPs are considered postgraduate education (Goode et al., 2018).

The future will see more customization of NRPs for specialty areas and with standardization to evidence-based curriculum. There will be residency tracts for a wide range of nursing specialties. Academic partnerships will lead to more innovative curriculum that will support early success in the role and opportunities for lifelong learning. Residencies for APRNs will increase and residency tracts will emerge for wider range of roles and educational preparations (Bernard & Martyn, 2018).

It will be necessary to leverage technology to create a distance-accessible and social media-like environment to support younger NLRNs. Millennials are accustomed to using online chat and social media as a support network. The NRPs of the future will need to embrace technology to create virtual support in an attempt to recreate the supportive feedback that is experienced in small group settings.

Summary

Since Benner (1984) published her seminal work *From Novice to Expert: Excellence and Power in Nursing*, we have understood that the transition from advanced beginner to competent professional requires time to move through the stages of skill acquisition and exposure to clinical experiences. Today it appears that structured, evidence-based NRPs can fulfill the promise of supporting the NLRNs' journey from advanced beginner to competent professional. These programs have demonstrated that they can improve NLRN retention, satisfaction, competence, confidence, and leadership. Although the initial cost of NRPs is higher, these programs decrease overall cost by increasing nurse retention (Silvestre et al., 2017). More importantly, NRPs provide a means for strengthening the healthcare delivery system by strengthening nursing and ultimately fulfilling the mandate for a robust professional practice in all areas of nursing, including that of ambulatory care.

Case Study

Elizabeth is a BSN student eagerly anticipating her graduation in 6 months. She and her fellow students are interviewing for their first jobs after they successfully pass NCLEX. Elizabeth has completed three interviews and has pending job offers with different healthcare systems clinics. One is an academic medical practice with an accredited ambulatory NRP, the second is a large multispecialty practice in an urban setting offering sign-on bonuses to RNs, and her last offer is with a well-established clinic eager to begin hiring new graduate RNs.

1. Which offer should she most seriously consider and why?
2. Using QSEN as a guide, discuss key competencies Elizabeth should expect to develop in her new position.

Key Points for Review

- All professional nurses should seek practice environments that aspire to professional practice and achieve the expectations of society's expectations of nursing as a discipline.
- The behavioral tenets of professional nursing practice include evidence-based practice, research, and education.
- The organizational requirements for professional nursing practice include a PPE and a PPM, both guided by shared governance.
- The support for professional nursing practice comes from continued professional development including nurse residencies.
- The AMR is a good way to reinforce evidence-based practice and research.
- Professional development is a key requisite structure of an effective PPM.
- Professional development supports the advancement of knowledge, skills, attributes, and competencies needed to deliver contemporary, evidence-based nursing practice in any ambulatory nursing role.
- A comprehensive professional development model contains learning structures and processes that start in the academic setting, continue in the professional setting, and are inclusive of both individual and interprofessional teams and grounded in QSEN competencies.
- The future of professional development will contain expanded residencies and fellowships, innovative learning models with the introduction of technologic businesses into the healthcare industry, and the use of simulation to ensure nurses practice at the top of their licensure while leading healthcare reform.
- Ambulatory nursing leaders, as culture architects, have a unique set of core competencies that require intentional professional development to actualize leadership excellence.
- NRPs can improve NLRN retention, satisfaction, competence, confidence, leadership, and professional integration into practice.
- NRPs should be at least 9 to 12 months in length and have highly supportive preceptors.
- All NLRNs should be required to complete a residency program.

REFERENCES

Allen, J. W. (2016). Transitioning the RN to ambulatory care. *Nursing Administration Quarterly, 40*(2), 115–121. https://doi.org/10.1097/NAQ.0000000000000151

American Academy of Ambulatory Care Nursing. (2014). *Ambulatory nurse residency white paper—The need for an ambulatory nurse residency*. https://www.aaacn.org/sites/default/files/documents/white-paper.pdf

American Academy of Ambulatory Care Nursing. (2016). *Ambulatory care nurse sensitive indicator industry report: Meaningful measurement of nursing in the ambulatory individual care environment*. https://www.aaacn.org/NSIReport

American Academy of Ambulatory Care Nursing. (2018). *What is ambulatory care nursing*. https://www.aaacn.org

American Nurses Association. (2003). *Nursing's social policy statement* (3rd ed.). ANA Enterprise.

American Nurses Credentialing Center. (2017). *2019 Magnet application manual*. ANA Enterprise.

American Nurses Credentialing Center. (2018a). *Nursing skills competency program*. ANA Enterprise. https://www.nursingworld.org/organizational-programs/accreditation/nursing-skills-competency/

American Nurses Credentialing Center. (2018b). *Practice transition accreditation program*. ANA Enterprise. https://www.nursingworld.org/organizational-programs/accreditation/ptap/

American Organization for Nursing Leadership. (2015). *AONL, AONE nurse executive competencies*. Author. https://www.aonl.org/sites/default/files/aone/nec.pdf

Barnes, H. (2015). Exploring factors that influence nurse practitioner role transition. *The Journal of Nurse Practitioners, 11*(2), 178–183. https://doi.org/10.1016/j.nurpra.2014.11.004

Barnett, J. S., Minnick, A. F., & Norman, L. D. (2014). A description of U.S. post-graduation nurse residency programs. *Nursing Outlook, 62*(3), 174–184. https://doi.org/10.1016/j.outlook.2013.12.008

Benner, P. (1984). *From novice to expert*. Prentice Hall.

Benner, P., Sutphen, M., Leonard, V., & Day, L. (2010). *Educating nurses: A call for radical transformation*. Jossey-Bass; The Carnegie Foundation for the Advancement of Teaching.

Bernard, N., & Martyn, K. K. (2018). Start together, stay together: Nurse residencies of the future. *Nursing Administration Quarterly*, *42*(4), 318–323. https://doi.org/10.1097/NAQ.0000000000000310

Berwick, D. M., Nolan, T. W., & Whittington, J. (2008). The triple aim: Care, health, and cost. *Health Affairs*, *27*(3), 759–769. https://doi.org/10.1377/hlthaff.27.3.759

Blegan, M. A., Spector, N., Ulrich, B. T., Lynn, M. R., Barnsteiner, J., & Silvestre, J. (2015). Preceptor support in hospital transition to practice programs. *The Journal of Nursing Administration, 45*(12), 642–649. https://doi.org/10.1097/NNA.0000000000000278

Bleich, M. R. (2012). In praise of nursing residency programs. *American Nurse Today*, *7*(5), 47–49. https://www.myamericannurse.com/in-praise-of-nursing-residency-programs/

Bush, C. T., & Lowery, B. (2016). Postgraduate nurse practitioner education: Impact on job satisfaction. *The Journal of Nursing Administration, 12*(4), 226–234. https://doi.org/10.1016/j.nurpra.2015.11.018

Centers for Medicare and Medicaid Services. (1996). *National provider identifier standard.* https://www.cms.gov/Regulations-and-Guidance/Administrative-Simplification/NationalProvIdentStand/

Clavelle, J. T., Weston, M. J., Porter O'Grady, T., & Verran, J. A. (2016). Evolution of structural empowerment moving from shared to professional governance. *Journal of Nursing Administration, 46*(6), 308–312.

Cobb, S., Shine, C., Wolf, K., & Jadwin, A. (2018). Involving clinical nurses in evaluation of a professional practice model. *Journal of Nursing Administration, 48*(9), 466–468. https://doi.org/10.1097/NNA.0000000000000650

Committee on the Robert Wood Johnson Foundation Initiative on the Future of Nursing, at the Institute of Medicine, Robert Wood Johnson Foundation, & Institute of Medicine (U.S.). (2011). *The future of nursing: Leading change, advancing health.* National Academies Press.

Gilland, D., Muirhead, L., Toney, S., & Coburn, C. (2019). Building a workforce pipeline: Development of an ambulatory nurse residency program. *Nursing Management, 50*(7), 32–37. https://doi.org/10.1097/01.NUMA.0000558520.60241.1f

Goode, C. J., Glassman, K. S., Ponte, P. R., Krugman, M., & Peterman, T. (2018). Requiring a nurse residency for newly licensed registered nurses. *Nursing Outlook, 66*, 329–332. https://doi.org/10.1016/j.outlook.2018.04.004

Goode, C. J., Lynn, M. R., McElroy, D., Bednash, G. D., & Murray, B. (2013). Lessons learned from 10 years of research on a post-baccalaureate nurse residency program. *Journal of Nursing Administration, 43*(2), 73–79. https://doi.org/10.1097/NNA.0b013e31827f205c

Goode, C. J., Ponte, P. R., Havens, D. S. (2016). Residency for transition into practice: An essential requirement for new graduates from basic RN programs. *Journal of Nursing Administration, 46*(2), 82–86. https://doi.org/10.1097/NNA.0000000000000300

Higgins, M., Simpson, R., & Johnson, W. (2018). *What about big data and nursing*? American Nurse Today. https://www.americannursetoday.com/big-data-nursing

HITECH Act of 2009, 42 USC sec 139w-4(0)(2) (February 2009), sec 13301, subtitle B: Incentives for the Use of Health Information Technology.

Institute for Healthcare Improvement. (2009). *Initiatives—The IHI triple aim.* http://www.ihi.org/Engage/Initiatives/TripleAim/Pages/default.aspx

Institute of Medicine. (2011). *The future of nursing: Leading change, advancing health.* National Academies Press.

Ives Erickson, J. (2012). 200 years of nursing—A chief nurse's reflections on practice, theory, policy, education, and research. *Journal of Nursing Administration, 42*(1), 9–11. https://doi.org/10.1097/NNA.0b013e31823c1710

Ives Erickson, J. (2013). Influencing professional practice at the bedside. In J. Ives Erikson, D. A. Jones, & M. Ditomassi (Eds.), *Fostering nurse-led care* (pp. 1–19). Sigma Theta Tau.

Ives Erickson, J., & Ditomassi, M. (2011). Professional practice model: Strategies for translating models into practice. *Nursing Clinics of North America, 46*, 35–44. https://doi.org/10.1016/j.cnur.2010.10.011

Ives Erickson, J., & Ditomassi, M. (2012). Professional practice. In H. R. Feldman, G. R. Alexander, M. J. Greenberg, M. Jaffe-Ruiz, A. B. McBride, M. L. McClure, & T. D. Smith (Eds.), *Nursing leadership: A concise encyclopedia* (pp. 313–318). Springer Publishing Company.

Jamoom, E., Yang, N., & Hing, E. (2016). *Adoption of certified electronic health record systems and electronic information sharing in physician offices: United States, 2013 and 2014.* US Department of Health and Human Services, Centers for Disease Control and Prevention, National Center for Health Statistics. https://pubmed.ncbi.nlm.nih.gov/26828707/

Joseph, M., & Bogue, R. (2016). A theory-based approach to nursing shared governance. *Nursing Outlook, 64*, 339–351. https://doi.org/10.1016/j.outlook.2016.01.004

Kovner, C. T., Brewer, C. S., Fatehi, F., & Jun, J. (2014). What does nurse turnover rate mean and what is the rate? *Policy, Politics, & Nursing Practice, 15*(3-4), 64–71. https://doi.org/10.1177/1527154414547953

Kramer, M., Maguire, P., Halfer, D., Budin, W., Hall, D., Goodloe, L., Klaristenfeld, J., Teasley, S., Forsey, L., & Lemke, J. (2012). The organizational transformative power of nurse residency programs. *Nursing Administration Quarterly, 36*(2), 155–168. https://doi.org/10.1097/NAQ.0b013e318249fdaa

Levine, J. (2014). *Practice resources.* American Academy of Ambulatory Care Nurses. https://aaacn.org/practice-resources/white-papers

Li, Y., & Jones, C. B. (2013). A literature review of nursing turnover costs. *Journal of Nursing Management, 21*(3), 404–418. https://doi.org/10.1111/j.1365-2834.2012.01411.x

Lindrooth, R. C., Yakusheva, O., Fairman, J. A., Naylor, M. D., & Pauly, M. V. (2015). *Increasing the value of health care: The role of nurses* (pp. 1–7). University of Pennsylvania ScholarlyCommons.

Martinez-Gonzalez, N. A., Djalali, S., Tandjung, R., Huber-Geismann, F., Markun, S., Wensing, M., & Rosemann, T. (2014). Substitution of physicians by nurses in primary care: A systematic review and meta-analysis. *BMC Health Services Research, 14*(214), 1–17. https://doi.org/10.1186/1472-6963-14-214

Martsolf, G. R., Nguyen, P., Freund, D., & Poghosyan, L. (2017). What we know about postgraduate nurse practitioner residency and fellowship programs. *The Journal for Nurse Practitioners, 13*(7), 482–487. https://doi.org/10.1016/j.nurpra.2017.05.013

McClure, M., Poulin, M., Sovie, M. D., & Vandelt, M. A. (1983). *Magnet® hospitals attraction and retention of professional nurses.* ANA Enterprise.

McDonagh, K. J. (1990). *Nursing shared governance: Restructuring for the future.* KJ McDonagh & Associates, Inc.

Palmer, R. E., Carrell, D. S., Cronkite, D., Saunders, K., Gross, D. E., Masters, E., Donevan, S., Hylan, T. R., & Von Kroff, M. (2015). The prevalence of problem opioid use in individuals receiving chronic opioid therapy: Computer-assisted review of electronic health record clinical notes. *Pain, 156*(7), 1208–1214. https://doi.org/10.1097/j.pain.0000000000000145

Porter-O'Grady, T. (2017). A response to the question of professional governance versus shared governance. *Journal of Nursing Administration, 47*(2), 69–71. https://doi.org/10.1097/NNA.0000000000000439

Quality and Safety Education for Nurses. (2018). *Competencies*. https://qsen.org/competencies/pre-licensure-ksas/

Rondinelli, J. L., Omery, A. K., Crawford, C. L., & Johnson, J. A. (2014). Self-reported activities and outcomes of ambulatory staff registered nurses: An exploration. *The Permanente Journal, 18*(1), e108–e115. https://doi.org/10.7812/TPP/13-135

Rush, K. L., Adamack, M., Lilly, M., & Janke, R. (2013). Best practices of formal new graduate nurse transition programs: An integrative review. *International Journal of Nursing Studies, 50*(3), 345–356. https://doi.org/10.1016/j.ijnurstu.2012.06.009

Saunders, R., Dugmore, H., Seaman, K., Singer, R., & Lake, F. (2018). Interprofessional learning in ambulatory care. *The Clinical Teacher, 15*, 1–6. https://doi.org/10.1111/tct.12764

Shaw, M. C. (1993). The discipline of nursing: Historical roots, current perspectives, future directions. *Journal of Advanced Nursing, 18*, 1651–1656. https://doi.org/10.1046/j.1365-2648.1993.18101651.x

Silvestre, J. H., Ulrich, B. T., Johnson, T., Spector, N., & Blegan, M. (2017). A multisite study on a new graduate registered nurse transition to practice program: Return on investment. *Nursing Economics, 35*(3), 110–118. https://www.nursingeconomics.net/necfiles/2017/MJ17/110.pdf

Snavely, T. M. (2016). A brief economic analysis of the looming nursing shortage in the United States. *Nursing Economics, 34*(2), 98–100.

Spector, N., Blegen, M. A., Silvestre, J., Barnseiner, J., Lynn, M. R., Ulrich, B., Fogg, L., & Alexander, M. (2015). Transition to practice study in hospital settings. *Journal of Nursing Regulation, 5*(4), 24–38. https://doi.org/10.1016/S2155-8256(15)30031-4. https://www.journalofnursingregulation.com/article/S2155-8256(15)30031-4/fulltext

Spence Laschinger, H. K., Grau, A. L., Finegan, J., & Wilk, P. (2012). Predictors of new graduate nurses' workplace well-being: Testing the job demands-resources model. *Health Care Management Review, 37*(2), 175–186. http://doi.org/10.1097/HMR.0b013e31822aa456

Styles, M. M. (1990). Nurse practitioners creating new horizons for the 1990s. *The Nurse Practitioner, 15*(2), 48–57. https://doi.org/10.1097/00006205-199002000-00011

The Joint Commission. (2018). *Standards and National Individual Safety Goals®*. https://www.jointcommission.org/topics/hai_standards_and_npsgs.aspx

Timmons, E. J. (2016). The effects of expanded nurse practitioner and physician assistant scope of practice on the cost of Medicaid individual care. *Health Policy, 121*, 189–196. https://doi.org/10.1016/j.healthpol.2016.12.002

Ulrich, B., Krozek, C., Early, S., Ashlock, C. H., Africa, L. M., & Carman, M. L. (2010). Improving retention, confidence and competence of new graduate nurses: Results from a 10 year longitudinal database. *Nursing Economics, 28*(6), 363–367. https://www.nursingeconomics.net/necfiles/2017/MJ17/110.pdf

U.S. Health and Human Services. (2010). *Compilation of individual protection and affordable care act*. https://www.hhs.gov/healthcare/about-the-aca/index.html

Vizient Inc. (2017). *Vizient/AACN Nurse Residency Program*. Author.

Weathers, S. M., & Raleigh, E. D. H. (2013). 1-year retention rates and performance ratings: Comparing associate degree, baccalaureate, and accelerated baccalaureate degree nurses. *Journal of Nursing Administration, 43*(9), 468–474. https://doi.org/10.1097/NNA.0b013e3182a23d9f

Wojnar, D. M., & Whelan, E. M. (2017). Preparing nursing students for enhanced roles in primary care: The current state of prelicensure and RN-to-BSN education. *Nursing Outlook, 65*, 222–232. http://doi.org/10.1016/j.outlook.2016.10.006

Index

Note: Page numbers followed by *f* and *t* indicates figures and tables, respectively.

D

E

F

H

Q

R